Evidence-based Anticancer Complementary and Alternative Medicine

Volume 3

Series Editor
William C. S. Cho

For further volumes:
http://www.springer.com/series/8883

William C. S. Cho
Editor

Acupuncture and Moxibustion as an Evidence-based Therapy for Cancer

Springer

Editor
William C. S. Cho
Queen Elizabeth Hospital
Department of Clinical Oncology
Kowloon
Hong Kong SAR
China

ISSN 2211-0534 ISSN 2211-0542 (Electronic)
ISBN 978-94-007-4832-3 ISBN 978-94-007-4833-0 (eBook)
DOI 10.1007/978-94-007-4833-0
Springer Dordrecht Heidelberg London New York

Library of Congress Control Number: 2012947032

Springer is part of Springer Science+Business Media (www.springer.com)

Preface

In the recent decade, numerous experimental and clinical works investigating the efficacy and safety of acupuncture and moxibustion for cancer care have been published in medical journals, together with oceans of online articles. Although there is a lot of information on acupuncture and moxibustion, the scientific and medical communities are thrust for up-to-date and systematic sources that are supported by concrete laboratory evidences or clinical trials. Subsequent to our previous volumes entitled *Evidence-based Anticancer Materia Medica* and *Materia Medica for Various Cancers*, this volume steps up to gather leading oncologists, physicians and scientists in the field to discuss the application of acupuncture and moxibustion for the management of cancer. This book consists of fifteen chapters which address a range of important aspects that will impact on the application of acupuncture and moxibustion. An overview of the safety and side effects of acupuncture and moxibustion for cancer care are also covered. In addition, the integration of acupuncture with Western medicine in cancer treatment and recent clinical trials are included as well. This specialized volume delivers evidence-based information about acupuncture and moxibustion for cancer care that would be helpful to both medical professionals and cancer patients.

William C. S. Cho

Contents

Contributors

Hani Ashamalla Radiation Oncology Department, New York Methodist Hospital and Weill Medical College of Cornell University, Brooklyn, NY 11215, USA

Steven K. H. Aung Department of Medicine and Family Medicine, Faculty of Medicine and Dentistry, University of Alberta, 9904 106 Street NW, Edmonton, Alberta, AL T5K 1C4, Canada

Mitchell C. Benson Department of Medicine, Columbia University, 10th Floor, 161 Fort Washington Avenue, New York, NY 10032, USA

Jillian L. Capodice Department of Medicine, Columbia University, 10th Floor, 161 Fort Washington Avenue, New York, NY 10032, USA

Barrie Cassileth Integrative Medicine Service, Memorial Sloan-Kettering Cancer Center, 1429 First Avenue, New York, NY 10021, USA

Yi-Hung Chen Graduate Institute of Acupuncture Science, China Medical University, Taichung, Taiwan

Tae-Young Choi Medical Research Division, Korea Institute of Oriental Medicine, 461-24, Jeonmin-dong, Yuseong-gu, Daejeon 305-811, South Korea

Gary Deng Integrative Medicine Service, Memorial Sloan-Kettering Cancer Center, 1429 First Avenue, New York, NY 10021, USA

Darcy L. Dennis Department of Clinical Research, Vancouver Island Cancer Centre, BC Cancer Agency, 2410 Lee Avenue, Victoria, BC V8R 6V5, Canada

Edzard Ernst Complementary Medicine, Peninsula Medical School, University of Exeter, Exeter, UK

Paul R. Graves Radiation Oncology Department, New York Methodist Hospital and Weill Medical College of Cornell University, Brooklyn, NY 11215, USA

Sarah C. Greene Indiana University, 357 S. Landmark Ave. Suite B, Bloomington, IN 47403, USA

Aye A. Gyi Neurosurgery Department, School of Medical Science, Faculty of Health Sciences, The University of Adelaide, Adelaide, South Australia, Australia

Dawn L. Hershman Department of Medicine, Columbia University, 10th Floor, 161 Fort Washington Avenue, New York, NY 10032, USA

Mark I. Johnson Faculty of Health and Social Sciences, Leeds Metropolitan University, Leeds, UK

Peter Johnstone Chair of the Department of Radiation Oncology, 535 Barnhill Drive RT041, Indianapolis, IN 46202, USA

Tae-Hun Kim Medical Research Division, Korea Institute of Oriental Medicine, 461-24, Jeonmin-dong, Yuseong-gu, Daejeon 305-811, South Korea

Malini M. Khanna Department of Physical Medicine and Rehabilitation, Perelman School of Medicine, University of Pennsylvania, 3400 Spruce Street/5 Gates, Philadelphia, PA 19104, USA

Rie Konno Joanna Briggs Institute, Faculty of Health Sciences, The University of Adelaide, Adelaide, South Australia, Australia

Lixing Lao Center for Integrative Medicine, School of Medicine, University of Maryland, Rm 8-22, MSTF, 685 West Baltimore Street, Baltimore, MD 21201, USA

Myeong Soo Lee Medical Research Division, Korea Institute of Oriental Medicine, 461-24 Jeonmin-dong, Yuseong-gu, Daejeon 305-811, South Korea

Jan T. W. Lim Department of Radiation Oncology, Faculty of Surgery, University of British Columbia, Vancouver Island Cancer Centre, BC Cancer Agency, 2410 Lee Avenue, Victoria, BC V8R 6V5, Canada

Jaung-Geng Lin School of Chinese Medicine, China Medical University, Taichung, Taiwan

Jun J. Mao Department of Family Medicine and Community Health, Abramson Comprehensive Cancer Center, Perelman School of Medicine, University of Pennsylvania, 3400 Spruce Street/2 Gates, Philadelphia, PA 19104, USA

Adriana C. Nicolussi College of Nursing at Ribeirão Preto, University of Sao Paulo, Ribeirão Preto, SP, Brazil

Liyoko Okino College of Nursing at Ribeirão Preto, University of Sao Paulo, Ribeirão Preto, SP, Brazil

Carole A. Paley Airedale NHS Foundation Trust, Ward 12, Research Office, Skipton Road, Steeton, Keighley, West Yorkshire, BD20 6TD, UK

Faculty of Health and Social Sciences, Leeds Metropolitan University, Leeds, UK

Francesco C. Peluso State University of New York Downstate Medical Center, Brooklyn, NY, USA

Stephen M. Sagar Departments of Oncology and Medicine, McMaster University; Juravinski Cancer Centre, 699 Concession Street, Hamilton, ON L8V 5C2, Canada

Namie O. Sawada College of Nursing at Ribeirão Preto, University of Sao Paulo, Ribeirão Preto, SP, Brazil

David Seto Department of Medicine, Weill Cornell Medical College, New York, NY, USA

Jennifer A. Stone Department of Radiation Oncology, School of Medicine, Indiana University, 357 S. Landmark Ave. Suite B, Bloomington, IN 47403, USA

Raimond K. Wong Departments of Oncology and Medicine, McMaster University; Juravinski Cancer Centre, 699 Concession Street, Hamilton, ON L8V 5C2, Canada

Ruixin Zhang Center for Integrative Medicine, School of Medicine, University of Maryland, Rm 8-22, MSTF, 685 West Baltimore Street, Baltimore, MD 21201, USA

Chapter 1
An Overview of Acupuncture and Moxibustion for Cancer Care

Tae-Young Choi, Myeong Soo Lee and Edzard Ernst

Abstract Acupuncture and moxibustion are frequently used in palliative and supportive cancer care. Many clinical trials have been conducted, and their results have been evaluated in numerous systematic reviews (SRs). The objective of this chapter is to provide an overview of these SRs. Fourteen databases were searched from their inception through November 2011. Study selection, data extraction, and validations were performed independently by two reviewers. The quality of SRs was assessed using The Overview Quality Assessment Questionnaire. We identified 14 relevant SRs: 11 SRs relating to acupuncture, 2 SRs relating to acupressure and 1 SR related to moxibustion met our inclusion criteria. The adverse events observed among cancer patients included hot flashes, chemotherapy-induced nausea and vomiting (CINV), leucopenia, xerostomia and pain. The indications supported by reasonably good evidence were CINV and cancer pain. This chapter concluded that CINV and cancer pain are the only indications for acupuncture, acupressure or moxibustion currently supported by concrete evidence. Future studies should be of high quality with a particular emphasis on designing adequate control interventions.

1.1 Introduction

Cancer is a leading cause of death worldwide, accounting for 7.6 million deaths (approximately 13% of all deaths in 2008) (Jemal et al. 2011). The estimated 5-year survival rate for all cancers has risen to approximately 66% (American Cancer Society 2012a,b). Cancer survivors experience a wide range of symptoms during and following the completion of treatment, and some of these symptoms may persist for years or even decades. While pharmacologic treatments relieve many symptoms, they may have negative side effects (Cassileth et al. 2007; Wesa et al. 2008).

M. S. Lee (✉) · T.-Y. Choi
Medical Research Division, Korea Institute of Oriental Medicine, 461-24, Jeonmin-dong, Yuseong-gu, Daejeon 305-811, South Korea
e-mail: drmslee@gmail.com

E. Ernst
Complementary Medicine, Peninsula Medical School, University of Exeter, Exeter, UK

W. C. S. Cho (ed.), *Acupuncture and Moxibustion as an Evidence-based Therapy for Cancer*, Evidence-based Anticancer Complementary and Alternative Medicine 3,
DOI 10.1007/978-94-007-4833-0_1, © Springer Science+Business Media Dordrecht 2012

During the last two decades, the use of complementary and alternative medicine (CAM), including acupuncture, as an adjunctive therapy for cancer-related symptoms and for improving a patient's quality of life has increased (Richardson et al. 2000). Several studies have shown rates of CAM use for cancer ranging from 34–91% in the USA (Dean-Clower et al. 2010). The usage of CAM therapies may be higher among those with more advanced cancer or significant cancer therapy-related symptoms (Bardia et al. 2007). The widespread use of CAM by cancer patients is attributed to their hope of improving survival, reducing recurrence, reducing the side effects of surgery and chemotherapy, and also treating physical and psychosocial issues. CAM is often administered to treat nausea and vomiting, fatigue, pain and other symptoms. Most cancer patients employ CAM as an adjunct rather than an alternative to conventional oncological care (Levinson et al. 2000; Beinfield and Korngold 2003).

However, the clinical effectiveness of CAM remains uncertain (Alimi et al. 2003; Vickers et al. 2004; American Society of Clinical Oncology 2006), and many experts doubt its biological plausibility.

Acupuncture and its variants are commonly used to control the symptoms of cancer patients, and some evidence suggests that it can play an important role in the support care for cancer-related conditions (Konkimalla and Efferth 2008).

The National Institutes of Health (NIH) Consensus Development Conference in 1997 stated that acupuncture is an effective treatment modality, particularly for nausea and vomiting induced by chemotherapy and for the relief of pain (NIH Consensus Statement 1998). The American Cancer Society informs patients that, "Acupuncture is simple, and often works. It has few side effects or complications, and the cost is low. For these reasons, "It can be a good choice for some problems" (American Cancer Society). The frequency of acupuncture use among cancer patients ranges between 1.2 and 31% (Filshie and Hester 2006; Gansler et al. 2008).

Numerous clinical trials of acupuncture for cancer care have emerged; however, their results are contradictory. Systematic reviews (SRs) summarizing this evidence may provide clarification. To date, several such articles have been published. Unfortunately, their conclusions are also conflicting.

Thus, this overview is aimed at summarizing and critically evaluating all SRs on acupuncture, acupressure and moxibustion as a symptomatic treatment for cancer patients. Our ultimate goal is to provide clinicians with clearer guidance as to the value of these approaches.

1.2 Methods

1.2.1 Data Sources

The following databases were searched from the date of their inception to November 27, 2011, without language restrictions: Medline, EMBASE, AMED, CINHAL, the Cochrane Library, six Korean Medical Databases (Korean Studies Information,

DBPIA, Korea Institute of Science and Technology Information, Korea Education and Research Information Service, KoreaMed and Korean National Assembly Library) and the China National Knowledge Infrastructure (CNKI). In addition, our extensive departmental files were searched by hand. The keywords used in the search were (systematic review OR meta-analysis) AND (acupuncture OR acupressure OR moxa OR moxibustion) AND (cancer OR tumor OR carcinoma). Articles were included if they related to a formal SR or meta-analysis on any type of acupuncture, acupressure or moxibustion as a symptomatic treatment for any type of cancer condition. Reviews, comments and overviews without a systematic methods section were excluded.

1.2.2 Study Selection

All systematic reviews were included if they investigated patients with cancer who received acupuncture, acupressure or moxibustion. Reviews that were not systematic were excluded. There were no language restrictions. Two review authors (TYC and MSL) independently reviewed the articles according to predefined criteria, including conditions, number of primary studies, methodological quality of the primary studies, conclusion of each SR, and data related to the search. Any disagreement between review authors was resolved by discussion, and, if necessary, by the other author.

1.2.3 Data Extraction

All clinical endpoints were considered, but the main outcome measures were the effectiveness of acupuncture, moxibustion or acupressure for the treatment of symptoms in cancer patients and cancer survivors. Two independently trained review authors extracted data for each eligible trial. Disagreements were resolved by a discussion between the authors to reach a consensus. If there was no agreement, a third review author acted as the arbitrator.

1.2.4 Assessment of the Quality of SRs

The Overview Quality Assessment Questionnaire (OQAQ) was used to evaluate the methodological quality of all included SRs (Oxman and Guyatt 1991; Jadad and McQuay 1996). In the OQAQ, the score ranges from 1 to 7. A score of 3 or less was considered as indicative of major flaws, whereas a score of 5 or more suggested only minor flaws. The two authors performed these assessments independently, and discrepancies were settled by discussion.

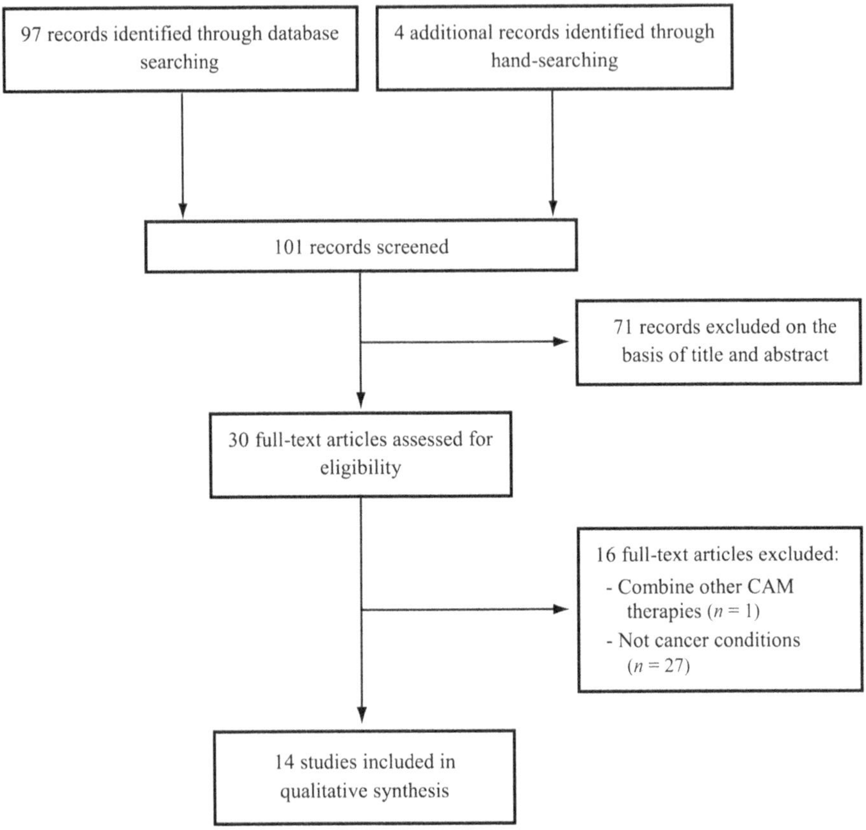

Fig. 1.1 Flow chart of the publication selection process. *CAM* complementary and alternative medicine

1.3 Results

Our searches generated 101 articles, and 14 SRs met our inclusion criteria (Fig. 1.1, Table 1.1 (Klein and Griffiths 2004; Jedel 2005; Lee et al. 2005, 2008, 2009a,b, 2010; Ezzo et al. 2006; Lu et al. 2007; Chao et al. 2009; Hollis 2010; O'Sullivan and Higginson 2010; Peng et al. 2010; Paley et al. 2011). They address a range of different symptoms among cancer patients including chemotherapy-induced nausea and vomiting (CINV) (Klein and Griffiths 2004; Ezzo et al. 2006; Lee et al. 2008, 2010), chemotherapy-induced neutropenia (Lu et al. 2007), cancer pain (Lee et al. 2005; Hollis 2010; Peng et al. 2010; Paley et al. 2011), xerostomia (Jedel 2005; O'Sullivan and Higginson 2010) and hot flashes (Lee et al. 2009a,b). Four studies originated from the UK (Klein and Griffiths 2004; Lee et al. 2005; O'Sullivan and Higginson 2010; Paley et al. 2011), 3 from the US (Ezzo et al. 2006; Lu et al. 2007; Hollis 2010), 4 from Korea (Lee et al. 2008, 2009a,b, 2010), one from Taiwan

Table 1.1 Systematic reviews (SRs) of acupuncture, moxibustion or acupressure for supportive cancer care

References/ country	Condition	Intervention	No. of primary studies	Methodological quality of primary studies[b]	Meta-analysis	Conclusion (quote)[b]	Quality of SR OQAQ[a]	Authors' result[b]
Chao et al. (2009) Taiwan	Therapy-related adverse effects in breast cancer patients	Acupuncture point stimulating therapies	26 studies (18 RCTs/8 CCTs)	Mostly poor	None	No conclusive remarks can be made	6	+/−
Lee et al. (2009a) Korea	Hot flashes in breast cancer patients	Acupuncture	6 studies (6 RCTs)	Mostly good	Acupuncture *vs* sham acupuncture; response rate post-treatment (3 RCTs): RR 1.91, 95% CI 0.10 to 3.71, $p = 0.02$, I^2 76%; response rate during treatment period (3 RCTs): RR 3.09, 95% CI −0.04 to 6.23, $p = 0.25$, $I^2 = 28\%$	The evidence is not convincing	6	−
Lee et al. (2009b) Korea	Hot flashes in prostate cancer patients	Acupuncture	6 studies (1 RCT/ 5 UOS)	Mostly poor	None	The evidence is not convincing	6	−
Lu et al. (2007) US	CT-induced leucopenia	Acupuncture	11 studies (11 RCTs)	Poor	Acupuncture-point stimulation (all types) *vs* control (all types), acute vomiting (7 RCTs): RR 1.22, 95% CI 0.64 to 1.81, $p < 0.05$, $I^2 = 81\%$	Studies may lead to false positive estimation	4	+/−

Table 1.1 (continued)

References/country	Condition	Intervention	No. of primary studies	Methodological quality of primary studies[b]	Meta-analysis	Conclusion (quote)[b]	Quality of SR OQAQ[a]	Authors' result[b]
Ezzo et al. (2006) US	CT-induced nausea and vomiting	Acupuncture point stimulating therapies	11 studies (11 RCTs)	Variable	Acupuncture-point stimulation (all types) *vs* control (all types), acute vomiting (9 RCTs): RR −0.82, 95% CI 0.69 to 0.99, $p = 0.84$, $I^2 = 0\%$; needle acupuncture *vs* control, acute vomiting (4 RCTs): RR 0.74, 95% CI 0.58 to 0.94, $p = 0.014$, $I^2 = 24\%$; electroacupuncture *vs* control, acute vomiting (3 RCTs): RR 0.77, 95% CI 0.61 to 0.97, $p = 0.026$, $I^2 = 40\%$; acupressure *vs* control, acute nausea-severity (1 RCT): SMD 0.02, 95% CI 0.42 to 0.46, $p = 0.92$	Suggests a biologic effect of acupoint stimulation	7	+

Table 1.1 (continued)

References/ country	Condition	Intervention	No. of primary studies	Methodological quality of primary studies[b]	Meta-analysis	Conclusion (quote)[b]	Quality of SR OQAQ[a]	Authors' result[b]
Klein (2004) UK	CT-induced nausea and vomiting	Acupressure	2 studies (2 RCTs)	Variable	None	Acupressure may decrease nausea	3	+
Lee et al. (2008) Korea	CT-induced nausea and vomiting	Acupressure	10 studies (10 RCTs)	Variable	None	Acupressure should be strongly recommended	1	+
Lee et al. (2010) Korea	CT-induced nausea and vomiting (cancer in general)	Moxibustion	5 studies (5 RCTs)	Poor	Moxa plus CT *vs* CT; response rate (4 RCTs): RR 1.04, 95% CI 0.94 to 1.15, $p = 0.43$, $I^2 = 26\%$; side effects (2 RCTs): RR 0.38, 95% CI 0.22 to 0.65, $p = 0.0005$, $I^2 = 0\%$	The evidence is limited to suggest moxibustion is an effective supportive cancer care in nausea and vomiting	5	+
Jedel (2005) Sweden	Xerostomia	Acupuncture	3 studies (3 RCTs)	Mostly poor	None	There is no evidence for the efficacy of acupuncture	6	–
O'Sullivan (2010) UK	Xerostomia	Acupuncture	3 studies (3 RCTs)	None	None	Limited evidence suggests that acupuncture is beneficial	6	+/–
Lee et al. (2005) UK	Cancer pain	Acupuncture	7 studies (3 RCTs/ 4 UOS)	Mostly poor	None	The notion that acupuncture is effective is not supported by rigorous clinical trials	6	–

Table 1.1 (continued)

References/ country	Condition	Intervention	No. of primary studies	Methodological quality of primary studies[b]	Meta-analysis	Conclusion (quote)[b]	Quality of SR OQAQ[a]	Authors' result[b]
Peng et al. (2010) China	Cancer pain	Acupuncture	7 studies (7 RCTs)	Mostly poor	None	Acupuncture is effective for pain relief	5	+
Hollis (2010) US	Cancer pain	Acupuncture	2 studies (3 RCTs/ 2 UOS)	Variable	None	Causality cannot be inferred	3	+/−
Paley et al. (2011) UK	Cancer pain	Acupuncture	3 studies (3 RCT)	Variable	Auricular acupuncture *vs* placebo, pain on VAS at 2 months (1 RCT): RR 0.82, 95% CI 1.36 to 0.28; acupuncture *vs* placebo ear seeds, pain on VAS at 2 months (1 RCT): RR 1.06, 95% CI 1.61 to 0.51; placebo acupuncture *vs* placebo ear seeds, pain on VAS at 2 months (1 RCT): RR 0.13, 95% CI 0.65 to 0.38	We concluded that there was insufficient evidence to judge whether acupuncture is effective in relieving cancer-related pain in adults	7	+

CCT non-randomized controlled trial, *CT* chemotherapy, *RCT* randomized controlled trial, *RR* relative risk, *SMD* standard mean difference, *SR* systematic review, *UOS* uncontrolled observational study, *VAS* visual analogue scale

[a]Overview Quality Assessment Questionnaire (OQAQ) the overall score ranges from 1 to 7, OQAQ ≤ 3 having extensive or major flaws, OQAQ ≥ 5 having minor or minimal flaws

[b]This score relied on the original authors' judgment, + overall positive, − failed to show effectiveness, +/− unclear

(Chao et al. 2009), one from China (Peng et al. 2010) and one from Sweden (Jedel 2005). Five SRs arrived at positive conclusions (Klein and Griffiths 2004; Ezzo et al. 2006; Lee et al. 2010; Peng et al. 2010; Paley et al. 2011). Most of the SRs were of good quality, but all were based on primary studies of poor quality (Table 1.1 and 1.2).

1.3.1 Chemotherapy-Induced Nausea and Vomiting

Based on the included reviews, acupuncture (Ezzo et al. 2006), acupressure (Klein and Griffiths 2004; Lee et al. 2008) and moxibustion (Lee et al. 2010) reduce CINV.

Ezzo et al. (2006) evaluated the efficacy of acupuncture-point stimulation on acute and delayed CINV in cancer patients. Eleven studies (n = 1,247) were included in the meta-analysis. Overall, the combined effect of all interventions reduced the incidence of acute vomiting (risk ratio (RR) = 0.82; 95% confidence interval (CI) 0.69 to 0.99; $p = 0.84$), but not of severe acute or delayed nausea compared to controls. Needle acupuncture reduced acute vomiting (RR = 0.74; 95% CI 0.58 to 0.94; $p = 0.014$) but not the severity of acute nausea. Electroacupuncture reduced acute vomiting (RR = 0.77; 95% CI 0.61 to 0.97; $p = 0.026$), but manual acupuncture did not (delayed symptoms were not reported). Acupressure reduced the mean acute nausea-severity (standard mean difference = 0.02; 95% CI −0.42 to 0.46; $p = 0.92$) but not acute vomiting or delayed symptoms. Non-invasive electrostimulation generated no benefits for any outcome measure. All trials used concomitant pharmacologic anti-emetics, and all, except the electroacupuncture trials, used state-of-the-art anti-emetics. However, this review complements data on post-operative nausea and vomiting suggesting a biological effect of acupuncture-point stimulation.

Klein and Griffiths (2004) assessed the effectiveness of acupressure in the form of SeaBand for the relief of treatment-related nausea and vomiting. The use of acupressure plus standard care was compared with standard care alone. Adult patients receiving cancer chemotherapy were monitored for the frequency and severity of nausea or vomiting. This SR identified two RCTs (n = 482) that compared acupressure to no such intervention. One RCT reported significant differences over the 10-day follow-up period in favor of acupressure in terms of both the experience ($p < 0.01$) and the intensity of nausea ($p < 0.04$) but not regarding the Chemotherapy Problem Checklist related to nausea ($p = 0.845$). The other RCT reported no significant effects ($p > 0.05$) on vomiting, delayed nausea or anti-emetic use, but there was a significant ($p < 0.05$) benefit in the acupressure group with regard to early nausea (0.4 points on a 7-point scale). These results therefore suggest that acupressure may decrease nausea among patients undergoing chemotherapy.

Lee et al. (2008) conducted an SR evaluating the effects of acupressure combined with anti-emetics for CINV. Ten RCTs were included (n = 1,464). Four of seven acupressure band RCTs demonstrated the positive effects of acupressure, whereas three acupressure band trials yielded negative results. All studies with negative results had methodological weaknesses. One quasi-experimental and two randomized finger

Table 1.2 Overview Quality Assessment Questionnaire (OQAQ) assessment of reporting characteristics

References	1 Were the search methods reported?	2 Was the search comprehensive?	3 Were the inclusion criteria reported?	4 Was selection bias avoided?	5 Were the validity criteria reported?	6 Was validity assessed appropriately?	7 Were the methods used to combine studies reported?	8 Were the findings combined appropriately?	9 Were the conclusions supported by the reported data?	10 Overall score
Chao et al. (2009)	2	2	2	0	2	2	2	2	2	6
Lee et al. (2009a)	2	2	2	0	2	2	2	2	2	6
Lee et al. (2009b)	2	2	2	0	2	2	2	2	2	6
Lu et al. (2007)	2	2	2	0	2	2	0	0	1	4
Ezzo et al. (2006)	2	2	2	2	2	2	2	2	2	7
Klein (2004)	2	2	2	1	2	2	0	0	1	3
Lee et al. (2008)	2	1	0	0	0	0	0	1	1	1
Lee et al. (2010)	2	2	2	0	0	2	2	2	2	5
Jedel (2005)	2	2	2	0	2	2	2	2	2	6
O'Sullivan et al. (2010)	2	2	2	0	2	2	2	2	2	6
Lee et al. (2005)	2	2	2	0	2	2	2	2	2	6
Peng et al. (2010)	2	2	2	0	2	2	0	2	2	5
Hopkins (2010)	2	2	2	0	1	1	0	2	2	3
Paley et al. (2011)	2	2	2	2	2	2	2	2	2	7

Overview Quality Assessment Questionnaire (OQAQ) the overall score ranges from 1 to 7, OQAQ ≤ 3 having extensive or major flaws, OQAQ ≥ 5 having minor or minimal flaws acupressure trials demonstrated positive effects of acupressure. The overall effect of acupressure was suggestive but not conclusive.

Lee et al. (2010) published an SR investigating the effects of moxibustion for supportive cancer care. Five RCTs (n = 301) compared the effects of moxibustion with conventional therapy. Four RCTs failed to show favorable effects on the response rate compared with chemotherapy (n = 229, RR 1.04, 95% CI 0.94 to 1.15, p = 0.43). Two RCTs assessing the occurrence of adverse effects of chemotherapy demonstrated the positive effects of moxibustion. A meta-analysis generated a favorable effect on the frequency of CINV (n = 80, RR 0.38, 95% CI 0.22 to 0.65, p = 0.0005, heterogeneity: $\chi^2 = 0.18$, $p = 0.67$, $I^2 = 0\%$). All studies had a high risk of bias, and thus the overall result was inconclusive.

In summary, the evidence is positive for acupuncture as a treatment for CINV. For other acupuncture-related interventions, the evidence is less certain.

1.3.2 *Chemotherapy-induced Neutropenia*

Lu et al. (2007) conducted an SR assessing the effectiveness of acupuncture for chemotherapy-induced leukopenia. Eleven RCTs with cancer patients (n = 682) who were undergoing or had just completed chemotherapy or chemoradiotherapy were included. They were randomized to either acupuncture therapy or standard care. The median sample size of each comparison group was 45, and the median trial duration was 21 days. The frequency of the acupuncture treatment was once a day, with a median of 16 sessions in each trial. In the seven trials in which white blood cell (WBC) counts were available, acupuncture use was associated with an increase in leukocyte counts in patients during chemotherapy or chemoradiotherapy, with a weighted mean difference of 1,221 WBC/μL (95% CI 636 to 1,807; $p < 0.0001$). The poor quality of the primary data prevented firm conclusions about the value of acupuncture for this indication.

In summary, the evidence fails to show definitively that acupuncture is effective for this indication.

1.3.3 *Cancer Pain*

Lee et al. (2005) conducted an SR summarizing the evidence for acupuncture for cancer-related pain. Of the seven studies included (n = 368), one high-quality RCT of ear acupuncture reported statistically significant pain relief in comparison with placebo ear acupuncture. All the other studies were either not blinded (n = 2) or uncontrolled (n = 4). A visual analog scale (VAS) and the patient's verbal assessment were used as primary pain-related outcome measures. The authors concluded that the notion of acupuncture as an effective analgesic adjunctive method for cancer patients is not supported by sound evidence.

Peng et al. (2010) published an SR of seven RCTs testing the effects of acupuncture on cancer pain. They compared acupuncture with placebo, Western drugs, Chinese herbal medicines, or acupuncture therapy plus drug treatments. The high-quality trial showed that auricular acupuncture therapy was significantly superior to placebo in alleviating pain. This SR therefore arrived at positive conclusions.

Hollis (2010) conducted an SR and meta-analysis of three studies investigating the effect of acupuncture treatment as a treatment modality for cancer pain. A synthesis of the current evidence revealed a lack of level I and II evidence. The majority of the evidence is level III or lower; therefore, the conclusions of this SR are not positive.

Paley et al. (2011) conducted an SR evaluating the efficacy of acupuncture for the relief of cancer-related pain in adults. Three RCTs ($n = 204$) were included. One high-quality study investigated the effect of auricular acupuncture compared with auricular acupuncture at placebo points with non-invasive vaccaria ear seeds attached at placebo points. There was a high risk of bias in both studies because of the low methodological quality. One study comparing acupuncture with medication concluded that both methods were effective in controlling pain, although acupuncture was the most effective. The second study compared acupuncture, point-injection and medications in participants with stomach cancer. Long-term pain relief was reported for both acupuncture and point-injection compared with medications administered during the last 10 days of treatment. Although both studies support the use of acupuncture, they should be interpreted with caution due to their methodological limitations, small sample size, poor reporting and inadequate analyses. Therefore, there is insufficient evidence to determine whether acupuncture is effective in treating cancer pain in adults.

In summary, these SRs do not arrive at uniform conclusions. The studies of better quality tend to be negative or cautious about the value of acupuncture or related interventions for reducing cancer pain. It therefore follows that the best current evidence fails to convincingly demonstrate the effectiveness of acupuncture for this indication.

1.3.4 Xerostomia

Jedel (2005) conducted an SR to assess the efficacy of acupuncture in the management of xerostomia. Three RCTs ($n = 79$) met the criteria for inclusion, and a criteria list was used to assess the quality of these studies, which turned out to be variable. The results of the trials were equally variable ranging from positive to negative. This SR therefore produced little evidence for the effectiveness of acupuncture in the management of xerostomia.

O'Sullivan and Higginson (2010) published an SR of three RCTs ($n = 108$) investigating the effectiveness and safety of acupuncture in radiation-induced xerostomia (RIX) in patients with head and neck cancer (HNC). Two trials compared acupuncture with sham acupuncture, and one compared acupuncture with standard care. The outcome measurements included salivary flow rates (SFRs) in two trials and subjective questionnaires in three. All three trials reported significant reductions in xerostomia *vs* the baseline SFR ($p < 0.05$); one reported greater effects for stimulated SFR in the intervention group ($p < 0.01$). A subjective assessment reported significant differences between true acupuncture and control treatment in two trials ($p < 0.02$–0.05). This limited evidence therefore suggests that acupuncture might be beneficial for RIX.

In summary, these SRs generated somewhat contradictory findings. The value of acupuncture as a treatment for xerostomia is therefore not firmly established.

1.3.5 Hot Flashes

Lee et al. (2009a) conducted an SR evaluating the effectiveness of acupuncture for hot flashes in patients with breast cancer. Six studies ($n = 281$) were included in the meta-analysis. The RCTs compared true acupuncture with sham acupuncture, another active treatment or no treatment. Three RCTs compared the effects of manual acupuncture with those of sham acupuncture. One RCT demonstrated favorable effects of acupuncture in reducing the frequency of hot flashes, while two RCTs failed to do so. The meta-analysis showed significant effects of acupuncture compared with sham acupuncture ($n = 189$, weighted mean difference 3.09, 95% CI −0.04 to 6.23, $p = 0.05$), but marked heterogeneity was observed in this model ($\chi^2 = 8.32$, $p = 0.02$, $I^2 = 76\%$). One RCT compared the effects of electroacupuncture with hormone replacement therapy. Hormone therapy was more effective than electroacupuncture. Another RCT compared acupuncture with venlafaxine and reported no significant differences between the groups. The authors concluded that there is inadequate evidence to suggest that acupuncture is an effective treatment for hot flashes in patients with breast cancer.

Lee et al. (2009b) tested the effects of acupuncture as a treatment for hot flashes in prostate cancer (PC) patients. Six studies ($n = 132$) met the inclusion criteria. One RCT compared the effects of manual acupuncture with acupuncture plus electroacupuncture. The other five studies were uncontrolled observational studies that were open to a range of biases. The authors concluded that there is no strong evidence to suggest acupuncture is an effective treatment for hot flashes in patients with PC.

In summary, these SRs fail to generate good evidence for acupuncture as treatment for cancer-related hot flashes.

1.3.6 Treating the Adverse Effects of Conventional Cancer Therapies

Chao et al. (2009) conducted an SR evaluating the evidence for acupoint stimulation in the management of therapy-related adverse events in breast cancer. This SR identified clinical trials that were designed to examine the efficacy of acupressure, acupuncture, or acupoint stimulation for the management of adverse events associated with breast cancer treatment. Twenty-six trials (18 RCTs and eight CCTs) satisfied the inclusion criteria. They assessed the application of acupoint stimulation on six disparate conditions related to anticancer therapies, including vasomotor syndrome, CINV, lymphedema, post-operation pain, aromatase inhibitor-related joint pain and leukopenia. The modalities of acupoint stimulation used included traditional acupuncture, acupressure, electroacupuncture, and the use of magnetic devices on acupuncture points. The methodological quality of the trials was assessed using a modified Jadad scale. Overall, 23 trials (88%) reported positive outcomes for at least one of the conditions examined. Three high-quality trials suggested that acupoint stimulation on Neiguan (PC6) was beneficial to CINV. In summary, apart from the evidence relating to CINV, there is little evidence to suggest that acupuncture is effective in reducing the adverse effects of oncological treatments.

In conclusion, numerous systematic reviews have recently become available, but evidence of the effectiveness of acupuncture or moxibustion for the symptomatic treatment or prevention of cancer symptoms is mixed, e.g. CINV is sometimes positively judged and sometimes not. Further limitations of our overview are the potentially poor quality of the primary data and the poor reporting of results, which were highly heterogeneous in virtually every respect. In the future, the areas that warrant further investigation include the efficacy of acupuncture or moxibustion interventions utilizing rigorous RCT designs.

1.4 Discussion

Our overview shows that several SRs on acupuncture, moxibustion or acupressure therapies have been published. Given that most of them were published recently, the scientific interest in CAM therapies seems to be growing. Many of the reviews were of poor quality, based on few and often less than rigorous clinical trials, and arrived at overall positive conclusions.

There were four reviews that focused on the treatment of CINV (Jedel 2005; Ezzo et al. 2006; Lee et al. 2008, 2010) (Table 1.3). They are all positive, but unfortunately they were based on primary studies that were mostly of poor quality.

Four systematic reviews on the treatment of cancer pain have been published (Lee et al. 2005; Hollis 2010; Peng et al. 2010; Paley et al. 2011) (Table 1.3). They were of relatively high quality and included seven mostly rigorous trials (Paley et al. 2011). Lee et al. (2005) concluded that "the evidence is negative", while Peng et al. (2010) and Paley et al. (2011) reported that "the evidence is positive". Hollis (2010) concluded that "the evidence is not consistent". The evidence is thus not conclusive. More well-designed trials using rigorous methodology are required to determine the effectiveness of acupuncture interventions for managing cancer pain.

For the treatment of hot flashes, there were two published SRs (Lee et al. 2009a, 2009b): one on breast cancer in women and one on prostate cancer in men. Both were

Table 1.3 Indications evaluated by multiple systematic reviews

Symptoms	Number of SRs	Direction of results			Overall effects	Comments
		+	+/−	−		
Chemotherapy induced nausea and vomiting	4	4	0	0	+	All the SRs are of high quality, the Cochrane review is positive
Xerostomia	2	0	1	1	+/−	A recent SR cannot confirm the effectiveness of alternative treatment
Cancer pain	4	2	1	1	+/−	The evidence is mixed

SR systematic review, + positive conclusion, − negative conclusion, +/− conclusion that was neither positive nor negative

low-quality studies that reported negative results and were mostly based on poor-quality primary studies. The evidence is thus inadequate to recommend acupuncture as an effective treatment for hot flashes in breast cancer and prostate cancer patients.

The other two SRs investigated chemotherapy-induced leucopenia (Lu et al. 2007) and xerostomia (Jedel 2005; O'Sullivan and Higginson 2010) (Table 1.3). Both were of poor quality and relied on a small number of flawed studies. Thus, the value of acupuncture is not well documented for either of these conditions.

Overall, the effectiveness of acupuncture, moxibustion and acupressure for the symptomatic treatment of cancer is currently not well documented. This is in sharp contrast to the many claims made by the proponents of these modalities.

Relatively encouraging evidence was found for the use of these tools in treating nausea and vomiting in cancer patients (Klein and Griffiths 2004; Ezzo et al. 2006; Lee et al. 2008, 2010). Unfortunately, these SRs were mostly based on poor quality primary studies. Thus, there is considerable uncertainty about the value of acupuncture, moxibustion and acupressure therapies for these indications.

Adverse events were reported in two SRs (Chao et al. 2009; Lee et al. 2009a). Chao et al. (2009) reported that the adhesive for the acu-magnet device and the electrocurrent stimulation generated a few side effects, including skin irritation and a shock sensation. Lee et al. (2009a) reported mild adverse events for acupuncture, such as distress, fatigue, a hematoma at the insertion site and a few second transient increase in vasomotor symptoms. However, there were no serious adverse events that required medical management.

Most SRs of acupuncture, moxibustion or acupressure therapies have stressed that their conclusiveness was limited by the often poor quality of the primary data. Our analysis confirms this impression. Many of the primary acupuncture, moxibustion or acupressure therapy trials originate in China (data not shown). Vickers et al. (1998) demonstrated that virtually 100% of Chinese acupuncture trials are positive. This disturbing finding casts considerable doubt on the reliability of these studies and limits the conclusions that can be drawn from many of the SRs included in this overview. Systematic reviews have been criticized for being unable to provide specific guidance. However, even if uncertainty persists, SRs have the important function of highlighting these concerns. Thus, as mentioned above, our overview highlights areas of research that require further clinical trials.

Our overview has several important limitations. Although our search strategy was thorough, it is possible that some relevant articles were missed. By evaluating systematic reviews rather than clinical trials, important details of the primary studies may have been lost. Most importantly, the poor quality of the primary data and the systematic reviews was a major weakness. Collectively, these limitations limit the conclusions that can be drawn.

Future RCTs of acupuncture-type therapies for supportive cancer care should adhere to the accepted standards of clinical trial methodology. The studies included in this review demonstrate a number of problems that have been previously noted by other reviews that examined the efficacy of acupuncture-type therapies. Furthermore, even though it is difficult to blind subjects to treatment, the use of examiner blinding and allocation concealment are important for reducing bias.

1.5 Conclusion

CINV and cancer pain are the only indications for acupuncture, acupressure or moxibustion currently supported by sound evidence. Future studies should be of high quality with a particular emphasis on designing adequate control interventions. In conclusion, numerous systematic reviews have recently become available, but evidence of the effectiveness of acupuncture or moxibustion for symptomatic treatment or for the prevention of cancer symptoms is mixed, e.g. CINV is sometimes positively judged and sometimes not. Further limitations of our overview are the potential poor quality of the primary data and the poor reporting of results, which were highly heterogeneous in virtually every respect. The areas that warrant further investigations include the efficacy of acupuncture or moxibustion interventions using a rigorous RCT design.

Acknowledgment MSL and TYC were supported by the KIOM (K11111 and C12080).

References

Alimi, D., Rubino, C., Pichard-Léandri, E., Fermand-Brulé, S., Dubreuil-Lemaire, M.L., Hill, C. (2003) Analgesic effect of auricular acupuncture for cancer pain: a randomized, blinded, controlled trial. *Journal of Clinical Oncology*, *15*, 4120–4126.

American Cancer Society (2012a). Acupuncture. http://www.cancer.org/Treatment/TreatmentsandSideEffects/ComplementaryandAlternativeMedicine/ManualHealingandPhysicalTouch/acupuncture. Accessed 12 Sep 2012.

American Cancer Society (2012b). Cancer facts & fig. 2012. http://www.cancer.org/acs/groups/content/@epidemiologysurveilance/documents/document/acspc-031941.pdf. Accessed 12 Sep 2012.

American Society of Clinical Oncology, Kris, M.G., Hesketh, P.J., Somerfield, M.R., Feyer, P., Clark-Snow, R., et al (2006) American Society of Clinical Oncology guideline for antiemetics in oncology: update 2006. *Journal of Clinical Oncology, 24*, 2932–2947.

Bardia, A., Greeno, E., Bauer, B.A. (2007) Dietary supplement usage by patients with cancer undergoing chemotherapy: does prognosis or cancer symptoms predict usage? *The Journal of Supportive Oncology*, *5*, 195–198.

Beinfield, H., Korngold, E. (2003) Chinese medicine and cancer care. *Alternative Therapies in Health and Medicine*, 9, 38–52.

Cassileth, B.R., Deng, G.E., Gomez, J.E., Johnstone, P.A., Kumar, N., Vickers, A.J. (2007) Complementary therapies and integrative oncology in lung cancer: ACCP evidence-based clinical practice guidelines (2nd edition). *Chest*, *132*, 340–354.

Chao, L.F., Zhang, A.L., Liu, H.E., Cheng, M.H., Lam, H.B., Lo, S.K. (2009) The efficacy of acupoint stimulation for the management of therapy-related adverse events in patients with breast cancer: a systematic review. *Breast Cancer Research and Treatment, 118*, 255–267.

Dean-Clower, E., Doherty-Gilman, A.M., Keshaviah, A., Baker, F., Kaw, C., Lu, W., et al (2010) Acupuncture as a palliative therapy for physical symptoms and quality of life for advanced cancer patients. *Integrated Cancer Therapies*, *9*, 158–167.

Ezzo, J.M., Richardson, M.A., Vickers, A., Allen, C., Dibble, S.L., Issell, B.F., et al (2006) Acupuncture-point stimulation for chemotherapy-induced nausea or vomiting. *Cochrane Database of Systematic Reviews (Online)*, *19*, CD002285.

Filshie, J., Hester, J. (2006) Guidelines for providing acupuncture treatment for cancer patients–a peer-reviewed sample policy document. *Acupuncture in Medicine*, *24*, 172–182.

Gansler, T., Kaw, C., Crammer, C., Smith, T. (2008) A population-based study of prevalence of complementary methods use by cancer survivors: a report from the American Cancer Society's studies of cancer survivors. *Cancer*, *113*, 1048–1057.

Hollis, A.S. (2010) Acupuncture as a treatment modality for the management of cancer pain: the state of the science. *Oncology Nursing Forum*, *37*, E344–348.

Jadad, A.R., McQuay, H.J. (1996) Meta-analyses to evaluate analgesic interventions: a systematic review of their methodology. *Journal of Clinical Epidemiol*, *49*, 235–243.

Jedel, E. (2005) Acupuncture in xerostomia: a systematic review. *Journal of Oral Rehabilitation*, *32*, 392–396.

Jemal, A., Bray, F., Center, M.M., Ferlay, J., Ward, E., Forman, D. (2011) Global Cancer Statistics. *CA: A Cancer Journal for Clinicians*, *61*, 69–90.

Klein, J., Griffiths, P. (2004) Acupressure for nausea and vomiting in cancer patients receiving chemotherapy. *British Journal of Community Nursing*, *9*, 383–388.

Konkimalla, V.B., Efferth, T. (2008) Evidence-based Chinese medicine for cancer therapy. *Journal of Ethnopharmacology*, *116*, 207–210.

Lee, H., Schmidt, K., Ernst, E. (2005) Acupuncture for the relief of cancer-related pain-a systematic review. *European Journal of Pain, 9*, 437–444.

Lee, J., Dodd, M., Dibble, S., Abrams, D. (2008) Review of acupressure studies for chemotherapy-induced nausea and vomiting control. *Journal of Pain and Symptom Management*, *36*, 529–544.

Lee, M.S., Choi, T.Y., Park, J.E., Lee, S.S., Ernst, E. (2010) Moxibustion for cancer care: a systematic review and meta-analysis. *BMC Cancer*, *10*, 130–138.

Lee, M.S., Kim, K.H., Choi, S.M., Ernst, E. (2009a) Acupuncture for treating hot flashes in breast cancer patients: a systematic review. *Breast Cancer Research and Treatment*, *115*, 497–503.

Lee, M.S., Kim, K.H., Shin, B.C., Choi, S.M., Ernst, E. (2009b) Acupuncture for treating hot flushes in men with prostate cancer: a systematic review. *Supportive Care in Cancer*, *17*, 763–770.

Levinson, W., Gorawara-Bhat, R., Lamb, J. (2000) A study of patient clues and physician responses in primary care and surgical settings. *JAMA*, *284*, 1021–1027.

Lu, W., Hu, D., Dean-Clower, E., Doherty-Gilman, A., Legedza, A.T., Lee, H.,et al (2007) Acupuncture for chemotherapy-induced leukopenia: exploratory meta-analysis of randomized controlled trials. *Journal of the Society for Integrative Oncology*, *5*, 1–10.

NIH Consensus Statement. (1998) Acupuncture. *JAMA, 280*, 1518–1524.

O'Sullivan, E.M., Higginson, I.J. (2010) Clinical effectiveness and safety of acupuncture in the treatment of irradiation-induced xerostomia in patients with head and neck cancer: a systematic review. *Acupuncture in Medicine Society, 28*, 191–199.

Oxman, A.D., Guyatt, G.H. (1991) Validation of an index of the quality of review articles. *Journal of Clinical Epidemiology, 44*, 1271–1278.

Paley, C.A., Johnson, M.I., Tashani, O.A., Bagnall, A.M. (2011) Acupuncture for cancer pain in adults. *Cochrane Database of Systematic Reviews, 19*, CD007753.

Peng, H., Peng, H.D., Xu, L., Lao, L.X. (2010) Efficacy of acupuncture in treatment of cancer pain: a systematic review. *Journal of Chinese Integrative Medicine, 8*, 501–509.

Richardson, M.A., Sanders, T., Palmer, J.L., Greisinger, A., Singletary, S.E. (2000) Complementary/alternative medicine use in a comprehensive cancer center and the implications for oncology. *Journal of Clinical Oncology, 18*, 2505–2514.

Vickers, A., Goyal, N., Harland, R., Rees, R. (1998) Do certain countries produce only positive results? A systematic review of controlled trials. *Controlled Clinical Trials, 19*, 159–166.

Vickers, A.J., Straus, D.J., Fearon, B., Cassileth, B.R. (2004) Acupuncture for postchemotherapy fatigue: a Phase II study. *Journal of Clinical Oncology, 22*, 1731–1735.

Wesa, K., Gubili, J., Cassileth, B. (2008) Integrative oncology: complementary therapies for cancer survivors. *Hematology/Oncology Clinics of North America, 22*, 343–353.

Chapter 2
The Mechanistic Studies of Acupuncture and Moxibustion

Jaung-Geng Lin and Yi-Hung Chen

Abstract Many preclinical and clinical studies have demonstrated that acupuncture results in multiple biological responses. Manual acupuncture (MA) and electro-acupuncture are capable of triggering a chain of events that can be understood through controlled experiments. The best-known mechanism is *via* endogenous opiates and their receptors. Different kinds of endogenous opiates, such as β-endorphin, enkephalin, endomorphin and dynorphin, reportedly act as frequency-dependent factors in electroacupuncture. While low-frequency electroacupuncture (2 Hz) accelerates the release of β-endorphin and enkephalin in the central nervous system (CNS), high-frequency electroacupuncture (100 Hz) accelerates the release of dynorphin. Notably, some researchers have found that there are different responses to acupuncture in normal and hyperalgesic animal models. Importantly, the frequency-dependent phenomenon may not be apparent in hyperalgesic animals. Serotonin is thought to have a role in acupuncture analgesia, with evidence suggesting that serotonin and its related descending inhibitory pathway regulate a hyperalgesic effect through the enkephalin interneurons located in the spinal cord. This chapter discusses the mechanisms of acupuncture analgesia and the mechanism of acupuncture in inflammation, insomnia, nausea and vomiting and drug addiction. It also discusses some mechanistic studies of acupuncture conducted by our research group. Recent mechanistic studies of moxibustion are also summarized.

2.1 Introduction

Traditional Chinese acupuncture has a history of over 3,500 years. Acupuncture has recently increased in popularity and is becoming more widespread throughout some Western countries. It is described as a "complementary medicine", showing efficacy in the treatment of many conditions and resulting in fewer side effects compared with other medical procedures, such as surgery or pharmaceuticals (Wu 1996). Notably,

Y.-H. Chen (✉)
Graduate Institute of Acupuncture Science, China Medical University, Taichung, Taiwan
e-mail: yihungchen@mail.cmu.edu.tw

J.-G. Lin (✉)
School of Chinese Medicine, China Medical University, Taichung, Taiwan
e-mail: jglin@mail.cmu.edu.tw

W. C. S. Cho (ed.), *Acupuncture and Moxibustion as an Evidence-based Therapy for Cancer*, Evidence-based Anticancer Complementary and Alternative Medicine 3,
DOI 10.1007/978-94-007-4833-0_2,

the World Health Organization (WHO) has published a guidance on the efficacy of acupuncture in the cure or relief of 64 different clinical conditions of acute and chronic pain, including for example fatigue, nausea, arthritis, and digestive problems (WHO 2003).

Two different strategies are employed by acupuncture therapy: manual acupuncture (MA) and electroacupuncture. Electroacupuncture is a modified form of the traditional MA. The advantage of electroacupuncture is in its combined therapeutic effects of transcutaneous electric nerve stimulation (TENS) and MA. Most studies use electroacupuncture because electroacupuncture can be standardized by frequency, voltage, wave form, length, etc. However, although standardization is essential for modern research, some experts do not agree that electroacupuncture can be a substitution for MA (Lin and Chen 2008).

2.2 General Concepts of the Mechanism of Acupuncture

Many studies in animals and humans have demonstrated that acupuncture can cause multiple biological responses (Wang et al. 2001). From the neurophysiologic point of view, the mechanical action of needling or its electrical equivalent, i.e. electroacupuncture, triggers a chain of events that can be understood through controlled experiments. For example, needling may cause receptors to send neural impulses to the spinal cord or act on ascending pathways to the brain, and cause the release of neurotransmitters that subsequently modulate functions in the brain as well as in the periphery (Sun and Li 2001; Liu et al. 2004; Middlekauff et al. 2004).

A recent review attests to substantial evidence in regard to the involvement of the nervous system in acupuncture analgesia (Han 2011). Studies have shown that application of MA to one acupoint (e.g. LI4) induces a gradual increase in skin pain threshold that reaches a plateau at 30 min, is maintained for at least 50 min, and fades after removal of the needle with a half-life of 15–17 min (Research Group of Acupuncture Anesthesia 1973). This characteristic time-dependent analgesic effect is totally abolished when the local anesthetic procaine is infused deep into the acupoint at the muscle and tendon layer, whereas subcutaneous application of procaine has no such effect, which highlights the importance of nerve innervations distributed in the deeper structures of the acupoint. The effect was present in hemiplegic patients when the needle was inserted in the healthy side, but was absent in the paralytic side of the body (Research Group of Acupuncture Anesthesia 1973).

The effects of acupuncture have now been extensively studied. This chapter concerns the mechanism of acupuncture on analgesia, inflammation, insomnia, nausea and vomiting, drug addiction, and the mechanism of moxibustion. It also discusses some mechanistic studies of acupuncture conducted by our group.

2.3 The Mechanism of Acupuncture Analgesia

2.3.1 *Endorphins Theory*

Endogenous opiates are considered to play important roles in acupuncture analgesia (AA). In early studies, naloxone, an antagonist to opiate (a morphine-like substrate), was found to attenuate the analgesic action of acupuncture in humans (Mayer et al. 1977) and mice (Pomeranz and Chiu 1976). This evidence suggested the release of a morphine-like substrate in the central nervous system (CNS) was a possible mechanism. In the early 1980s, β-endorphin and enkephalin were purified and it was suggested that they play important roles in AA. Elevated levels of endorphin have been identified in cat cerebrospinal fluid (CSF) after auricular electroacupuncture (Pert et al. 1981), while in humans, elevated levels of CSF, β-endorphin (Clement-Jones et al. 1980) and plasma enkephalin (Kiser et al. 1983) have been observed after acupuncture. Subsequently, the relationship between AA and different endogenous opiates has been examined. Pomeranz and colleagues first described the possibility that different mechanisms of analgesia exist, in their investigations into different frequencies of electroacupuncture application (Cheng and Pomeranz 1979), which inspired further research. The most widely recognized research group comprises Dr Han and colleagues (Chen and Han 1992), whose experiments in electroacupuncture analgesia have clarified that frequency is a basic determinant for secretion of different endogenous opiates. They found that lower frequency (2 Hz) electroacupuncture analgesia is mediated by μ- and δ-opioid receptors and that higher frequency (100 Hz) electroacupuncture analgesia is mediated by the κ-opioid receptor. They concluded that 2 Hz electroacupuncture stimulates the release of β-endorphin, enkephalin and endomorphin (Han et al. 1999; Huang et al. 2000) within the CNS network and that 100 Hz electroacupuncture releases dynorphin (Han 2003).

More recent research has focused on the antihyperalgesic effects of acupuncture in inflammatory animal models (Koo et al. 2002; Sekido et al. 2003; Huang et al. 2004; Lao et al. 2004). Injured neurons express increased numbers of peptides (substance P, somatostatin and calcitonin gene-related peptide) related to pain transmission, a phenomenon commonly referred to as neuronal plasticity (Hokfelt 1991). With persistent inflammation, neuronal plasticity causes hyperalgesia (hyperexcitable to pain). Research groups led by Berman and Zhang identified that AA differs between chronic pain animal models (induced by persistent inflammation) and normal animal models. They concluded that in hyperalgesic rats, both lower (10 Hz) and higher (100 Hz) frequency electroacupuncture decreased paw withdrawal latency through μ- and δ-opioid receptors (Zhang et al. 2004a). Conversely, in normal animals, only lower frequency electroacupuncture, not higher frequency electroacupuncture, is mediated through the μ- and δ-opioid receptors. Higher frequency electroacupuncture elicits analgesic effects *via* the κ-opioid receptor (Han 2003). These researchers have demonstrated the existence of different mechanisms in various animal models. In peripheral inflamed tissue, immune cells express endogenous opiates and bind with opioid receptors on peripheral afferent nerves (Stein 1995). This binding of opiates and their receptors can inhibit the transmission of noxious signals from the peripheral nerve system (PNS) to the CNS. Local peripheral opioid receptors on nerve endings are upregulated during inflammation and these peripheral receptors are likely to be more responsive than those central receptors to AA (Sekido et al. 2003). Sekido's research (2003) established that local blockade, rather than systemic blockade, of opioid receptors decreased the analgesic effect of electroacupuncture. Evidence for a neuroimmune link has informed recent debate concerning whether endogenous opiates act as neurotransmitters or hormones: endorphins are capable of functioning as neurotransmitters in the CNS and as hormones within peripheral tissue. Given these complexities, AA cannot be explained by any single mechanism.

2.3.2 Serotonin and the Descending Pain Inhibitory Pathway Theory

Our research group focuses on the role of central monoamimergic systems in AA, with a particular emphasis on serotonin (5-hydroxytryptamine, 5-HT), speculated to be an analgesic transmitter in an early study, which demonstrated an increase in the threshold of tail pressure pain in Sprague-Dawley (SD) rats after application of 2 Hz electroacupuncture (Cheng et al. 1979). This analgesic effect diminished after injection with the serotonin synthesis inhibitor, p-chlorophenylalanine (Tsai et al. 1989a). Thus, serotonin is thought to have a role in AA. Evidence suggests that serotonin levels increase in the spinal cord (Tsai et al. 1989b) and that its precursor (5-hydroxytryptophan) responds to enhanced analgesia at 2 Hz electroacupuncture (Chang et al. 2004). In order to elucidate those receptor subtypes that serotonin acts upon at different frequencies of electroacupuncture, we used antagonists for 5-HT_{1a}, 5-HT_2 and 5-HT_3 receptor subtypes to analyze electroacupuncture-related changes in analgesic effects. It has been found that electroacupuncture analgesia is blocked by 5-HT_{1a} and 5-HT_3 antagonists at both low and high frequencies, whereas electroacupuncture analgesia is enhanced by 5-HT_2 antagonism at a high frequency (100 Hz) (Chang et al. 2004). These results suggest the importance of the serotoninergic pathway in AA and are supported by later studies (Baek et al. 2005; Kim et al. 2005).

There are many serotonin-releasing nuclei (serotoninergic neurons) in the CNS, one of which is the nucleus raphe magnus (NRM). Positioned in the lower brainstem (from lower pons to medulla), the NRM is associated with the descending pain inhibitory pathway. As the axons of these serotoninergic neurons terminate at the level of the spinal cord, they are termed the serotoninergic raphe-spinal neurons. Electroacupuncture activates these neurons (Liu et al. 1986). Serotonin is released from the terminals of the serotoninergic raphe-spinal neurons and then binds to the receptors on the surface of the inhibitory interneurons. There are several 5-HT receptor subtypes. The 5-HT_1 and 5-HT_3 subtypes are located in the dorsal horn of the spinal cord and their agonists have been found to reduce pain (Danzebrink and Gebhart 1991; Eide and Hole 1993). The 5-HT_{1a} subtype is also an autoreceptor within the NRM.

The binding of serotonin to its receptor can activate the inhibitory interneurons in the spinal cord, which contain enkephalin (enkephalinergic interneurons). Enkephalin and μ/δ-opioid receptors are thought to play important roles in inhibiting pain sensation signals. These enkephalinergic interneurons presynaptically block the signal transmission of peripheral nociception by releasing enkephalin. Electroacupuncture, at both lower and higher frequencies, can activate the abovementioned mechanism.

2.3.3 *Acupuncture and the Adenosine Receptor*

Goldman et al. (2010) found that adenosine, a neuromodulator with anti-nociceptive properties, was released during acupuncture in mice and that its anti-nociceptive actions required adenosine A_1 receptor expression. Direct injection of an adenosine A_1 receptor agonist replicated the analgesic effect of acupuncture. Inhibition of enzymes involved in adenosine degradation potentiated the acupuncture-elicited increase in adenosine, as well as its anti-nociceptive effect. These observations indicate that adenosine mediates the effects of acupuncture and that interfering with adenosine metabolism may prolong the clinical benefit of acupuncture (Goldman et al. 2010). This is the first report to show involvement of the adenosine receptor in the effects of acupuncture.

A schematic diagram indicating the mechanisms of acupuncture/Electroacupuncture-induced analgesia is shown in Fig. 2.1.

2.4 Acupuncture and Inflammation

It has been shown that long-term electroacupuncture reduces the activities of T and B cells in the lymph nodes of collagen-induced arthritic mice (Yim et al. 2007). In another study (Yu et al. 1998), the activity of splenic natural killer (NK) cells in mice was enhanced after long-term electroacupuncture. The apparent immune modulating effect of electroacupuncture is eliminated by β-endorphin antagonist (naloxone) injection. In a hyperalgesic animal model, inflammatory responses (edema and hyperalgesia) are reduced by electroacupuncture (Zhang et al. 2004b, 2005; Choi et al. 2005). This effect may be explained by endogenous opiates: injection of naloxone at the site of injury can attenuate the anti-inflammatory action caused by electroacupuncture. Therefore, it has been suggested that peripheral opioid receptors play a role in the anti-inflammatory action (Sekido et al. 2003). However, the immediate anti-inflammatory effect of electroacupuncture persists after intraperitoneal injection of naloxone. Using different study protocols, the anti-inflammatory effect of electroacupuncture was shown to act *via* a non-opioid mechanism in the CNS (Sekido et al. 2003; Zhang et al. 2004b). This conflicting evidence demonstrates that different mechanisms are involved in the long-term and immediate anti-inflammatory effects of

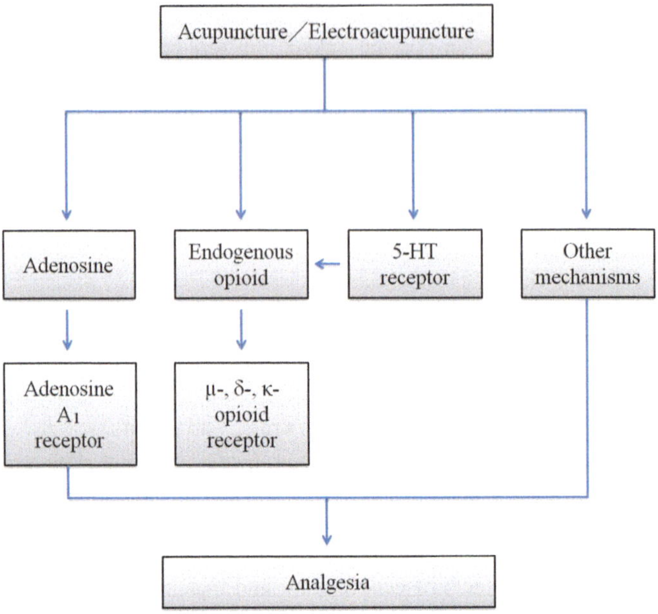

Fig. 2.1 Schematic diagram showing the mechanisms of acupuncture/electroacupuncture-induced analgesia

electroacupuncture. A schematic diagram indicating the mechanisms of acupuncture/electroacupuncture-induced anti-inflammatory effects is shown in Fig. 2.2.

2.5 Acupuncture and Immunomodulation

Electroacupuncture can modulate the imbalance between the innate and acquired immune systems. Electroacupuncture has been shown to have the ability to adjust the pattern of leukocytes (granulocytes and lymphocytes) in human subjects (Mori et al. 2002). Several lines of evidence indicate that this effect is associated with the hypothalamus-pituitary-adrenal (HPA) axis (Son et al. 2002; Chiu et al. 2003; Lao et al. 2004; Lee et al. 2004; Sung et al. 2004). Notably, hypothalamic messenger RNA (mRNA) expression of proinflammatory cytokines induced by lipopolysaccharide stimulation is reduced by electroacupuncture (Son et al. 2002). It has been reported that lower frequency electroacupuncture (4 Hz) produces less of an analgesic effect in animals that have undergone pituitary gland removal (Pomeranz et al. 1977). A schematic diagram indicating the mechanisms of acupuncture/electroacupuncture-induced immunomodulation is shown in Fig. 2.3.

Fig. 2.2 Schematic diagram showing the mechanisms of acupuncture/electro-acupuncture-induced anti-inflammatory effects

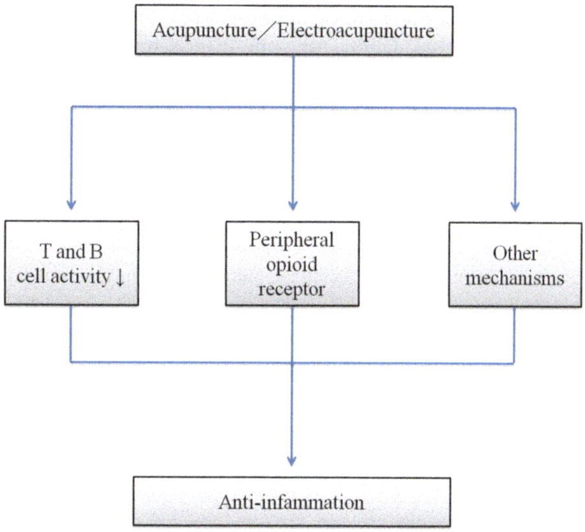

Fig. 2.3 Schematic diagram showing the mechanisms of acupuncture/electro-acupuncture-induced immunomodulative effects

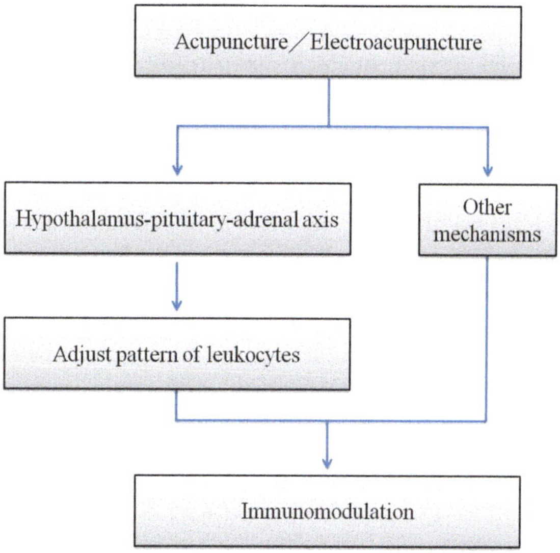

2.6 Acupuncture and Insomnia

Hyperarousal is associated with pathophysiology involving both the CNS and the ANS (Bonnet and Arand 1997; Richardson 2007; Roth et al. 2007). Acupuncture is potentially a unique method for insomnia intervention because of its direct effects on the ANS (Huang et al. 2011). Certainly, acupuncture has been shown to influence some known indicators of autonomic activities, such as blood pressure (Tam and Yiu 1975; Williams et al. 1991; Sugiyama et al. 1995), pupil size (Ohsawa et al. 1997), skin conductance, thermographic skin temperature measurements (Ernst and Lee 1985; Hsieh et al. 1999), microneurographic evaluation of muscle sympathetic nerve activities (Sugiyama et al. 1995; Knardahl et al. 1998), heart rate and/or pulse rate (Nishijo et al. 1997; Hsieh et al. 1999), and heart rate variability (Haker et al. 2000; Li et al. 2003b; Hsu et al. 2006; Litscher 2007).

At different acupoints, acupuncture can account for different effects on the ANS. For example, acupoints Ximen (PC4) (Nishijo et al. 1997), Dazhui (GV14) and Neiguan (PC6) (Li et al. 2003b), as well as Sishencong (EX-HN1) (Wang et al. 2002), are all capable of increasing parasympathetic while simultaneously suppressing sympathetic activities (Haker et al. 2000), whereas stimulation of the auricular Lung (Haker et al. 2000) significantly increases parasympathetic activity without affecting sympathetic activity. Moreover, whereas Quchi (LI11) (Haker et al. 2000) activates both parasympathetic and sympathetic activities, Zusanli (ST-36) increases segmental sympathetic vasomotor activity with central sympathetic inhibition (Sugiyama et al. 1995).

The caudal nucleus tractus solitarius (NTS) may be activated by acupuncture, since the NTS is located in the dorsomedial medulla oblongata and receives afferents primarily from the vagus and glossopharyngeal nerves (Cottle 1964; Cheng et al. 2011). Ascending projections from the NTS have been traced through the lateral and dorsal tegmentum and periventricular gray zone up to the rostral pons and midbrain, terminating in the parabrachial nucleus, which in turn projects to the thalamus, hypothalamus, preoptic area, bed nucleus of the stria terminalis, amygdala and the frontal cortex; regions commonly belonging to the visceral-limbic forebrain (Norgren 1978; Ryan 1985). Recently, studies have suggested the existence of neurons in the NTS that are involved in generating sleep. Furthermore, microinjection of morphine into the NTS provokes an enhancement of slow-wave sleep (SWS) and this effect is blocked by naloxone (Reinoso-Barbero and de Andres 1995), suggesting the somnogenic effect of the opioidergic system in the NTS. Yi and colleagues (2004) demonstrated that activation of the cholinergic system in the caudal NTS of the medulla oblongata mediates the enhancement of non-rapid eye movement (NREM) sleep induced by electroacupuncture stimulation of Anmian (EX17) acupoints. Electroacupuncture may also increase β-endorphin concentrations in the NTS and subsequently alter sleep, since the NTS area is one of the anatomically distinct β-endorphin pathways in the brain that is influenced by electroacupuncture (Bronstein et al. 1993). It is believed that mechanisms of electroacupuncture-induced NREM sleep enhancement may be mediated, in part, by cholinergic activation, stimulation of the opioidergic neurons to increase the concentrations of β-endorphin and the involvement of the μ-opioid receptors (Cheng et al. 2011).

A more recent study (Cheng et al. 2012) has demonstrated that high-frequency (100 Hz) electroacupuncture at the Anmian acupoint enhanced SWS during the dark period, but exhibited no direct effect on REM sleep. High-frequency electroacupuncture-induced SWS enhancement was dose-dependently blocked by microinjection of naloxone or a κ-opioid receptor antagonist (nor-binaltrophimine) into the caudal NTS, whereas no such effect was seen after administration of a μ-opioid receptor antagonist (naloxonazine) nor after a δ-opioid receptor antagonist (natrindole), suggesting that NTS κ-opioid receptors play a role in SWS enhancement induced by high-frequency electroacupuncture. These results and those from previous studies depict the opioid mechanisms of electroacupuncture-induced sleep. A schematic diagram showing the mechanisms of acupuncture/electroacupuncture-induced insomnia intervention is shown in Fig. 2.4.

2.7 Acupuncture and Nausea and Vomiting

Nausea and vomiting is primarily controlled by the vomiting center, an area in the brainstem in the dorsolateral reticular formation of the medulla. This center is influenced by afferent stimuli from the CNS including the cerebral cortex, vestibular and cerebellar nuclei and the chemoreceptor trigger zone. The chemoreceptor trigger zone is close to the area postrema on the floor of the fourth ventricle. The chemoreceptor trigger zone is very sensitive to stimuli from chemoreceptors and pressure receptors in the gut, and to circulating chemicals like opioids or other emetic drugs. Histamine, serotonin-dopamine, acetylcholine, and opioid receptors are all found in the chemoreceptor trigger zone.

Streitberger et al. (2006) have reviewed the mechanism underlying acupuncture at Neiguan (PC6) against nausea and vomiting. They propose that several mechanisms of action are responsible for the effect of PC6 on nausea and vomiting, as follows:

1. PC6 works through neurotransmitters. Many experimental studies have shown that acupuncture influenced the endogenous opioid system (Han and Terenius 1982) as well as serotonin transmission *via* activation of serotonergic and noradrenergic fibers (Mao et al. 1980; Takeshige et al. 1992).
2. Acupuncture at PC6 affects the smooth muscle of the gut (Hu et al. 1995; Stern et al. 2001).
3. Acupuncture at PC6 affects the somatovisceral reflex. Electrostimulation at PC6 inhibited the rate of transient lower esophageal sphincter relaxations triggered by gastric distension in healthy volunteers, while sham acupuncture had no such effect (Zou et al. 2005). In contrast to findings from Tatewaki et al. (2005), this effect was not inhibited by naloxone, which thus suggests a non-opioid mechanism is involved. Zou and colleagues speculated the possible involvement of a somatovisceral reflex, which has been previously demonstrated to affect gastric motility in rats (Sato et al. 1993).
4. PC6 works through sensory input inhibition. According to this theory, when sensory input from gastric distension is inhibited, it leads to an inhibition of the frequency of transient lower esophageal sphincter relaxations. Because acupuncture has no influence on the residual lower esophageal sphincter pressure or on the duration of lower esophageal sphincter relaxations, it seems unlikely that acupuncture acts primarily on the efferent motor pathway (Zou et al. 2005).
5. PC6 stimulates a somatosympathetic reflex that induces gastric relaxation. The reflex centre is within the medulla, and the ventrolateral medulla neurons may play an important role (Tada et al. 2003).

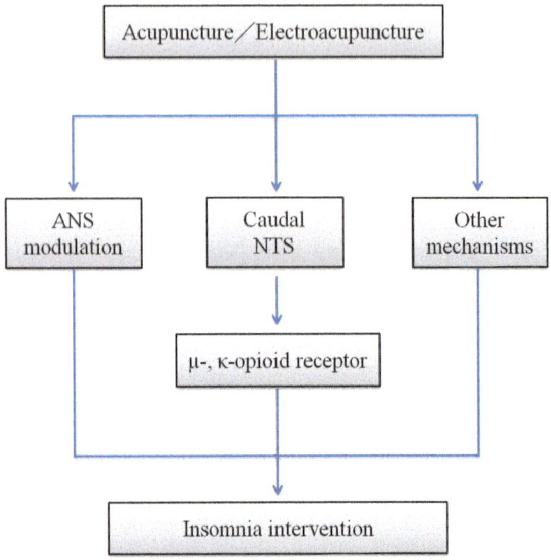

Fig. 2.4 Schematic diagram showing the mechanisms of acupuncture/electro-acupuncture-induced insomnia intervention

6. PC6 can increase vagal modulation. Huang et al. (2005) proposed that vagal modulation could be examined through heart rate variability analysis. When normalized high-frequency power was used to measure vagal modulation, normalized high-frequency power increased in the PC6 group but not in the sham acupuncture or no-treatment groups. Similar results were observed for acupuncture at PC6 in combination with a second acupuncture point LI4 compared to a sham procedure (Li et al. 2005).
7. PC6 may influence the cerebellar vestibular neuromatrix. According to functional magnetic resonance imaging (fMRI) data, acupuncture at PC6 selectively activates the left superior frontal gyrus, anterior cingulated gyrus and dorsomedial nucleus of the thalamus, whereas sham acupuncture or tactile stimulation fails to do so (Yoo et al. 2004).

2.8 Acupuncture and Drug Addiction

The application of acupuncture in opiate addiction originated from a serendipitous observation by Dr. Wen in 1972, who reported that acupuncture combined with electrical stimulation at four body points and two ear points relieved the symptoms of opioid withdrawal in persons with opiate addiction (Cui et al. 2008).

This method was later adopted in many clinical settings in Western countries, using a protocol developed in 1985 by Dr. M. Smith, the head of the US National Acupuncture Detoxification Association (NADA). The NADA protocol describes the insertion of five needles without the use of electrical stimulation bilaterally into the outer ear or auricle at points termed the sympathetic, shenmen, kidney, lung, and liver.

The NADA protocol advises that five-point auricular acupuncture relieves withdrawal symptoms, prevents symptoms of craving, and increases patient participation rates in long-term treatment programs (McLellan et al. 1993). Auricular acupuncture is the most common form of acupuncture treatment for substance addiction in both the US and the UK (Margolin 2003; D'Alberto 2004).

The mesolimbic dopamine system originates in the ventral tegmental area (VTA) and projects to regions that include the nucleus accumbens and prefrontal cortex, which are believed to play a pivotal role in the development of opiate addiction (Yang et al. 2008a). Opiate abuse-induced changes in the levels of dopamine in the brain are associated with feelings of well-being and pleasure, providing positive reinforcement of continued opiate abuse (Weiss et al. 1992; Peoples et al. 1998). Conversely, withdrawal from chronic opiate administration reduces dopamine outflow in the nucleus accumbens (Diana et al. 1996; Rossetti et al. 1999). Opioid withdrawal causes dysphonia and significant distress, a state that addicts seek to avoid and one that can be a major motive for continuing opiate use (i.e. negative reinforcement) (Wise et al. 1995; Weiss and Porrino 2002).

Early studies demonstrated the involvement of κ-opioid receptors underlying the effects of acupuncture on morphine addiction. In 1993, Han and Zhang (1993) reported the effectiveness of electroacupuncture in the morphine abstinence syndrome in a rat experimental model. The authors found that 100 Hz electroacupuncture produced a statistically significant suppression of wet shakes, teeth chattering, escape attempts, weight loss, and penile licking ($p < 0.05$) whereas 2 Hz electroacupuncture produced a mild but significant suppression in escape attempts and wet shakes. These results suggest that 100 Hz electroacupuncture was far more effective than 2 Hz electroacupuncture in suppressing withdrawal syndrome. Further studies have suggested that electroacupuncture suppresses the opiate withdrawal syndrome by activating κ-opioid receptors and dynorphin release (Wen and Ho 1982; Han and Zhang 1993; Green and Lee 1988; Wu et al. 1999a; Cui et al. 2000).

Moreover, acupuncture affects the reinforcing effects of morphine. The method of conditioned place preference (CPP) is a commonly used animal model of drug craving (Markou et al. 1993). Wang et al. (2000) reported that morphine-induced place preference in rats is significantly suppressed by frequencies of 2 and 2/100 Hz, but not by 100 Hz. However, Shi et al. (2003) showed that 100 Hz electroacupuncture significantly attenuated morphine-induced CPP, and this effect was completely blocked by δ- and κ-opioid receptor antagonists, suggesting that the anti-craving effects induced by 100 Hz electroacupuncture are mediated by the activation of δ- and κ-opioid receptors.

In 2008, Yang et al. (2008a) reviewed the possible mechanism underlying the effectiveness of acupuncture in the treatment of drug addiction and provided clear evidence for the biological effects underlying the use of acupuncture to treat drug abuse. This review provided a hypothetical model for the effects of acupuncture on dopamine release in the nucleus accumbens. Regarding positive reinforcement, acupuncture treatment activates $GABA_B$ receptors on the dopamine cell body and activates presynaptic κ-opioid receptors in the nucleus accumbens through dynorphin neurons, resulting in decreased dopamine release. Regarding negative reinforcement, acupuncture treatment stimulates enkephalin neurons in the hypothalamus and interacts with μ-opioid receptors to inhibit ventral tegmental area GABAergic interneurons and thus increases dopamine release in the nucleus accumbens (Yang et al. 2008a).

In summary, neurochemical and behavioral evidence has shown that acupuncture helps reduce the effects of positive and negative reinforcement involved in opiate addiction, by modulating mesolimbic dopamine neurons. Moreover, several brain neurotransmitter systems involving opioids and GABA have been implicated in the modulation of dopamine release by acupuncture. A schematic diagram indicating the mechanisms of acupuncture/electroacupuncture-induced beneficial effects on positive and negative reinforcement involved in opiate addiction is shown in Fig. 2.5.

2.9 The Cerebral Cortex Plays an Important Role in the Physiological Mechanism of Acupuncture

Electrophysiological recordings, including evoked potential recordings, blink reflex and H reflex recordings, have been widely used for particular purposes. These signals are stable and the sources are easily identified, making them suitable for use in studying the mechanism of acupuncture, as shown in studies by Professor Ching-Liang Hsieh at China Medical University.

2.9.1 The Auditory Endogenous Potential, P300

The auditory endogenous potential, P300, is a positive reflection wave with a latency of 300–400 ms. P300 activity originates from multiple cerebral areas (Neshige and Luders 1988, 1992; Tarkka et al. 1995, 1996). It is a reliable method for evaluating recognition of a stimulus by the cerebral cortex. We therefore investigated the physiological mechanism and response to acupuncture stimulation using the acupoints formula. The observation that acupuncture stimulation of both Zusanli (ST36) acupoints decreased P300 amplitudes suggested involvement of the cerebral cortex when simultaneous sensations are received from both acupoints. No such changes were observed in the non-acupoint assessment, which has been suggested to be related to so-called acupoint specificity (Hsieh et al. 1998).

2.9.2 Sympathetic Skin Response and Somatosensory Evoked Potentials

In order to study the physiological mechanism of acupuncture stimulation, palm recordings of sympathetic skin response (SSR) were evoked by electrical stimulation of the right median nerve in 13 normal adult volunteers. Median nerve-evoked short-latency somatosensory evoked potential (SEP) recordings were taken at least

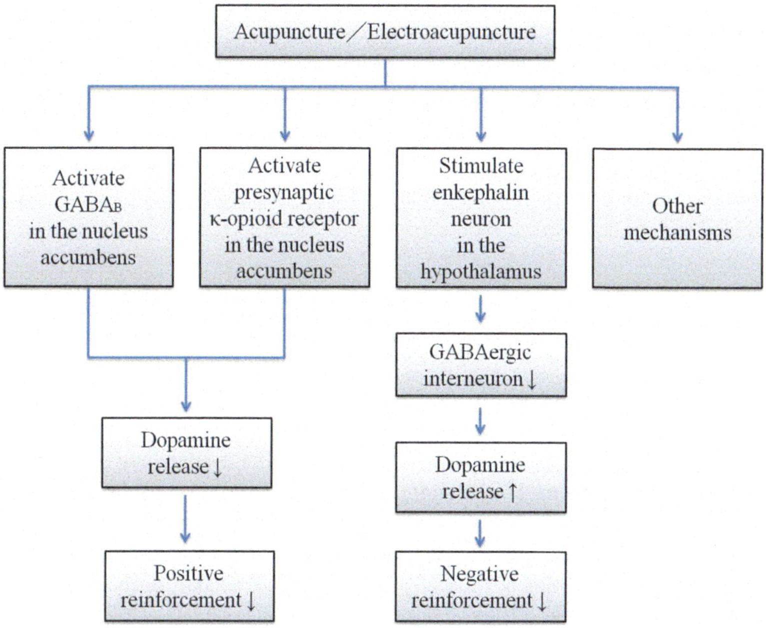

Fig. 2.5 Schematic diagram showing the mechanisms of acupuncture/electroacupuncture-induced beneficial effects on positive and negative reinforcement involved in opiate addiction

one week after SSR recordings. Latency and amplitude calculations suggest that acupuncture stimulation of both ST36 acupoints inhibited SSRs, which implies that the cerebral cortex contributes at least in part to this inhibition (Hsieh 1998).

2.10 Intermittent-alternating Mode of Administering Electroacupuncture Stimulation Postpones the Development of Electroacupuncture Tolerance

As mentioned above, electroacupuncture produces analgesia that is mediated by a variety of central neurochemical substances including opioid peptides, and different electroacupuncture frequencies accelerate the release of different types of opioid peptides in the CNS. However, no matter which frequency is applied, prolonged electroacupuncture stimulation over several hours inevitably leads to a decrease in the analgesic effect, a phenomenon known as "tolerance to electroacupuncture analgesia," or "electroacupuncture tolerance", which hinders the use of "electroacupuncture anesthesia" during major surgery. Clinical experience has revealed that the effect of electroacupuncture analgesia can last longer if electroacupuncture is applied intermittently.

We attempted to change the parameters and mode of stimulation in order to avoid, or at least postpone, the development of electroacupuncture tolerance. Electroacupuncture stimulation was applied to the bilateral ST36 and Sanyinjiao (SP6) acupoints in rats, using a simultaneous mode (S mode) on both legs or an alternating mode (A mode) between the legs. A similar degree of analgesic effect was obtained with both modes of stimulation. However, whereas tolerance usually developed within 5 h in the S mode, it was postponed for 10 h in the A mode. It is therefore recommended that the alternating mode rather than the simultaneous mode be used for treating chronic pain patients, in order to postpone or avoid electroacupuncture tolerance without affecting the potency of electroacupuncture-induced analgesia (Lin et al. 1993).

2.11 Effects of Acupuncture on Exercise Physiology

In addition to analgesia, acupuncture is able to modulate body functions, such as heart rate and blood pressure, improve coronary artery blood flow, and lower fat and cholesterol levels. It can also be used to improve gas metabolism and pulmonary respiratory function (Plummer 1981; Chang 1982; Liu 1990). Our group has compared the effects of acupuncture at the PC6 and ST36 acupoints with those of acupuncture at non-acupoints on cardiopulmonary function. Healthy male volunteers were divided into three groups (16 subjects in each). Group 1 was treated with acupuncture at PC6 and ST36; Group 2 was treated with acupuncture at non-acupoints; Group 3 received no treatment. In the acupuncture groups, significant decreases were observed in resting heart rate and carbon dioxide production, as well as a slight decrease in oxygen consumption. These results provide further support for the hypothesis that acupuncture can decrease the resting heart rate and carbon dioxide production, and thus lower the metabolic rate (Lin et al. 1996).

We also investigated whether ear acupuncture affects exercise-induced heart rate responses. Twelve healthy male subjects were included. Small objects (seeds, small steel balls, etc.) were taped to ear acupoints in each subject. Measurement of 75% VO_2 maximum was performed with and without ear point pressing. We found that (1) ear point pressing significantly increased oxygen consumption at rest and during exercise, but not after exercise, (2) ear point pressing significantly decreased the heart rate while resting but values did not differ significantly during and after exercise, (3) ear point pressing significantly lowered the rate of perceived exertion at 10 and 15 min, but not significantly after 5 min of exercise. These results indicate that ear point pressing may enhance exercise performance by virtue of its beneficial effects on physiological responses (Lin et al. 1995).

2.12 Acupuncture fMRI Experiment

The brain controls many functional subsystems within the body and helps regulate homeostatic balance. The brain may be responsible for transducing the needle stimulus into signals aimed at maintaining homeostatic balance within and across functional subsystems. Noninvasive functional neuroimaging provides a means for observing acupuncture effects within the human brain and for better understanding as to how multiple bodily functions may be modified simultaneously (Dhond et al. 2007).

MRI can measure regional change in blood oxygenation level-dependent (BOLD) contrast, caused by increased neuronal activity during a specific task. Thus, fMRI permits non-invasive mapping of brain activity during various specific tasks (Kwong et al. 1992). Recently, fMRI has been used to map the sites of brain activation during acupuncture. In their acupuncture fMRI experiment providing stimulus to the Zhiyin (BL67) acupoint, Cho et al. (1998) presented the first evidence revealing the neurological effects induced by acupuncture, which were equivalent to increasing BOLD signal intensity in the primary visual cortex upon passive light stimulation. This discovery encourages further research using functional neuroimaging techniques into defining the neural correlates of acupuncture stimulus. In almost identical settings to the study conducted by Cho et al. (1998), Siedentopf and colleagues (2002) successfully induced activations in the primary visual cortex by stimulating the BL67 acupoint with laser acupuncture. Li and colleagues (2003a) were also able to successfully provoke visual activations, by applying electroacupuncture to more than one acupoint (connecting positive electrodes to the Shugu (BL65) and BL67 acupoints and negative electrodes to the Kinlun (BL60) and Zutonggu (BL66) acupoints) along the same meridian. However, when Gareus and colleagues (2002) used almost identical settings to those employed by Cho et al., with the only difference being that the acupuncture stimulus was applied to the Guangming (GB37) acupoint instead of to BL67, they failed to find any acupuncture-related brain activities. It is noted that Cho et al. (2006) retracted their article of 1998 which presented the first evidence in 2006. In other similar studies, researchers have reported activations in only the hypothalamus in addition to the pain matrix (M1/S1, anterior cingulate cortex, amygdala, hippocampus, superior temporal gyrus, insula, etc) instead of the brain areas supposedly associated with the stimulated acupoints (Wu et al. 1999b, (2002; Hsieh et al. 2001).

As mentioned previously, due to inherent difficulties in conducting fMRI experiments with the acupuncture paradigm (for example, long carryover effects as characterized by Ho et al. (2008)) as well as in the analyzing of fMRI data, results from previous acupuncture fMRI studies have been inconclusive. The true hemodynamic BOLD responses in relation to acupuncture stimuli will only be defined when the experimental paradigms successfully avoid all confounding factors associated with acupuncture stimuli, and when data analysis methods account for the substantial inter-subject variability. Therefore, in one study, we specifically modeled acupuncture stimulus-induced BOLD responses according to each individual-subject data set. fMRI data were analyzed using the general linear model (GLM) as implemented in Statistical Parametric Mapping 2 (SPM2) with a predefined BOLD time course, with additional time-to-onset shifts. This study firstly revealed the wide variability of acupuncture-induced BOLD onset responses across subjects and, more importantly, demonstrated an approach that accurately defined the true BOLD onsets for each individual subject (Ho et al. 2009).

2.13 Investigations into Safe Needling Depths of Acupoints

If the depth of acupoint insertion extends beyond its safe level, especially in the areas of the neck, chest and back, serious adverse events such as pneumothorax and internal organ damage may occur (Chung et al. 2003). Although ancient Chinese medical literature and modern acupuncture textbooks state needling depths for acupoints, there is scant mention of their safe depths. Our group initially conducted adult autopsies to study the safe needling depths of acupoints of the human back Bladder Meridian; we later studied the safe needling depths of acupoints on the human chest and back using computed tomography (CT) scanning (Lin 1982, 1991). Similarly, Prof Yan's group (Shao et al. 2007) at Shanghai University of Traditional Chinese Medicine (TCM) studied safe needling depths in adult autopsies, and Prof Li's group (Li et al. 2004) at Heilongjiang University of TCM has used CT scanning and adult autopsies to study safe needling depths for a few acupoints.

We conducted a meta-analysis of the published evidence concerning acupoint needling depths, with the aim of providing a uniform guidance. We suggest that CT or MRI be used to measure acupoint needling depths in the living human body. The data can then be subjected to statistical analysis, using methods including multiple regression analysis, to calculate safe needling depths (Chou et al. 2011; Lin et al. 2011). Our group's CT scanning results indicate safe needling depths for acupoints in the back and chest for different-sized people, i.e. normal, over- and under-weight adults, and for sex differences (Tables 2.1–2.4) (Lin 2011).

2.14 The Mechanism of Moxibustion

Moxibustion is a traditional Chinese medical intervention that involves the burning of moxa (i.e. *Artemisia vulgaris* or mugwort) at the acupuncture points. One form of moxibustion applies it directly to the skin surface at the acupuncture point, whereas the indirect form of moxibustion places insulating materials (i.e. ginger, salts) between the moxa cone and the skin (WHO 2007).

Unlike acupuncture stimulation, which involves thrusting or twisting needles, resulting in various biochemical reactions that can produce effects throughout the body, moxibustion uses heat stimulation at various temperature levels from mild skin warming to tissue damage from burning. Therapeutic indications for moxibustion include stomach pain, nausea, dyspepsia, dysmenorrhea, knee osteoarthritis, diarrhea, asthma, stroke, cancer and hypertension, and others (Yao 1985).

Lee et al. (2010) conducted a systematic review of moxibustion for cancer care and concluded that there is no convincing evidence for the effectiveness of moxibustion. However, two RCTs demonstrate that moxibustion as an adjunctive therapy is more effective for reduction of chemotherapy-related side effects, specifically nausea and vomiting, than chemotherapy alone (Chen et al. 2000; Kim et al. 2009).

The mechanisms of acupuncture have been extensively studied, whereas those of moxibustion have been less well studied: recent evidence is summarized below:

Table 2.1 Mean values with 95% confidence intervals for needling depths of acupoints in the chest in different-sized male subjects

Acupoints	Overweight adults Mean ± 95% CI	Normal adults Mean ± 95% CI	Underweight adults Mean ± 95% CI	F
Tiantu (CV22)	3.94 ± 0.19	2.87 ± 0.26	2.34 ± 0.65	19.61*
Xuanji (CV21)	0.94 ± 0.11	0.64 ± 0.10	2.30 ± 0.10	38.22*
Huagai (CV20)	0.89 ± 0.11	0.057 ± 0.10	0.25 ± 0.10	39.46*
Zigong (CV19)	0.89 ± 0.11	0.60 ± 0.10	0.29 ± 0.10	35.79*
Yutang (CV18)	0.88 ± 0.14	0.53 ± 0.10	0.28 ± 0.09	31.32*
Danzhong (CV17)	0.86 ± 0.11	0.52 ± 0.11	0.25 ± 0.09	36.96*
Zhongting (CV16)	0.95 ± 0.14	0.56 ± 0.13	0.34 ± 0.11	25.57*
Shufu (KI27)	4.19 ± 0.46	3.29 ± 0.48	2.32 ± 0.49	16.20*
Yuzhong (KI26)	2.98 ± 0.27	2.20 ± 0.25	1.50 ± 0.27	34.18*
Shencang (KI25)	2.59 ± 0.21	2.00 ± 0.21	1.26 ± 0.22	42.93*
Lingxu (KI24)	2.56 ± 0.17	2.13 ± 0.23	1.49 ± 0.19	32.09*
Shenfeng (KI23)	2.47 ± 0.17	1.96 ± 0.17	1.44 ± 0.17	40.78*
Bulang (KI22)	2.33 ± 0.15	1.95 ± 0.17	1.46 ± 0.15	33.64*
Qihu (ST13)	5.24 ± 0.48	4.15 ± 0.55	2.88 ± 0.47	23.71*
Kufang (ST14)	3.82 ± 0.36	3.10 ± 0.31	2.02 ± 0.29	32.21*
Wuyi (ST15)	3.11 ± 0.27	2.64 ± 0.52	1.38 ± 0.17	26.51*
Yingchuang (ST16)	2.78 ± 0.21	2.35 ± 0.53	1.33 ± 0.22	19.52*
Ruzhong (ST17)	2.59 ± 0.19	2.07 ± 0.38	1.23 ± 0.20	27.28*
Rugen (ST18)	2.27 ± 0.16	1.78 ± 0.22	1.19 ± 0.20	33.89*
Tianchi (PC1)	2.64 ± 0.21	2.25 ± 0.72	1.18 ± 0.21	11.97*
Yunmen (LU1)	6.73 ± 0.55	5.14 ± 0.57	3.26 ± 0.79	32.78*
Zhongfu (LU2)	5.05 ± 0.62	3.69 ± 0.47	2.20 ± 0.70	24.06*
Zhourong (SP20)	3.71 ± 0.50	2.70 ± 0.35	1.68 ± 0.51	21.06*
Xiongxiang (SP19)	3.15 ± 0.37	2.26 ± 0.23	1.53 ± 0.43	23.38*
Tianxi (SP18)	2.88 ± 0.29	2.05 ± 0.25	1.32 ± 0.19	40.68*
Shidou (SP17)	2.61 ± 0.21	1.91 ± 0.22	1.28 ± 0.18	45.01*
Zhejin (GB23)	3.48 ± 0.39	2.43 ± 0.26	1.73 ± 0.37	28.00*
Yuanye (GB22)	4.52 ± 0.41	3.07 ± 0.34	2.20 ± 0.33	43.58*

The definitions for "Overweight adults", "Normal adults" and "Underweight adults" are following the guidance of the Department of Health, Taiwan: "The suggested ideal body weight of Taiwanese people". As such, readers from outside Taiwan should bear in mind that ideal body weights differ between countries. The specified needling depths in the table are a suggested guide only. The data are extracted from JG Lin's Review on the History and Practice of the Needling Depth of Acupoints (2011), National Research Institute of Chinese Medicine (Chinese), Taipei, Taiwan. According to "The suggested ideal body weight of Taiwanese people", ideal body weights are calculated as follows: Males: The ideal body weight is 62 kg for a height of 170 cm. For every increase or decrease by 1 cm in height, the ideal body weight increases or decreases accordingly by 0.6 kg; Females: The ideal body weight is 52 kg for a height of 158 cm. For every increase or decrease by 1 cm in height, the ideal body weight increases or decreases accordingly by 0.5 kg; The normal range varies from between −10% and 10% outside the ideal body weight. Excess body weight for height than the normal range is defined as overweight, while body weight falling below the normal range is defined as underweight

X ± 1.96 SD: 95% confidence interval (CI), X: mean depth, units are provided in centimeters

F is the statistic for One-way ANOVA

*$p < 0.01$

Table 2.2 Mean values with 95% confidence intervals for needling depths of acupoints in the chest in different-sized female subjects

Acupoints	Overweight adults Mean ± 95% CI	Normal adults Mean ± 95% CI	Underweight adults Mean ± 95% CI	F
Tiantu (CV22)	4.46 ± 0.42	3.69 ± 0.46	3.01 ± 0.80	7.39*
Xuanji (CV21)	1.37 ± 0.27	1.03 ± 0.25	0.41 ± 0.33	9.81*
Huagai (CV20)	1.18 ± 0.29	0.88 ± 0.23	0.49 ± 0.38	5.24*
Zigong (CV19)	1.32 ± 0.24	0.97 ± 0.19	0.50 ± 0.40	9.73*
Yutang (CV18)	1.42 ± 0.25	1.00 ± 0.20	0.56 ± 0.46	9.89*
Danzhong (CV17)	1.55 ± 0.23	1.07 ± 0.22	0.71 ± 0.57	8.63*
Zhongting (CV16)	1.75 ± 0.003	1.41 ± 0.32	0.90 ± 0.76	4.17*
Shufu (KI27)	4.31 ± 0.72	3.36 ± 0.47	2.23 ± 0.46	9.90*
Yuzhong (KI26)	2.93 ± 0.44	2.46 ± 0.33	1.53 ± 0.55	9.31*
Shencang (KI25)	2.69 ± 0.39	2.29 ± 0.29	1.53 ± 0.46	8.35*
Lingxu (KI24)	2.70 ± 0.35	2.40 ± 0.26	1.69 ± 0.57	7.19*
Shenfeng (KI23)	2.89 ± 0.32	2.46 ± 0.24	1.79 ± 0.60	9.52*
Bulang (KI22)	2.95 ± 0.30	2.49 ± 0.23	1.79 ± 0.45	11.15*
Qihu (ST13)	4.73 ± 0.77	3.75 ± 0.57	2.46 ± 1.10	8.14*
Kufang (ST14)	3.51 ± 0.51	3.04 ± 0.45	2.06 ± 1.07	5.52*
Wuyi (ST15)	3.05 ± 0.52	2.72 ± 0.38	1.76 ± 0.82	5.61*
Yingchuang (ST16)	2.94 ± 0.47	2.66 ± 0.37	1.90 ± 0.78	4.08*
Ruzhong (ST17)	2.91 ± 0.42	2.58 ± 0.33	1.93 ± 0.62	4.73*
Rugen (ST18)	2.92 ± 0.40	2.44 ± 0.31	1.69 ± 0.56	9.45*
Tianchi (PC1)	3.34 ± 0.69	2.86 ± 0.37	1.89 ± 0.73	5.37*
Yunmen (LU1)	5.84 ± 0.79	4.42 ± 0.76	3.51 ± 1.59	6.52*
Zhongfu (LU2)	4.43 ± 0.55	3.74 ± 0.47	2.81 ± 1.45	5.39*
Zhourong (SP20)	3.82 ± 0.59	3.49 ± 0.46	2.37 ± 1.15	4.72*
Xiongxiang (SP19)	3.70 ± 0.53	3.31 ± 0.42	2.23 ± 0.82	6.40*
Tianxi (SP18)	3.41 ± 0.53	3.06 ± 0.44	2.07 ± 0.79	5.25*
Shidou (SP17)	3.34 ± 0.53	2.80 ± 0.40	1.83 ± 0.72	7.49*
Zhejin (GB23)	3.63 ± 0.57	3.43 ± 0.43	2.24 ± 0.99	5.24*
Yuanye (GB22)	4.06 ± 0.64	3.72 ± 0.54	2.39 ± 1.08	5.48*

The definitions for "Overweight adults", "Normal adults" and "Underweight adults" are following the guidance of the Department of Health, Taiwan: "The suggested ideal body weight of Taiwanese people". As such, readers from outside Taiwan should bear in mind that ideal body weights differ between countries. The specified needling depths in the table are a suggested guide only. The data are extracted from JG Lin's Review on the History and Practice of the Needling Depth of Acupoints (2011), National Research Institute of Chinese Medicine (Chinese), Taipei, Taiwan
X ± 1.96 SD: 95% confidence interval (CI), X: mean depth, units are provided in centimeters
F is the statistic for One-way ANOVA
$*p < 0.01$

- Increasing spinal cord concentrations of dynorphin and endomorphin.
- Decreasing the relative hypothalamic CRH mRNA expression level.
- Reducing 5-hydroxytryptamine concentrations in the colon.
- Antitumor effects.
- Regulating of renal function and hormone secretion with body fluid metabolism.
- Causing mast cell degranulation.
- Immunomodulation.

Table 2.3 Mean values with 95% confidence intervals for needling depths of acupoints in the back from different-sized male subjects

Acupoints	Overweight adults Mean ± 95% CI	Normal adults Mean ± 95% CI	Underweight adults Mean ± 95% CI	F
Dazhui (GV14)	6.76 ± 0.41	5.39 ± 0.40	4.81 ± 0.54	20.90*
Taodao (GV13)	6.35 ± 0.40	5.24 ± 0.40	4.66 ± 0.47	17.03*
Shenzhu (GV12)	5.39 ± 0.37	4.79 ± 0.35	4.10 ± 0.34	14.13*
Shendao (GV11)	4.86 ± 0.32	4.30 ± 0.30	3.65 ± 0.23	18.95*
Lingtai (GV10)	4.88 ± 0.32	4.27 ± 0.30	3.56 ± 0.21	22.69*
Zhiyang (GV9)	4.86 ± 0.33	4.20 ± 0.27	3.47 ± 0.19	27.32*
Jianzhongshu (SI15)	7.43 ± 0.50	6.47 ± 0.59	5.77 ± 0.70	8.18*
Dazhu (BL11)	6.98 ± 0.54	6.19 ± 0.49	5.36 ± 0.79	7.33*
Fengmen (BL12)	6.21 ± 0.50	5.53 ± 0.47	5.08 ± 0.77	3.95*
Feishu (BL13)	5.70 ± 0.49	5.15 ± 0.48	4.67 ± 0.66	3.73*
Jueyinshu (BL14)	5.37 ± 0.47	4.76 ± 0.41	4.39 ± 0.57	4.42*
Xinshu (BL15)	5.04 ± 0.67	4.54 ± 0.43	4.27 ± 0.50	2.25*
Dushu (BL16)	5.18 ± 0.47	4.52 ± 0.48	4.13 ± 0.45	5.34*
Geshu (BL17)	5.30 ± 0.47	4.55 ± 0.46	4.18 ± 0.47	6.28*
Jianwaishu (SI14)	6.05 ± 0.39	5.39 ± 0.43	5.00 ± 0.63	4.79*
Fufen (BL41)	5.10 ± 0.45	4.37 ± 0.37	4.38 ± 0.59	3.40*
Pohu (BL42)	4.40 ± 0.37	3.75 ± 0.35	3.56 ± 0.50	5.06*
Gaohuang (BL43)	3.98 ± 0.35	3.34 ± 0.35	2.98 ± 0.41	7.99*
Shentang (BL44)	3.75 ± 0.36	2.98 ± 0.30	2.57 ± 0.35	13.39*
Yixi (BL45)	3.70 ± 0.46	2.76 ± 0.28	2.28 ± 0.37	16.03*
Geguan (BL46)	3.66 ± 0.45	2.63 ± 0.28	2.33 ± 0.36	15.08*
Quyuan (SI13)	5.36 ± 0.32	4.76 ± 0.35	4.31 ± 0.42	8.78*

The definitions for "Overweight adults", "Normal adults" and "Underweight adults" are following the guidance of the Department of Health, Taiwan: "The suggested ideal body weight of Taiwanese people". As such, readers from outside Taiwan should bear in mind that ideal body weights differ between countries. The specified needling depths in the table are a suggested guide only. The data are extracted from JG Lin's Review on the History and Practice of the Needling Depth of Acupoints. Taipei: National Research Institute of Chinese Medicine (Chinese), Taipei, Taiwan.
X ± 1.96 SD: 95% confidence interval (CI), X: mean depth, units are provided in centimeters
F is the statistic for One-way ANOVA
*$p < 0.01$

- Decreasing gastric injury and apoptosis of gastric mucosal cells while increasing mucosal expression of transforming growth factor (TGF)-α and heat shock protein 70 (Hsp70) .
- Increases hepatic Hsp70 expression and protects the liver from ischemia-reperfusion injury.
- Inhibiting sphincter of Oddi (SO) and internal anal sphincter motility through nitrergic neural release of NO.
- Cardioprotection through electroacupuncture and by local somatothermal stimulation.

Table 2.4 Mean values with 95% confidence intervals for needling depths of acupoints in the back in different-sized female subjects

Acupoints	Overweight adults Mean ± 95% CI	Normal adults Mean ± 95% CI	Underweight adults Mean ± 95% CI	F
Dazhui (GV14)	6.37 ± 0.71	5.21 ± 0.70	4.35 ± 0.19	5.91*
Taodao (GV13)	6.01 ± 0.45	4.97 ± 0.58	4.13 ± 0.88	8.58*
Shenzhu (GV12)	5.36 ± 0.35	4.40 ± 0.39	3.60 ± 0.64	15.31*
Shendao (GV11)	5.01 ± 0.38	3.97 ± 0.30	3.40 ± 0.64	18.12*
Lingtai (GV10)	4.89 ± 0.35	3.83 ± 0.28	3.28 ± 0.63	21.03*
Zhiyang (GV9)	4.90 ± 0.41	3.86 ± 0.29	3.37 ± 0.67	15.06*
Jianzhongshu (SI15)	6.62 ± 0.48	5.87 ± 0.62	4.15 ± 1.36	10.43*
Dazhu (BL11)	6.42 ± 0.53	5.39 ± 0.62	4.27 ± 0.96	8.77*
Fengmen (BL12)	5.83 ± 0.39	4.78 ± 0.61	4.13 ± 1.08	6.97*
Feishu (BL13)	5.32 ± 0.38	4.43 ± 0.46	4.03 ± 0.97	6.66*
Jueyinshu (BL14)	5.07 ± 0.47	4.25 ± 0.43	3.73 ± 0.87	6.40*
Xinshu (BL15)	4.91 ± 0.51	3.97 ± 0.32	3.63 ± 0.88	8.36*
Dushu (BL16)	4.90 ± 0.49	3.86 ± 0.30	3.63 ± 0.80	10.35*
Geshu (BL17)	4.91 ± 0.47	3.92 ± 0.37	3.58 ± 0.92	8.57*
Jianwaishu (SI14)	5.57 ± 0.41	4.91 ± 0.48	3.85 ± 0.81	8.83*
Fufen (BL41)	4.85 ± 0.31	4.07 ± 0.42	3.07 ± 0.85	12.60*
Pohu (BL42)	4.35 ± 0.28	3.53 ± 0.31	2.60 ± 0.74	19.67*
Gaohuang (BL43)	3.96 ± 0.32	3.15 ± 0.31	2.30 ± 0.61	18.00*
Shentang (BL44)	3.67 ± 0.35	2.75 ± 0.27	2.02 ± 0.48	21.33*
Yixi (BL45)	3.59 ± 0.37	2.56 ± 0.23	1.88 ± 0.54	24.99*
Geguan (BL46)	3.59 ± 0.40	2.53 ± 0.28	1.78 ± 0.49	22.77*
Quyuan (SI13)	5.16 ± 0.37	4.32 ± 0.39	3.08 ± 0.58	18.83*

The definitions for "Overweight adults", "Normal adults" and "Underweight adults" are following the guidance of the Department of Health, Taiwan: "The suggested ideal body weight of Taiwanese people". As such, readers from outside Taiwan should bear in mind that ideal body weights differ between countries. The specified needling depths in the table are a suggested guide only. The data are extracted from JG Lin's Review on the History and Practice of the Needling Depth of Acupoints (2011), National Research Institute of Chinese Medicine (Chinese), Taipei, Taiwan

X ± 1.96 SD: 95% confidence interval (CI), X: mean depth, units are provided in centimeters

F is the statistic for One-way ANOVA

*$p < 0.01$

2.14.1 Increasing Spinal Cord Concentrations of Dynorphin and Endomorphin

Liu et al. (2010) reported that moxibustion can significantly enhance the pain threshold of rats with chronic visceral hyperalgesia, and that this effect may be closely related to increased spinal cord concentrations of dynorphin and endomorphin. The moxibustion was applied bilaterally to the Tianshu (ST25) and Shangjuxu (ST37) acupoints, using a fine moxibustion stick with the smoldered end held 2 cm away from the acupoints, once daily for 10 min each time, 7 times in total. Moxibustion significantly decreased visceral pain caused by colorectal distension in the rat model and also increased spinal cord concentrations of dynorphin and endomorphin.

2.14.2 Decreasing the Relative Hypothalamic CRH mRNA Expression Level

In another study (Zhou et al. 2011), bilateral moxibustion at the ST25 and ST37 acupoints significantly decreased visceral sensitivity to colorectal distension in rats and also decreased the hypothalamic CRH mRNA expression level relative to control levels.

2.14.3 Reducing 5-Hydroxytryptamine Concentrations in the Colon

Zhou et al. (2009) evaluated the effects of moxibustion on rectal sensory thresholds and analyzed its possible mechanisms in the treatment of chronic visceral hypersensitivity in rats. Moxibustion at ST25 (bilateral) increased the pain threshold and restored normal sensitivity by reducing 5-hydroxytryptamine concentrations in the rat colon.

2.14.4 Antitumor Effects

Qiu et al. (2004) investigated the effects of moxibustion on serum interleukin (IL)-2 and IL-12 levels, as well as on NK cell and ascitic tumor cell activities, in tumor-bearing H22 mice. They found that moxibustion can inhibit tumor growth, in direct relation to the increase in serum IL-2 and IL-12 levels and the enhancing NK cell activities.

2.14.5 Regulating of Renal Function and Hormone Secretion with Body Fluid Metabolism

Lee et al. (1997) investigated the effects of moxibustion at the meridian points Xinshu (BL15) and Xiaochangshu (BL27), in regard to renal function, systolic blood pressure, plasma levels of renin activity, aldosterone and atrial natriuretic peptide, in spontaneously hypertensive rats. Their results showed that urine volume increased significantly after moxibustion at BL15, but decreased after BL27 application. Urinary excretion of Na^+ decreased after moxibustion at both meridian points. Systolic blood pressure decreased after moxibustion at BL15, whereas no such effect was observed at BL27. Plasma levels of aldosterone and renin activity increased significantly, but levels of atrial natriuretic peptide decreased significantly, after moxibustion at BL15. Plasma levels of aldosterone and atrial natriuretic peptide increased significantly after moxibustion at BL27. These results suggest that moxibustion at BL15 and BL27 relates to the regulation of renal function and hormone secretion with body fluid metabolism (Lee et al. 1997).

2.14.6 Causing Mast Cell Degranulation

Shi et al. (2011) investigated the effects of moxibustion on the morphology and function of mast cells at ST25 in rats with trinitrobenzene sulfonic acid-induced colitis. They observed an improvement in colonic injury in the moxibustion group and a markedly higher degranulation ratio of mast cells at the ST25 acupoint in the moxibustion group than in the control group. These data suggest that moxibustion exerted its effect on healing-impaired colonic mucosa by increasing the degranulation ratio of local mast cells, but had little effect on their morphology.

2.14.7 Immunomodulation

Yamashita et al. (2001) measured human peripheral lymphocyte subpopulations after direct moxibustion using moxa cones the size of a half-rice grain. They found that after direct moxibustion, the NK cell percentage decreased and CD4/CD8 ratio increased significantly. In rabbits, the CD4/CD8 ratio was significantly increased and recovered at between 24 and 72 h after treatment. These results revealed that direct moxibustion has at least a transient influence on the immune system.

2.14.8 Decreasing Gastric Injury and Apoptosis of Gastric Mucosal Cells While Increasing Mucosal Expression of TGF-α and Hsp70

Chang et al. (2007) observed the effects of pre-moxibustion on apoptosis and proliferation of gastric mucosal cells in rats with stress-induced ulcers, and analyzed the relationship between those effects and the expression of Hsp70. They found that moxibustion at the ST36 and Liangmen (ST21) points significantly decreased gastric injury and apoptosis of gastric mucosal cells, while it markedly increased the mucosal expression of TGF-α and Hsp70 as well as the proliferation of gastric mucosal cells. Their results suggested that the protective effects are closely related to its actions in promoting the synthesis of TGF-α and proliferation of gastric mucosal cells, suppressing gastric mucosal cell apoptosis, and upregulating Hsp70 expression.

2.14.9 Increases Hepatic Hsp70 Expression and Protects the Liver from Ischemia-Reperfusion Injury

One study was designed to test the hypothesis that hepatic Hsp70 could be induced by local somatothermal stimulation in the right seventh intercostal nerve territory and that preconditioning rats with local somatothermal stimulation would protect the liver from subsequent ischemia-reperfusion injury. The study concluded that mild local heat stress (one dose) on the right seventh intercostal nerve territory upregulated hepatic gene expression of Hsp70 and protected the liver from subsequent ischemia-reperfusion injury. Therefore, local somatothermal stimulation might be appropriate in patients facing ischemia-reperfusion challenge of the liver (Lin et al. 2001).

2.14.10 Inhibiting Sphincter of Oddi (SO) and Internal Anal Sphincter Motility through Nitrergic Neural Release of Nitric Oxide (NO)

NO is a recognized signal transduction mechanism and plays a role in killing victim cells (Änggård 1994; Nathan and Xie 1994). NO also plays a role in the gastrointestinal system and acts as a neurotransmitter in nonadrenergic, noncholinergic (or "nitrergic") neurons of the peripheral nervous system (Bredt et al. 1990; Bult et al. 1990; Änggård 1994).

To examine the way in which local somatothermal stimulation inhibits the function of the SO in humans and in animals with different types of SO, Chiu et al. (1998) measured SO activity with continuously perfused open-tip manometric methods in anesthetized cats and rabbits. Local somatothermal stimulation was achieved by applying an electroheating rod 0.5 cm away from the skin area near the right subcostal region. The local heat-induced SO relaxation was not inhibited by pretreatment with atropine, propranolol, phentolamine or anti-cholecystokinin octapeptide, but was almost completely blocked by infiltration of local anesthetics. Pretreatment with a NO synthesis inhibitor also blocked the relaxation, which was reversed by pretreatment with L-arginine, but not by D-arginine. The inhibition of SO motility by local heat in rabbits was also blocked by pretreatment with L-NAME, and this blockade was reversed by L-arginine. Application of local heat in patients demonstrated obvious inhibitory SO responses. These observations indicated that local somatothermal stimulation inhibits SO motility in animals through the activation of heat-sensitive NO-mediated neural release.

Another study was performed to examine how local somatothermal stimulation inhibits functioning of the internal anal sphincter. Local somatothermal stimulation was achieved by applying an electroheating rod 1 cm away from the skin area at the right popliteal region. The responses were further manipulated by pretreating the rabbits with agonists or antagonists linked to NO synthesis. The results revealed that local somatothermal stimulation inhibited internal anal sphincter motility through the activation of nonadrenergic noncholinergic neural release of NO (Jiang et al. 2000).

2.14.11 Proteomic Analysis Finds Different Myocardial Protective Mechanisms for Median Nerve Stimulation by Electroacupuncture and by Local Somatothermal Stimulation

It is reported that ischemia-reperfusion injury of the heart can be attenuated by application of median nerve stimulation (MNS) through either electroacupuncture or local somatothermal stimulation (Lin et al. 2001). A study in rats investigated the differences in myocardial protein expression between each MNS application method (Tsou et al. 2004). MNS in response to electroacupuncture followed by a 30 min rest period or by three doses of local somatothermal stimulation resulted in cardioprotection against ischemia-reperfusion injury. However, the myocardial protein expression profiles differed markedly between the electroacupuncture and the local somatothermal stimulation groups. Thus, MNS produced by electroacupuncture and by local somatothermal stimulation attenuates ischemia-reperfusion injury in rat hearts through different protective mechanisms (Tsou et al. 2004).

2.15 Ginger Moxibustion

There are various ways of practicing moxibustion. Commonly used techniques involve burning a moxa stick directly over the skin at an acupuncture point (Cardini and Weixin 1998). However, indirect moxibustion places insulating materials such as monkshood cake or sliced ginger or garlic between the body and a burning moxa cone (Shen et al. 2006).

The therapeutic effects of ginger moxibustion are superior to those of acupuncture treatment for the treatment of cervical vertigo (Xiaoxiang 2006). Ginger moxibustion is also reported to produce reliable effects in the treatment of chemotherapy-induced leukopenia (Zhao et al. 2007). Few mechanistic studies of indirect moxibustion exist. One study reported moxibustion may act by producing modest thermal action and a sympathetic vibration at the skin surface (Shen et al. 2006). Another study reported that ginger moxibustion is effective in relieving abdominal pain in patients with primary dysmenorrhea. It is thought that this effect may be associated with the lowering of plasma endothelin-1 levels and elevations in serum NO (Yang et al. 2008b).

Acknowledgments We are grateful to Ms. Iona MacDonald for her help in proofreading the English of the manuscript and to Ms. Ya-Ting Wu and Ms. Rong-Wei Wong for their assistance in collating the literatures.

References

Änggård, E. (1994). Nitric oxide: mediator, murderer, and medicine. *The Lancet, 343*, 1199–1206.

Baek, Y. H., Choi, D. Y., Yang, H. I., & Park, D. S. (2005). Analgesic effect of electroacupuncture on inflammatory pain in the rat model of collagen-induced arthritis: mediation by cholinergic and serotonergic receptors. *Brain Research, 1057*, 181–185.

Bonnet, M. H., & Arand, D. L. (1997). Hyperarousal and insomnia. *Sleep Medicine Reviews, 1*, 97–108.

Bredt, D. S., Hwang, P. M., & Snyder, S. H. (1990). Localization of nitric oxide synthase indicating a neural role for nitric oxide. *Nature, 347*, 768–770.

Bronstein, D. M., Day, N. C., Gutstein, H. B., Trujillo, K. A., & Akil, H. (1993). Pre- and post-translational regulation of beta-endorphin biosynthesis in the CNS: effects of chronic naltrexone treatment. *Journal of Neurochemistry, 60*, 40–49.

Bult, H., Boeckxstaens, G. E., Pelckmans, P. A., Jordaens, F. H., Maercke, Y. M. V., & Herman, A.G. (1990). Nitric oxide as an inhibitory non-adrenergic non-cholinergic neurotransmitter. *Nature, 345*, 346–347.

Cardini, F., & Weixin, H. (1998). Moxibustion for correction of breech presentation: a randomized controlled trial. *JAMA: The Journal of the American Medical Association, 280,* 1580–1584.

Chang, F. C., Tsai, H. Y., Yu, M. C., Yi, P. L., & Lin, J. G. (2004). The central serotonergic system mediates the analgesic effect of electroacupuncture on ZUSANLI (ST36) acupoints. *Journal of Biomedical Science, 11*, 179–185.

Chang, H. T. (1982). Roles of acupuncture in medicine. *The American Journal of Chinese Medicine, 10*, 1–4.

Chen, K., Jiang, Y., & Wen, H. (2000). Clinical study on treatment of nasopharyngeal carcinoma by radio- and chemotherapy with supplementary moxibustion on Shenque point. *Zhongguo Zhong Xi Yi Jie He Za Zhi, 20*, 733–735.

Chen, X. H. & Han, J. S. (1992). Analgesia induced by electroacupuncture of different frequencies is mediated by different types of opioid receptors: another cross-tolerance study. *Behavioural Brain Research, 47*, 143–149.

Cheng, C. H., Yi, P. L., Lin, J. G., & Chang, F. C. (2011). Endogenous Opiates in the Nucleus Tractus Solitarius Mediate Electroacupuncture-induced Sleep Activities in Rats. *Evidence Based Complementary and Alternative Medicine, 2011*, 159209.

Cheng, C. H., Yi, P. L., Chang, H. H., Tsai, Y. F., & Chang, F. C. (2012). Kappa-opioid receptors in the caudal nucleus tractus solitarius (NTS) mediate 100 Hz electroacupuncture-induced sleep activities in rats. *Evidence Based Complementary and Alternative Medicine, 2012*, 715024.

Cheng, R., Pomeranz, B., & Yu, G. (1979). Dexamethasone partially reduces and 2% saline-treatment abolished electroacupunture analgesia: these findings implicate pituitary endorphins. *Life Sciences, 24*, 1481–1486.

Cheng, R. S., & Pomeranz, B. (1979). Electroacupuncture analgesia could be mediated by at least two pain-relieving mechanisms; endorphin and non-endorphin systems. *Life Sciences, 25*, 1957–1962.

Chiu, J. H., Chung, M. S., Cheng, H. C., Yeh, T. C., Hsieh, J. C., & Chang, C. Y., et al. (2003). Different central manifestations in response to electroacupuncture at analgesic and nonanalgesic acupoints in rats: a manganese-enhanced functional magnetic resonance imaging study. *The Canadian Journal of Veterinary Research, 67*, 94–101.

Chiu, J. H., Lui, W. Y., Chen, Y. L., & Hong, C. Y. (1998). Local somatothermal stimulation inhibits the motility of sphincter of Oddi in cats, rabbits and humans through nitrergic neural release of nitric oxide. *Life Sciences, 63*, 413–428.

Cho, Z. H., Chung, S. C., Jones, J. P., Park, J. B., Park, H. J., & Lee, H. J., et al. (1998). New findings of the correlation between acupoints and corresponding brain cortices using functional MRI. *Proceedings of the National Academy of Sciences of the United States of America, 95,* 2670–2673.

Cho, Z. H., Chung, S. C., Lee, H. J., Wong, E. K., & Min, B. I. (2006). Correction for Cho et al., New findings of the correlation between acupoints and corresponding brain cortices using functional MRI. *Proceedings of the National Academy of Sciences of the United States of America, 103,* 10527.

Choi, B. T., Kang, J., & Jo, U. B. (2005). Effects of electroacupuncture with different frequencies on spinal ionotropic glutamate receptor expression in complete Freund's adjuvant-injected rat. *Acta Histochemica, 107*, 67–76.

Chou, P. C., Chu, H. Y., & Lin, J. G. (2011). Safe needling depth of acupuncture points. *Journal of Alternative and Complementary Medicine, 17*, 199–206.
Chung, A., Bui, L., & Mills, E. (2003). Adverse effects of acupuncture. Which are clinically significant? *Canadian Family Physician, 49*, 985–989.
Clement-Jones, V., McLoughlin, L., Tomlin, S., Besser, G. M., Rees, L. H., & Wen, H. L. (1980). Increased beta-endorphin but not met-enkephalin levels in human cerebrospinal fluid after acupuncture for recurrent pain. *Lancet, 2*, 946–949.
Cottle, M. K. (1964). Degeneration Studies of Primary Afferents of IXth and Xth Cranial Nerves in the Cat. *The Journal of Comparative Neurology, 122*, 329–345.
Cui, C. L., Wu, L. Z., & Han, J. S. (2000). Spinal kappa-opioid system plays an important role in suppressing morphine withdrawal syndrome in the rat. *Neuroscience Letters, 295*, 45–48.
Cui, C. L., Wu, L. Z., & Luo, F. (2008). Acupuncture for the treatment of drug addiction. *Neurochemical Research, 33*, 2013–2022.
D'Alberto, A. (2004). Auricular acupuncture in the treatment of cocaine/crack abuse: a review of the efficacy, the use of the National Acupuncture Detoxification Association protocol, and the selection of sham points. *Journal of Alternative and Complementary Medicine, 10*, 985–1000.
Danzebrink, R. M., & Gebhart, G. F. (1991). Evidence that spinal 5-HT1, 5-HT2 and 5-HT3 receptor subtypes modulate responses to noxious colorectal distension in the rat. *Brain Research, 538*, 64–75.
Dhond, R. P., Kettner, N., & Napadow, V. (2007). Neuroimaging acupuncture effects in the human brain. *Journal of Alternative and Complementary Medicine, 13*, 603–616.
Diana, M., Pistis, M., Muntoni, A., & Gessa, G. (1996). Mesolimbic dopaminergic reduction outlasts ethanol withdrawal syndrome: evidence of protracted abstinence. *Neuroscience, 71*, 411–415.
Eide, P. K., & Hole, K. (1993). The role of 5-hydroxytryptamine (5-HT) receptor subtypes and plasticity in the 5-HT systems in the regulation of nociceptive sensitivity. *Cephalalgia, 13*, 75–85.
Ernst, M. & Lee, M. H. (1985). Sympathetic vasomotor changes induced by manual and electrical acupuncture of the Hoku point visualized by thermography. *Pain, 21*, 25–33.
Gareus, I.K., Lacour, M., Schulte, A. C., & Hennig, J. (2002). Is there a BOLD response of the visual cortex on stimulation of the vision-related acupoint GB 37? *Journal of Magnetic Resonance Imaging: JMRI, 15*, 227–232.
Goldman, N., Chen, M., Fujita, T., Xu, Q., Peng, W., & Liu, W., et al. (2010). Adenosine A1 receptors mediate local anti-nociceptive effects of acupuncture. *Nature Neuroscience, 13*, 883–888.
Green, P. G., & Lee, N. M. (1988). Dynorphin A-(1-13) attenuates withdrawal in morphine-dependent rats: effect of route of administration. *European Journal of Pharmacology, 145*, 567–272.
Haker, E., Egekvist, H., & Bjerring, P. (2000). Effect of sensory stimulation (acupuncture) on sympathetic and parasympathetic activities in healthy subjects. *Journal of Autonomic Nervous System, 79*, 52–59.
Han, J. S. (2003). Acupuncture: neuropeptide release produced by electrical stimulation of different frequencies. *Trends in Neurosciences, 26*, 17–22.
Han, J. S. (2011). Acupuncture analgesia: areas of consensus and controversy. *Pain, 152*, S41–48.
Han, J. S., & Terenius, L. (1982). Neurochemical basis of acupuncture analgesia. *Annual Review of Pharmacology Toxicology, 22*, 193–220.
Han, J. S. & Zhang, R. L. (1993). Suppression of morphine abstinence syndrome by body electroacupuncture of different frequencies in rats. *Drug and Alcohol Dependence, 31*, 169–175.
Han, Z., Jiang, Y. H., Wan, Y., Wang, Y., Chang, J. K., & Han, J. S. (1999). Endomorphin-1 mediates 2 Hz but not 100 Hz electroacupuncture analgesia in the rat. *Neuroscience Letters, 274*, 75–78.
Ho, T. J., Duann, J. R., Chen, C. M., Chen, J. H., Shen, W. C., & Lu, T. W., et al. (2008). Carryover effects alter FMRI statistical analysis in an acupuncture study. *The American Journal of Chinese Medicine, 36*, 55–70.

Ho, T. J., Duann, J. R., Chen, C. M., Chen, J. H., Shen, W. C., & Lu, T. W., et al. (2009). Temporally shifted hemodynamic response model helps to extract acupuncture-induced functional magnetic resonance imaging blood oxygenation-level dependent activities. *Chinese Medical Journal, 122*, 823–829.

Hokfelt, T. (1991). Neuropeptides in perspective: the last ten years. *Neuron, 7*, 867–879.

Hsieh, C. L. (1998). Modulation of cerebral cortex in acupuncture stimulation: a study using sympathetic skin response and somatosensory evoked potentials. *The American Journal of Chinese Medicine, 26*, 1–11.

Hsieh, C. L., Li, T. C., Lin, C. Y., Tang, N. Y., Chang, Q. Y., & Lin, J. G. (1998). Cerebral cortex participation in the physiological mechanisms of acupuncture stimulation: a study by auditory endogenous potentials (P300). *The American Journal of Chinese medicine, 26*, 265–274.

Hsieh, C. L., Lin, J. G., Li, T. C., & Chang, Q. Y. (1999). Changes of pulse rate and skin temperature evoked by electroacupuncture stimulation with different frequency on both Zusanli acupoints in humans. *The American Journal of Chinese Medicine, 27*, 11–18.

Hsieh, J. C., Tu, C. H., Chen, F. P., Chen, M. C., Yeh, T. C., & Cheng, H. C., et al. (2001). Activation of the hypothalamus characterizes the acupuncture stimulation at the analgesic point in human: a positron emission tomography study. *Neuroscience Letters, 307*, 105–108.

Hsu, C. C., Weng, C. S., Liu, T. S., Tsai, Y. S., & Chang, Y. H. (2006). Effects of electrical acupuncture on acupoint BL15 evaluated in terms of heart rate variability, pulse rate variability and skin conductance response. *The American Journal of Chinese Medicine, 34*, 23–36.

Hu, S., Stritzel, R., Chandler, A., & Stern, R. M. (1995). P6 acupressure reduces symptoms of vection-induced motion sickness. Aviation, Space, and Environmental Medicine, 66, 631–634.

Huang, C., Hu, Z. P., Long, H., Shi, Y. S., Han, J. S., & Wan, Y. (2004). Attenuation of mechanical but not thermal hyperalgesia by electroacupuncture with the involvement of opioids in rat model of chronic inflammatory pain. *Brain Research Bulletin, 63*, 99–103.

Huang, C., Wang, Y., Chang, J. K., & Han, J. S. (2000). Endomorphin and mu-opioid receptors in mouse brain mediate the analgesic effect induced by 2 Hz but not 100 Hz electroacupuncture stimulation. *Neuroscience letters, 294*, 159–162.

Huang, S. T., Chen, G. Y., Lo, H. M., Lin, J. G., Lee, Y. S., & Kuo, C. D. (2005). Increase in the vagal modulation by acupuncture at neiguan point in the healthy subjects. *The American Journal of Chinese Medicine, 33*, 157–164.

Huang, W., Kutner, N., & Bliwise, D. L. (2011). Autonomic activation in insomnia: the case for acupuncture. *JCSM: official publication of the American Academy of Sleep Medicine, 7*, 95–102.

Jiang, J. K., Chiu, J. H., & Lin, J. K. (2000). Local somatothermal stimulation inhibits motility of the internal anal sphincter through nitrergic neural release of nitric oxide. *Diseases of the Colon and Rectum, 43*, 381–388.

Kim, S. K., Park, J. H., Bae, S. J., Kim, J. H., Hwang, B. G., Min, B. I., et al. (2005). Effects of electroacupuncture on cold allodynia in a rat model of neuropathic pain: mediation by spinal adrenergic and serotonergic receptors. *Experimental Neurology, 195*, 430–436.

Kim, S. Y., Chae, Y., Lee, S. M., Lee, H., & Park, H. J. (2009). The Effectiveness of Moxibustion: An Overview During 10 Years. *Evidence Based Complementary Alternative Medicine, 2011*, 306515.

Kiser, R. S., Khatami, M. J., Gatchel, R. J., Huang, X. Y., Bhatia, K., & Altshuler, K. Z. (1983). Acupuncture relief of chronic pain syndrome correlates with increased plasma met-enkephalin concentrations. *Lancet, 2*, 1394–1396.

Knardahl, S., Elam, M., Olausson, B., & Wallin, B. G. (1998). Sympathetic nerve activity after acupuncture in humans. *Pain, 75*, 19–25.

Koo, S. T., Park, Y. I., Lim, K. S., Chung, K., & Chung, J. M. (2002). Acupuncture analgesia in a new rat model of ankle sprain pain. *Pain, 99*, 423–431.

Kwong, K. K., Belliveau, J. W., Chesler, D. A., Goldberg, I. E., Weisskoff, R. M., & Poncelet, B. P., et al. (1992). Dynamic magnetic resonance imaging of human brain activity during primary sensory stimulation. *Proceedings of the National Academy of Sciences of the United States of America, 89*, 5675–5679.

Lao, L., Zhang, R. X., Zhang, G., Wang, X., Berman, B. M., & Ren. K. (2004). A parametric study of electroacupuncture on persistent hyperalgesia and Fos protein expression in rats. *Brain Research, 1020*, 18–29.

Lee, H. J., Lee, B., Choi, S.H., Hahm, D. H., Kim, M. R., & Roh, P. U., et. al. (2004) Electroacupuncture reduces stress-induced expression of c-fos in the brain of the rat. *The American Journal of Chinese Medicine, 32*, 795–806.

Lee, H. S., Yu, Y. C., Kim, S. T., & Kim, K. S. (1997). Effects of moxibustion on blood pressure and renal function in spontaneously hypertensive rats. *The American Journal of Chinese Medicine, 25*, 21–26.

Lee, M. S., Choi, T. Y., Park, J. E., Lee, S. S., & Ernst, E. (2010). Moxibustion for cancer care: a systematic review and meta-analysis. *BMC Cancer, 10*, 130.

Li, G., Cheung, R. T., Ma, Q. Y., & Yang, E. S. (2003a). Visual cortical activations on fMRI upon stimulation of the vision-implicated acupoints. *Neuroreport, 14*, 669–673.

Li, Z., Jiao, K., Chen, M., & Wang, C. (2003b). Effect of magnitopuncture on sympathetic and parasympathetic nerve activities in healthy drivers–assessment by power spectrum analysis of heart rate variability. *European* Journal of Applied Physiology, *88*, 404–410.

Li, Y. D., Li J. N., Dong, H. Y., Zhang, C., & Dong, H. S. (2004). Applying the CT measures the urine bladder through the first side line seven caves enter the directional research in depth, angle in needle. *Journal of Clinical Acupuncture and Moxibustio, 20,* 47–51 (Chinese).

Li, Z., Wang, C., Mak, A. F., & Chow, D. H. (2005). Effects of acupuncture on heart rate variability in normal subjects under fatigue and non-fatigue state. *European Journal of Applied Physiology, 94,* 633–640.

Lin, J. G. (1982). Study on the safety depth of straight insertion at the acupuncture loci of the human back bladder meridian using the body modular inch. Taichung, Taiwan: China Medical University, Master thesis (Chinese).

Lin, J. G. (1991). Detecting the safety depth on chest and back loci by computer tomographic scanning. Taichung, Taiwan: China Medical University, Docter thesis (Chinese).

Lin J. G. (2011). Review on the History and Practice of the Needling Depth of Acupoints. Taipei: National Research Institute of Chinese Medicine (Chinese).

Lin, J. G. & Chen, W. L. (2008). Acupuncture analgesia: a review of its mechanisms of actions. *The American Journal of Chinese Medicine, 36*, 635–645.

Lin, J. G., Hao, T., Chen, X. H., & Han, J. S. (1993). Intermittent-alternating mode of administering electroacupuncture stimulation postpones the development of electroacupuncture tolerance. *American Journal of Acupuncture, 21*, 51–57.

Lin, J. G., Ho, S. J., & Lin. J. C. (1996). Effect of acupuncture on cardiopulmonary function. *Journal of Chinese Medicine, 109*, 482–485.

Lin, J. G., Lin, J. C., & Salashin, H. (1995). A study of effect of ear point pressing on physiological responses to exercise. *Journal of Chinese Medicine, 6*, 37–46.

Lin, Y. H., Chiu, J. H., Tung, H. H., Tsou, M. T., Lui, W. Y., & Wu, C. W. (2001). Preconditioning somatothermal stimulation on right seventh intercostal nerve territory increases hepatic heat shock protein 70 and protects the liver from ischemia-reperfusion injury in rats. *Journal of Surgery Research, 99*, 328–334.

Litscher, G. (2007). Bioengineering assessment of acupuncture, part 7: heart rate variability. *Critical Reviews in Biomedical Engineering, 35*, 183–195.

Liu, H. R., Qi, L., Wu, L. Y., Ma, X. P., Qin, X. D., & Huang, W. Y., et al. (2010). Effects of moxibustion on dynorphin and endomorphin in rats with chronic visceral hyperalgesia. *World Journal of Gastroenterology, 16*, 4079–4083.

Liu, J. H., Yan, J., Yi, S. X., Chang, X. R., Lin, Y. P., & Hu, J. M. (2004). Effects of electroacupuncture on gastric myoelectric activity and substance P in the dorsal vagal complex of rats. *Neuroscience Letters, 356*, 99–102.

Liu, X., Zhu, B., & Zhang, S. X. (1986). Relationship between electroacupuncture analgesia and descending pain inhibitory mechanism of nucleus raphe magnus. *Pain, 24*, 383–396.

Liu, Z. C. (1990). Regulatory effects of acupuncture and moxibustion on simple obese complicated with hypertension. *Zhong Xi Yi Jie He Za Zhi, 10*, 522–525, 515.

Mao, W., Ghia, J. N., Scott, D. S., Duncan, G. H., & Gregg, J. M. (1980). High versus low intensity acupuncture analgesia for treatment of chronic pain: effects on platelet serotonin. *Pain, 8*, 331–342.

Margolin, A. (2003). Acupuncture for substance abuse. *Current Psychiatry Reports, 5*, 333–339.

Markou, A., Weiss, F., Gold, L. H., Caine, S. B., Schulteis, G., & Koob, G. F. (1993). Animal models of drug craving. *Psychopharmacology, 112*, 163–182.

Mayer, D. J., Price, D. D., & Rafii, A. (1977). Antagonism of acupuncture analgesia in man by the narcotic antagonist naloxone. *Brain Research, 121*, 368–372.

McLellan, A. T., Grossman, D. S., Blaine, J. D., & Haverkos, H. W. (1993). Acupuncture treatment for drug abuse: a technical review. *Journal of Substance Abuse Treatment, 10*, 569–576.

Middlekauff, H. R., Shah, J. B., Yu, J. L., & Hui, K. (2004). Acupuncture effects on autonomic responses to cold pressor and handgrip exercise in healthy humans. *Clinical Autonomous Research, 14*, 113–118.

Mori, H., Nishijo, K., Kawamura, H., & Abo, T. (2002). Unique immunomodulation by electro-acupuncture in humans possibly via stimulation of the autonomic nervous system. *Neuroscience Letters, 320*, 21–24.

Nathan, C., & Xie, Q-W. (1994). Nitric oxide synthases: roles, tolls, and controls. *Cell, 78*, 915–918.

Neshige, R., & Luders, H. (1988). Identification of a negative bitemporal component (N300) of the event-related potentials demonstrated by noncephalic recordings. *Neurology, 38*, 1803–1805.

Neshige, R., & Luders, H. (1992). Recording of event-related potentials (P300) from human cortex. *Journal of Clinical Neurophysiology, 9*, 294–298.

Nishijo, K., Mori, H., Yosikawa, K., & Yazawa, K. (1997). Decreased heart rate by acupuncture stimulation in humans via facilitation of cardiac vagal activity and suppression of cardiac sympathetic nerve. *Neuroscience Letters, 227*, 165–168.

Norgren, R. (1978). Projections from the nucleus of the solitary tract in the rat. *Neuroscience, 3*, 207–218.

Ohsawa, H., Yamaguchi, S., Ishimaru, H., Shimura, M., & Sato, Y. (1997). Neural mechanism of pupillary dilation elicited by electro-acupuncture stimulation in anesthetized rats. *Journal of Autonomous Nerveous System, 64*, 101–106.

Peoples, L. L., Uzwiak, A. J., Guyette, F. X., & West, M. O. (1998). Tonic inhibition of single nucleus accumbens neurons in the rat: a predominant but not exclusive firing pattern induced by cocaine self-administration sessions. *Neuroscience, 86*, 13–22.

Pert, A., Dionne, R., Ng, L., Bragin, E., Moody, T. W., & Pert, C. B. (1981). Alterations in rat central nervous system endorphins following transauricular electroacupuncture. *Brain Research, 224*, 83–93.

Plummer, J. P. (1981). Acupuncture and homeostasis: physiological, physical (postural) and psychological. *The American Journal of Chinese Medicine, 9*, 1–14.

Pomeranz, B., Cheng, R., & Law, P. (1977). Acupuncture reduces electrophysiological and behavioral responses to noxious stimuli: pituitary is implicated. *Experimental Neurology, 54*, 172–178.

Pomeranz, B. & Chiu, D. (1976). Naloxone blockade of acupuncture analgesia: endorphin implicated. *Life Sciences, 19*, 1757–1762.

Qiu, X., Chen, K., Tong, L., Shu, X., Lu, X., & Wen, H. et al., (2004). Effects of moxibustion at shenque (CV 8) on serum IL-12 level and NK cell activities in mice with transplanted tumor. *Journal of Traditional Chinese Medicine, 24*, 56–58.

Reinoso-Barbero, F. & de Andres, I. (1995). Effects of opioid microinjections in the nucleus of the solitary tract on the sleep-wakefulness cycle states in cats. *Anesthesiology, 82*, 144–152.

Research Group of Acupuncture Anesthesia B M C. (1973). Effect of needling positions in acupuncture on pain threshold of human skin. *Zhonghua Yi Xue Za Zhi, 3*, 151–157.

Richardson, G. S. (2007). Human physiological models of insomnia. Sleep Medicine, 8(Suppl 4), S9–14.

Rossetti, Z. L., Isola, D., De Vry, J., & Fadda, F. (1999). Effects of nimodipine on extracellular dopamine levels in the rat nucleus accumbens in ethanol withdrawal. *Neuropharmacology, 38*, 1361–1369.

Roth, T., Roehrs, T., & Pies, R. (2007). Insomnia: pathophysiology and implications for treatment. *Sleep Medicine Reviews, 11*, 71–79.

Ryan, L. J. (1985). Cholinergic regulation of neocortical spindling in DBA/2 mice. *Experimental Neurology, 89*, 372–381.

Sato, A., Sato, Y., Suzuki, A., & Uchida, S. (1993). Neural mechanisms of the reflex inhibition and excitation of gastric motility elicited by acupuncture-like stimulation in anesthetized rats. *Neurosci Research, 18*, 53–62.

Sekido, R., Ishimaru, K., & Sakita, M. (2003). Differences of electroacupuncture-induced analgesic effect in normal and inflammatory conditions in rats. *The American journal of Chinese medicine, 31*, 955–965.

Shao, S. J., Zhang, J. H., & Dong, Y. (2007). Study on safe needling depth of risk acupoints: introduction to Yan Zhenguo's academic achievement. *Shanghai Journal of Acupuncture and Moxibustio, 21*, 9–11 (Chinese).

Shen, X., Ding, G., Wei, J., Zhao, L., Zhou, Y., & Deng, H. et al., (2006). An infrared radiation study of the biophysical characteristics of traditional moxibustion. *Complementary Therapies in Medicine, 14*, 213–219.

Shi, X. D., Ren, W., Wang,. G. B., Luo, F., Han, J. S., & Cui, C. L. (2003). Brain opioid-receptors are involved in mediating peripheral electric stimulation-induced inhibition of morphine conditioned place preference in rats. *Brain Research, 981*, 23–29.

Shi, Y., Qi, L., Wang, J., Xu, M. S., Zhang, D., & Wu, L. Y., et al. (2011). Moxibustion activates mast cell degranulation at the ST25 in rats with colitis. *World Journal of Gastroenterology, 17*, 3733–3738.

Siedentopf, C. M., Golaszewski, S. M., Mottaghy, F. M., Ruff, C. C., Felber, S., & Schlager, A. (2002). Functional magnetic resonance imaging detects activation of the visual association cortex during laser acupuncture of the foot in humans. *Neuroscience Letters, 327*, 53–56.

Son, Y. S., Park, H. J., Kwon, O. B., Jung, S. C., Shin, H. C., & Lim, S. (2002). Antipyretic effects of acupuncture on the lipopolysaccharide-induced fever and expression of interleukin-6 and interleukin-1 beta mRNAs in the hypothalamus of rats. *Neuroscience Letters, 319*, 45–48.

Stein, C. (1995). The control of pain in peripheral tissue by opioids. *The New England Journal of Medicine, 332*, 1685–1690.

Stern, R. M., Jokerst, M. D., Muth, E. R., & Hollis, C. (2001). Acupressure relieves the symptoms of motion sickness and reduces abnormal gastric activity. *Alternative Therapies in Health and Medicine, 7*, 91–94.

Streitberger, K., Ezzo, J., & Schneider, A. (2006). Acupuncture for nausea and vomiting: an update of clinical and experimental studies. *Autonomic Neuroscience, 129*, 107–117.

Sugiyama, Y., Xue, Y. X., & Mano, T. (1995). Transient increase in human muscle sympathetic nerve activity during manual acupuncture. *Japanese Journal Physiology, 45*, 337–345.

Sun, H. L. & Li, X. M. (2001). Clinical study on treatment of cerebral apoplexy with penetration needling of scalp acupoints tou xue tou ci zhi liao nao zu zhong lin chuang yan jiu. *Chinese Acupuncture and Moxibustion, 21*, 275–278.

Sung, H. J., Kim, Y. S., Kim, I. S., Jang, S. W., Kim, Y. R., & Na, D. S., et al. (2004). Proteomic analysis of differential protein expression in neuropathic pain and electroacupuncture treatment models. *Proteomics, 4*, 2805–2813.

Tada, H., Fujita, M., Harris, M., Tatewaki, M., Nakagawa, K., & Yamamura, T. et al. (2003). Neural mechanism of acupuncture-induced gastric relaxations in rats. *Digestive Diseases and Sciences, 48*, 59–68.

Takeshige, C., Sato, T., Mera, T., Hisamitsu, T., & Fang, J. (1992). Descending pain inhibitory system involved in acupuncture analgesia. *Brain Research Bulletin, 29*, 617–634.

Tam, K. C. & Yiu, H. H. (1975). The effect of acupuncture on essential hypertension. *American Journal of Chinese Medicine, 3*, 369–375.

Tarkka, I. M., Micheloyannis, S., & Stokic, D. S. (1996). Generators for human P300 elicited by somatosensory stimuli using multiple dipole source analysis. *Neuroscience, 75*, 275–287.

Tarkka, I. M., Stokic, D. S., Basile, L. F., & Papanicolaou, A. C. (1995). Electric source localization of the auditory P300 agrees with magnetic source localization. *Clinical Neurophysiology, 96*, 538–545.

Tatewaki, M., Strickland, C., Fukuda, H., Tsuchida, D., Hoshino, E., & Pappas, T. N. et al. (2005). Effects of acupuncture on vasopressin-induced emesis in conscious dogs. *American Journal of Physiology - Regulatory, Integrative and Comparative Physiology, 288*, R401–408.

Tsai, H. Y., Chen, Y. L., & Lin, J. G. (1989a). Effect of electroacupuncture analgesia on serotoninergic neurons in rat central nervous system. *Chinese Journal of Pharmacology, 52*, 123–126.

Tsai, M. Y., Lin, J. G., & Inoki, R. (1989b). Further evidence for possible analgesic mechanism of electroacupuncture: effect on neuropeptides and serotonergic neutons in rat spinal cord. *Japanese Journal of Pharmacology, 49*, 181–185.

Tsou, M. T., Ho, J. Y., Lin, C. H., & Chiu, J. H. (2004). Proteomic analysis finds different myocardial protective mechanisms for median nerve stimulation by electroacupuncture and by local somatothermal stimulation. *International Journal of Molecular Medicine, 14*, 553–563.

Wang, B., Luo, F., Xia, Y. Q., & Han, J. S. (2000). Peripheral electric stimulation inhibits morphine-induced place preference in rats. *Neuroreport, 11*, 1017–1020.

Wang, G., Jiang, N., & He, Z. (2001). Effects of scalp acupuncture on plasma ET-1, MDA and NO contents in the patient of cerebral infarction. *Chinese Acupuncture and Moxibustion, 21*, 241–242.

Wang, J. D., Kuo, T. B., & Yang, C. C. (2002). An alternative method to enhance vagal activities and suppress sympathetic activities in humans. *Autonomic Neuroscience, 100*, 90–95.

Weiss, F., Paulus, M. P., Lorang, M. T., & Koob, G. F. (1992). Increases in extracellular dopamine in the nucleus accumbens by cocaine are inversely related to basal levels: effects of acute and repeated administration. *Journal of Neuroscience, 12*, 4372–4380.

Weiss, F. & Porrino, L. J. (2002). Behavioral neurobiology of alcohol addiction: recent advances and challenges. *Journal of Neuroscience, 22*, 3332–3337.

Wen, H. L. & Ho, W. K. (1982). Suppression of withdrawal symptoms by dynorphin in heroin addicts. *European Journal of Pharmacology, 82*, 183–186.

WHO. (2003). Acpuncture: Review and analysis of reports on controlled clinical trials.

WHO. (2007). WHO International Standard Terminologies on Traditional Medicine in the Western Pacific Region. World Health Organization.

Williams, T., Mueller, K., & Cornwall, M. W. (1991). Effect of acupuncture-point stimulation on diastolic blood pressure in hypertensive subjects: a preliminary study. *Physical Therapy, 71*, 523–529.

Wise, R. A., Newton, P., Leeb, K., Burnette, B., Pocock, D., & Justice, J. B., Jr. (1995). Fluctuations in nucleus accumbens dopamine concentration during intravenous cocaine self-administration in rats. *Psychopharmacology (Berl), 120*, 10–20.

Wu, J. N. (1996) A short history of acupuncture. *Journal of Alternative Complementary Medicine, 2*, 19–21.

Wu, L. Z., Cui, C. L., Tian, J. B., Ji, D., & Han, J. S. (1999a). Suppression of morphine withdrawal by electroacupuncture in rats: dynorphin and kappa-opioid receptor implicated. *Brain Research, 851*, 290–296.

Wu, M. T., Hsieh, J. C., Xiong, J., Yang, C. F., Pan, H. B., & Chen, Y. C., et al. (1999b). Central nervous pathway for acupuncture stimulation: localization of processing with functional MR imaging of the brain–preliminary experience. *Radiology, 212*, 133–141.

Wu, M. T., Sheen, J. M., Chuang, K. H., Yang, P., Chin, S. L., & Tsai, C. Y., et al. (2002). Neuronal specificity of acupuncture response: a fMRI study with electroacupuncture. *NeuroImage, 16*, 1028–1037.

Xiaoxiang, Z. (2006). Jinger moxibustion for treatment of cervical vertigo—a report of 40 cases. *Journal of Traditional Chinese Medicine, 26*, 17–18.

Yamashita, H., Ichiman, Y., & Tanno, Y. (2001). Changes in peripheral lymphocyte subpopulations after direct moxibustion. *The American Journal of Chinese Medicine, 29*, 227–235.
Yang, C. H., Lee, B. H., & Sohn, S. H. (2008a). A possible mechanism underlying the effectiveness of acupuncture in the treatment of drug addiction. *Evidence Based Complementary Alternative Medicine, 5*, 257–266.
Yang, J. J., Sun, L. H., She, Y. F., Ge, J. J., Li, X. H., & Zhang, R. J. (2008b). Influence of ginger-partitioned moxibustion on serum NO and plasma endothelin-1 contents in patients with primary dysmenorrhea of cold-damp stagnation type. *Zhen Ci Yan Jiu, 33*, 409–412.
Yao, M. L. (1985). Introductory remarks on the clinical application of moxibustion. *Journal of Traditional Chinese Medicine, 5*, 220–222.
Yi, P. L., Tsai, C. H., Lin, J. G., Liu, H. J., & Chang, F. C. (2004). Effects of electroacupuncture at 'Anmian (Extra)' acupoints on sleep activities in rats: the implication of the caud al nucleus tractus solitarius. *Journal of Biomedical Science 11*, 579–590.
Yim, Y. K., Lee, H., Hong, K. E., Kim, Y. I., Lee, B. R., & Son, C. G., et al. (2007). Electro-acupuncture at acupoint ST36 reduces inflammation and regulates immune activity in Collagen-Induced Arthritic Mice. *Evidence Based Complementary Alternative Medicine, 4*, 51–57.
Yoo, S. S., Teh, E. K., Blinder, R. A., & Jolesz, F. A. (2004). Modulation of cerebellar activities by acupuncture stimulation: evidence from fMRI study. *NeuroImage, 22*, 932–940.
Yu, Y., Kasahara, T., Sato, T., Asano, K., Yu, G., & Fang, J., et al. (1998). Role of endogenous interferon-gamma on the enhancement of splenic NK cell activity by electroacupuncture stimulation in mice. *Journal of Neuroimmunology, 90,* 176–186.
Zhang, R. X., Lao, L., Wang, L., Liu, B., Wang, X., & Ren, K., et al. (2004a). Involvement of opioid receptors in electroacupuncture-produced anti-hyperalgesia in rats with peripheral inflammation. *Brain Research, 1020*, 12–17.
Zhang, R. X., Lao, L., Wang, X., Fan, A., Wang, L., & Ren, K., et al. (2005). Electroacupuncture attenuates inflammation in a rat model. *Journal of Alternative and Complementary Medicine, 11*, 135–142.
Zhang, S. P., Zhang, J. S., Yung, K. K., & Zhang, H. Q. (2004b). Non-opioid-dependent anti-inflammatory effects of low frequency electroacupuncture. *Brain Research Bulletin, 62*, 327–334.
Zhao, X. X., Lu, M., Zhu, X., Gao, P., Li, Y. L., & Wang, X. M., et al. (2007). Multi-central clinical evaluation of ginger-partitioned moxibustion for treatment of leukopenia induced by chemotherapy. *Zhongguo Zhen Jiu, 27*, 715–720.
Zhou, E. H., Liu, H. R., Wu, H. G., Shi, Y., Wang, X. M., & Tan, L. Y., et al. (2009). Suspended moxibustion relieves chronic visceral hyperalgesia via serotonin pathway in the colon. *Neuroscience Letters, 451*, 144–147.
Zhou, E. H., Wang, X. M., Ding, G. H., Wu, H. G., Qi, L., & Liu, H. R., et al. (2011). Suspended moxibustion relieves chronic visceral hyperalgesia and decreases hypothalamic corticotropin-releasing hormone levels. *World Journal of Gastroenterology, 17*, 662–665.
Zou, D., Chen, W. H., Iwakiri, K., Rigda, R., Tippett, M., & Holloway, R. H. (2005). Inhibition of transient lower esophageal sphincter relaxations by electrical acupoint stimulation. *American Journal of Physiology. Gastrointestinal and Liver Physiology, 289*, G197–201.

Chapter 3
Acupuncture for Cancer Pain

Carole A. Paley and Mark I. Johnson

Abstract Cancer pain is a major challenge in healthcare and many patients report unsatisfactory pain relief. Current pain relieving strategies include the use of opioid-based analgesia, bisphosphonates and radiotherapy. Although patients experience some pain relief, these interventions may produce unacceptable side-effects which inevitably affect the quality of life. Acupuncture represents a potentially valuable adjunct to existing strategies for pain relief and it is known to be relatively free of harmful side-effects. Acupuncture is used in palliative care settings for all types of cancer pain, but the evidence-base is sparse, inconclusive and there is very little evidence to show its effectiveness in relieving cancer-related pain. The aim of this chapter is to review the biological mechanisms underpinning acupuncture as a treatment for cancer pain using a Western medical acupuncture model, discuss the clinical indications for treatment, consider acupuncture techniques and safety issues, as well as review the current evidence for clinical efficacy. Directions for future research will also be discussed.

3.1 Introduction

Cancer-related pain remains a major challenge in modern healthcare and significant pain is not limited to the later stages of disease (Cleeland 2006). It has been reported that 40% of individuals with early or intermediate stage cancer and 90% of those with advanced cancer will experience moderate to severe pain (Laird and Colvin 2008). The European Pain in Cancer survey screened for patients experiencing cancer pain at least weekly. Of the 5,084 adult patients contacted for the survey, 56% experienced moderate to severe pain at least monthly and of those prescribed analgesics, 63% experienced breakthrough pain (Breivik et al. 2009). Late-stage cancer pain often has multiple causes, with bone destruction being a major cause of severe pain in 70% of patients (Cleeland 2006). Many patients report unsatisfactory pain relief, particularly

C. A. Paley (✉)
Airedale NHS Foundation Trust, Ward 12, Research Office, Skipton Road, Steeton, Keighley, West Yorkshire BD20 6TD, UK
e-mail: carolepaley2@btinternet.com

C. A. Paley · M. I. Johnson
Faculty of Health and Social Sciences, Leeds Metropolitan University, Leeds, UK

W. C. S. Cho (ed.), *Acupuncture and Moxibustion as an Evidence-based Therapy for Cancer*, Evidence-based Anticancer Complementary and Alternative Medicine 3,
DOI 10.1007/978-94-007-4833-0_3, © Springer Science+Business Media Dordrecht 2012

in cases of pain which is difficult to control, such as bone pain and neuropathic pain (Caraceni and Portenoy 1999; Diel 2006; Laird and Colvin 2008). Poorly controlled pain affects physical and psychological well-being leading to a decreased quality of life for the patient (Vallerand et al. 2007; van den Beuken-van Everdingen et al. 2007a,b).

There is evidence to suggest that acupuncture is widely used in palliative cancer care (Filshie 1990; Dillon and Lucas 1999; Leng 1999; Chang et al. 2011; Filshie and Rubens 2011) and large surveys show that a relatively high percentage of cancer patients use various complementary therapies for pain and other symptoms (Ernst 2003; Ernst et al. 2007; Eustachi et al. 2009). Nevertheless, there is relatively little evidence available to support the use of acupuncture specifically for cancer pain. There continues to be a debate about its efficacy and recent systematic reviews are inconclusive with any positive results overshadowed by the poor quality of the trials included in the reviews (Lee et al. 2005; Ernst and Lee 2010; Paley et al. 2011a; Peng et al. 2010).

Acupuncture is delivered by practitioners aligned to different philosophical approaches, most typically either the traditional Chinese Medicine (TCM) approach or the Western medical acupuncture (WMA) model. Practitioners in the West tend to select segmental points related to the affected region and symptoms and may also use some traditional points that are supported by research evidence. Manual acupuncture is the main technique in use, but a variety of other techniques are used to increase the intensity of stimulation (e.g. electroacupuncture), to enhance the effects of acupuncture in other ways (e.g. moxibustion) or to utilise micro-systems such as the ear (auricular acupuncture).

3.2 The Mechanisms of Acupuncture for Cancer Pain

Pain associated with cancer may be due to the growth of a tumor, neural impingement, metastatic spread, secondary to operative treatment or as a result of the cancer treatment itself. Bony metastases are the main cause of cancer pain and occur commonly in advanced prostate, breast, lung cancers and multiple myeloma (Lipton 2004; Diel 2006).

In recent years there has been much progress in our understanding of the pathophysiology of cancer bone pain and it is known that cancer-induced bone pain is a unique pain state, resulting from specific changes in the dorsal horn. These changes result in pain with characteristics of both neuropathic and nociceptive-type pain and unique characteristics of its own (Urch et al. 2003, 2005; Donovan-Rodriguez et al. 2005; Sevcik et al. 2005). In addition, bone metastases alter the proportion of nociceptive specific (NS) to wide-dynamic range (WDR) cells in the spinal cord from 74:26% (NS:WDR) to 53:47% respectively (Urch et al. 2003). Because the WDR cells start to interpret non-noxious stimuli as pain, this results in hypersensitivity to mechanical and thermal input (allodynia) and exaggerated responses to noxious input (hyperalgesia) (Clohisy and Mantyh 2003; Urch et al. 2003; Goblirsch et al.

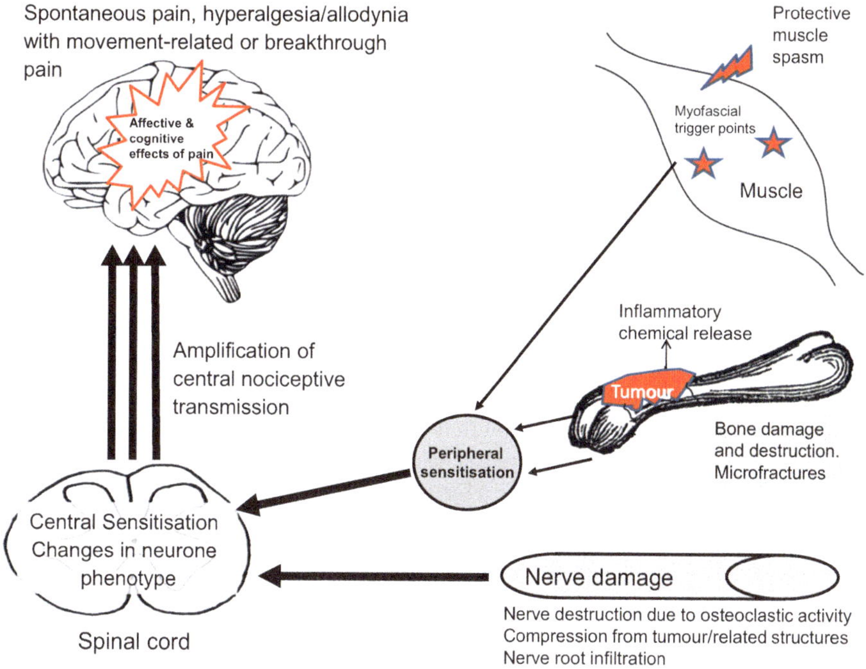

Fig. 3.1 The mechanisms of cancer-induced bone pain

2005). Figure 3.1 illustrates some of the mechanisms of pain resulting from bone metastases in cancer.

To date, there are few clinical studies on the effects of acupuncture on cancer-related pain. Consequently, we have to relate the findings of studies investigating the physiological effects of acupuncture using animal models of cancer pain to the human condition (Qi-Liang et al. 2006; Mao-Ying et al. 2006, 2008; Zhang et al. 2007, 2008; Rui-Xin et al. 2008). These studies suggest that a combination of mechanisms contribute to cancer-related pain and that interventions that reduce peripheral and central transmission and sensitisation of pain-related information are likely to relieve pain associated with cancer. A wealth of electrophysiological studies suggests that acupuncture acts to inhibit ongoing nociceptive transmission and sensitisation in the peripheral and central nervous system. The central mechanisms can be better understood by considering both the segmental and extra-segmental effects of acupuncture.

3.3 Segmental Analgesia and Desensitization

Acupuncture stimulates small myelinated Aδ fibres in muscle and skin which depress activity in the dorsal horn of the spinal cord. This results in the release of inhibitory neuromodulators such as enkephalin which depresses activity in nociceptive-specific

(NS) and wide-dynamic range (WDR) neurons (Thompson and Filshie 2005). It is claimed that it is necessary to retain the needles *in situ* for 10–20 min to ensure the release of enkephalin (White et al. 2008b). Long-term depression (LTD) of nociceptive transmission following Aδ fibre stimulation has been demonstrated in animal studies as continuing for hours after withdrawal of the stimulus (Sandkühler et al. 1997; Sandkühler 2000). Long-term depression of nociceptive transmission is particularly relevant for patients suffering from chronic cancer pain.

Continuous or repetitious stimulation of Aδ fibres using electrical currents has been shown to reduce dorsal horn sensitivity in rats (Sandkühler et al. 1997). Chemical mediators such as dynorphin, substance P and interleukin-1β—all known to facilitate persistent hyperalgesia—are suppressed by electroacupuncture (Zhang et al. 2007). However, it must be borne in mind that the doses of stimulation *via* electroacupuncture applied to animals in the laboratory represent 'ideal' conditions which might not be possible to attain in the clinic.

It is widely thought that it is possible to produce a long-term depression of nociceptive transmission in the dorsal horn for days or even weeks by manual acupuncture alone (Sandkühler 2000; Carlsson 2002). Recent studies using mice have shown that manual acupuncture with bi-directional stimulation (rotating the needle) stimulates connective tissue which generates a strong afferent input to the dorsal horn and is therefore likely produce a depressing effect (Langevin et al. 2006, 2007). The connective tissue fibres have been found to wind around the needle as it rotates, thus having a mechanical effect throughout the connective tissue matrix. It has also been suggested that the release of oxytocin in response to non-noxious sensory stimulation such as manual acupuncture may give rise to long-term elevations in pain threshold (Carlsson 2002). It is therefore likely that acupuncture should help to prevent allodynia and hyperalgesia resulting from central sensitisation.

The need for regular and repetitive stimulation of afferent Aδ fibres to achieve long-lasting analgesia is borne out by anecdotal evidence which suggests that patients with cancer pain need to be treated two or three times per week initially for optimal effects, particularly in cases of cancer-induced bone pain where pain relief is often achieved for a very short time (Filshie 1990).

3.4 Extra-Segmental Effects

Cumulative and sustained analgesic effects of acupuncture probably occur due to permanent changes in the endogenous opioid peptide mechanism (Clement-Jones et al. 1980; Guo et al. 1996). The release of β-endorphins results in the inhibition of pain transmission in the dorsal horn *via* the descending pain inhibitory system; an effect which is similar to the action of opioid drugs (Clement-Jones et al. 1980; Han 2004). This finding is supported by clinical trials which show that administration of the opioid antagonist naxolone reverses some of the pain-relieving effects of acupuncture (Mayer et al. 1977; Zhou et al. 1981; Han and Terenius 1982; Ceccherelli et al. 2002; Han 2003). When Zhou et al. (1981) injected the narcotic antagonist naloxone into discrete brain areas and assessed its effect on acupuncture analgesia in rabbits, it was concluded that nuclei accumbens, amygdala, habenula and periaquaductal grey are the strategic sites for endogenous opioids to exert their analgesic effect. Furthermore, cumulative stimulation of Aδ fibres results in the increased manufacture and storage of peptides and activates μ-opioid receptors thus prolonging the analgesic response to acupuncture (Guo et al. 1996; Ceccherelli et al. 2002).

Non-opioid systems also play an important part in acupuncture analgesia. Serotonin in the brainstem activates descending inhibitory systems resulting in the release of serotonin and noradrenaline in the dorsal horn which inhibit nociceptive transmission.

When an acupuncture needle is inserted into the skin, an immediate and powerful sympathetic response occurs within a segmental distribution. This sometimes results in striking effects such as flushed patches or sweating on the skin corresponding with the relevant dermatome. In the long-term, it also reduces pain perception by affecting activity in the hypothalamus (White et al. 2008c). This is a cumulative effect occurring over several treatments and it probably does not matter where the needles are inserted (Hopwood 2004). The effect of acupuncture on autonomic activity in the hypothalamus might explain why patients often feel relaxed or experience improved sleep quality after treatment. This in itself has a positive effect on quality of life as many patients with intractable cancer pain suffer from anxiety and impaired sleep (Portenoy and Lesage 1999; Theobald 2004).

Acupuncture can also produce a rapid analgesia *via* the application of strong stimulation that activates Aδ and C fibres to a part of the body which is outside the receptive field of the neurons causing the original pain. This so-called ‘counter irritation’ elicits a rapid widespread reduction in pain *via* diffuse noxious inhibitory controls (DNIC) (Willer et al. 1989; Bing et al. 1990; Le Bars et al. 1991) and can persist for several minutes. This strong stimulus may cause discomfort and supports claims that ‘de qi’ (needle sensation) is required for effective rapid acupuncture analgesia (Benham and Johnson 2009). It also supports claims that strong needle stimulation can be applied anywhere on the body to produce an analgesic effect (Campbell 2006a).

Brain imaging studies have shown that acupuncture affects the limbic system which modulates affective (emotional) responses to pain (Wu et al. 1999; Hui et al. 2000, 2005; MacPherson et al. 2008; Wang et al. 2008; Fang et al. 2009). The C fibre ‘tactile system’ is an important component of this response. Light touch stimulates mechanoreceptors in the skin and this induces a ‘limbic response’ which reduces perception of the unpleasantness of pain and increases the sense of well-being (Lund and Lundeberg 2006). This response can occur wherever the skin is stimulated and suggests that point specificity may not be as important for central pain modulation as it is in segmental acupuncture (Campbell 2006a; Aghabati et al. 2010). This also explains why other therapies involving light touch (e.g. massage, gentle mobilisations) have an anti-nociceptive effect (Lund et al. 2002; Campbell 2006b). The limbic response occasionally results in euphoria or other extremes of emotion (e.g. laughter or tears) (Campbell 1999). A positive feedback loop in the meso-limbic system results in a continuous outflow from descending inhibitory pathways and may help sustain analgesia (Han et al. 1986; Thompson and Filshie 2005).

3.5 Myofascial Trigger Points

Another manifestation of chronic pain is the presence of reactive muscle spasm which in turn causes additional pain and shortening of the muscle, affecting function (Gunn 1989). It has been suggested that myofascial trigger points (MTPs) perpetuate lower pain thresholds in uninjured tissues and that central sensitization may itself be maintained by the presence of MTPs (Freeman et al. 2009). In a recent study of chronic neck pain local anaesthetic was injected into MTPs which improved function and suggested that the eradication of MTPs using acupuncture may be a useful therapeutic tool (Freeman et al. 2009). The mechanism of acupuncture in deactivating myofascial trigger points is not fully understood, although it is likely that a combination of mechanical disruption and sensory stimulation helps to produce the often rapid and dramatic improvements which occur (Cummings and Baldry 2007). Where MTPs are present they are maintained by the continual release of acetylcholine (ACh) which results in a sustained contraction and increasing energy demands in the muscle but impeding the circulation. The effect of deactivating MTPs in terms of normalising muscle tone, restoring muscle balance and thus improving mobility and function has been noted in cancer patients and is an important therapeutic outcome (Filshie 2005).

3.6 Clinical Technique and Dosage

There continues to be a debate about the efficacy of acupuncture for any pain state (Ernst 2006). There is also a lack of agreement as to what constitutes an adequate dose of acupuncture, although this will necessarily depend upon the nature and source of the pain and how the patient responds to the treatment (White et al. 2008a). There are practical, peer-reviewed guidelines for providing acupuncture for cancer patients, which include criteria for acupuncture practice, indications, contraindications and treatment guidelines (Filshie and Hester 2006). The safety aspects of these guidelines are summarised in the following section. To our knowledge, there has been no published research investigating dose of acupuncture for cancer pain.

Manipulation of dosage may include the location and number of points, the amount of needle stimulation and the duration and frequency of treatment. One systematic review which defined an adequate dose of acupuncture for chronic pain conditions recommended that acupuncture should be performed at least once per week for six treatments (Ezzo et al. 2000). This was based on a review including 51 randomised controlled trials which were scored for methodological quality using a validated method (Jadad et al. 1996). After adjusting for study quality, six or more treatments were associated with positive outcomes ($p = 0.05$). Another systematic review including 13 randomised controlled trials of acupuncture for chronic knee pain suggested that an 'adequate' dose of acupuncture should consist of at least 6 weekly treatments using four or more points for a duration of 20 min or more (White et al. 2007). As discussed earlier, sustained, repetitive stimulation of needles inserted in a segmental distribution for 10–20 min may result in sustained analgesia *via* depression of nociceptive transmission in the spinal cord. Where rapid analgesia is required, for example, in breakthrough cancer pain, strong stimulation techniques which elicit diffuse noxious inhibitory controls might be effective although there is no published research supporting this.

The treatment of myofascial trigger points in cancer must be treated with caution because muscle spasm is often a protective function and when it occurs around a potentially unstable spine, release of the trigger point could potentially result in a lowering of muscle tone, sufficient to cause spinal instability (Filshie and Hester 2006; Cummings and Baldry 2007). Nevertheless, muscle spasm and trigger points cause additional pain and loss of normal function, affecting mobility and quality of life (Gunn 1989; Twycross 1995) and eliminating them can improve function and help restore normal movement where there has previously been restriction.

Auricular acupuncture is also used to elicit autonomic effects (Haker et al. 2000; Gao et al. 2008) and may be useful for pain relief although the precise mechanisms of this type of acupuncture remain unclear (Harding et al. 2009). One RCT has found that auricular acupuncture was effective for cancer pain relief (Alimi et al. 2003) (refer to section 'Clinical Research Evidence') and auricular acupuncture has been successfully used for some of the other distressing vasomotor symptoms associated with cancer and its treatment such as hot flashes, nausea and breathlessness (Filshie et al. 1996, 2005; Filshie and Hester 2006; Filshie and Rubens 2011). Auricular acupuncture is based on the assumption that all internal organs are represented on the ear, but unfortunately so many different auricular maps exist that there is little agreement as to point location (Gori and Firenzuoli 2007; Usichenko et al. 2008).

3.7 Safety and Adverse Events

Although studies have shown acupuncture to be relatively safe from serious adverse effects (MacPherson et al. 2001; White et al. 2001) practitioners should liaise closely with the medical team and be aware that serious adverse events, though relatively rare, continue to be reported (Ernst et al. 2011). Acupuncture is not contraindicated in cancer provided that practitioners are aware of the precautions and relative contraindications and they follow the available safety guidelines (Filshie and Hester 2006; AACP 2007). Acupuncture can be carried out in conjunction with other treatments for pain and can be used to supplement other complementary therapies and enhance exercise programmes, where appropriate, thus promoting functional independence. It is important, however, that practitioners have a good understanding of the overall condition and current management of their patients before using acupuncture.

Absolute contraindications to acupuncture include:

- Severe immuno-suppression;
- Extreme needle phobia;

- Severe clotting dysfunction and/or an unstable International Normalized Ratio (INR) on anti-coagulants;
- Presence of a factor 2/prothrombin deficiency.

Relative contraindications and precautions include:

- Insertion of needles into a lymphodaemic limb;
- Insertion of needles into a tumor;
- Insertion of needles into an infected area;
- Insertion of needles in and around a potentially unstable spine.

Care must also be taken if a patient is suspected of or known to be a strong reactor to acupuncture (Campbell 1999). In addition, electroacupuncture is contraindicated where a cardiac pacemaker is present (Cummings 2011). There is also a potential risk that some patients with incurable, but painful, conditions such as cancer may be looking at acupuncture as a 'cure' so practitioners must encourage patients to continue with prescribed medication.

3.8 Clinical Research Evidence

Three systematic reviews (Lee et al. 2005; Peng et al. 2010; Paley et al. 2011a) of acupuncture for cancer-related pain have been conducted and all three identified only one high quality study (Alimi et al. 2003). A recent Cochrane review (Paley et al. 2011a,b) on acupuncture for cancer pain conducted by our team identified 253 published references from six electronic databases, but only three studies met the review criteria (Table 3.1) and only one was judged to be of sufficient methodological quality (Alimi et al. 2003). Alimi included 90 adult participants with cancer pain randomized to one of three groups: auricular acupuncture ($n = 29$), placebo auricular acupuncture (on placebo points) ($n = 30$) and ear seeds (on placebo points) ($n = 31$). Pain scores on a visual analogue scale (VAS) and average electrical potential differences were taken at 30 and 60 days. The reported results showed a significant decrease in pain intensity of 36% (58–37 mm on VAS) from baseline at 2 months in the acupuncture group with an insignificant change in the group having acupuncture at placebo points (58–55 mm on VAS). The differences between the acupuncture and placebo acupuncture groups was statistically significant ($p < 0.0001$). Pain scores at 30 days were also lower in the true acupuncture group than either of the other two groups. The main criticisms of this research were the relatively small sample size and the unblinding effect of using ear seeds as these had to be applied using tape. Two low-quality studies which met the criteria for the review gave positive results in favour of acupuncture for cancer pain (Dang and Yang 1998; Chen et al. 2008), but these were judged to have methodological limitations, small sample sizes, poor reporting and inadequate analysis of the data. Meta-analysis was not appropriate due to heterogeneity of the included data. The Cochrane review concluded that there was insufficient evidence to provide a judgement on whether acupuncture was effective for treating cancer pain.

Table 3.1 Cochrane review: summary of included studies. (Paley et al. 2011a)

Author (year)	Design	Groups and interventions	Pain outcome measures	Secondary outcomes	Pain results
Alimi et al. (2003)	RCT, $n = 90$ Single-blind Three groups	Auricular acupuncture ($n = 29$) Auricular acupuncture at placebo points ($n = 30$) Auricular seed at placebo points ($n = 31$)	Pain intensity on VAS at D30 and D60	Average electrical potential difference at D30 and D60	Pain intensity on VAS significantly decreased in acupuncture group compared with placebo at both D30 and D60
Chen et al. (2008)	RCT, $n = 66$ Three groups Two subgroups for each group	Three groups: mild, moderate and severe pain. Each group randomly subdivided into two subgroups: acupuncture group and medication group	Analgesic effect: complete relief, average relief, partial relief, no relief	None reported	General effectiveness (%) in acupuncture group: mild pain = 100%, mod pain = 94.4%, severe pain = 91.7% In medication group: mild pain = 75%, mod pain = 89.5%, severe pain = 88.9% Groups compared for general effectiveness: acupuncture = 94.1%, medication = 87.5%
Dang and Yang (1998)	RCT, $n = 48$ Four groups	Three pain groups randomly divided into: FN, PI and WM (medication) groups One control group of normal subjects	Treatment effectiveness % score based on three categories: markedly effective, improved, ineffective Categories include pain, vigor, sleep and appetite	Plasma leucine enkephalin concentration Quality of life Chemotherapeutic reaction E-rosette forming cell rate (%) Leukocyte count	After 2 months: total effective rates of analgesia were around 81% for FN, PI and WM groups; and the markedly effective scores were FN 48.8%, PI 51.9% and WM 33.8%

D30/60 day 30/60, *FN* filiform needle, *PI* point injection, *RCT* randomised controlled trial, *VAS* visual analogue scale, *WM* Western medicine

Another systematic review (Bardia et al. 2006) examined the effectiveness of various complementary and alternative medicine therapies for cancer related pain, including acupuncture, but was unable to evaluate the efficacy of acupuncture because of insufficient good quality evidence. Eighteen randomised controlled trials were included in the review which concluded that hypnosis, imagery, support groups, acupuncture, and healing touch seemed promising, but none could be recommended because of a paucity of rigorous trials. Meta-analysis was not carried out. The only high-quality acupuncture study identified was that of Alimi et al. (2003) as described above. Other studies published since then were inconclusive. Mehling et al. (2007) reported that a combination of massage and acupuncture reduced pain and depressive mood when added to usual care in 138 postoperative cancer patients, although differences in outcome were small. Patients were randomly assigned to receive massage and acupuncture ($n = 93$) or to receive usual care only ($n = 45$). Participants in the intervention group experienced a decrease of 1.4 points on a 0–10 pain scale, compared to 0.6 in the control group ($p = 0.038$), and a decrease in depressive mood of 0.4 +/− 0.7 (on a scale of 1–5) compared to 0.01 +/− 0.5 in the control group ($p = 0.003$). Wong and Sager (2006) reported that acupuncture reduced chemotherapy induced peripheral neuropathic pain in five patients. Minton and Higginson (2007) attempted to undertake a single-blind RCT of electroacupuncture on cancer-related neuropathic pain but only three patients completed the study.

There is clearly a need for more high quality trials to provide evidence for the efficacy and effectiveness of acupuncture in treating cancer pain (Ernst et al. 2007; Ernst and Lee 2010). Particular attention should be paid to aspects of treatment such as dose, clinical technique and the need of this patient group and to the standard and methodological quality of study design.

3.9 Summary

Evidence for the use of acupuncture to relieve cancer pain is relatively sparse but the physiological rationale is persuasive. Acupuncture is known to reduce central sensitisation and to depress transmission of nociceptive information in the dorsal horn. It is likely that regular treatments reduce ongoing nociceptive transmission and sensitisation and up regulate the opioid peptide system. The release of myofascial trigger points may also help to lower central sensation. Additionally, the effect of acupuncture on the limbic system in the brain may modulate emotional responses to pain and render it more tolerable. Future research must focus upon well-designed randomised controlled clinical trials using human subjects and focus in particular upon aspects of needle placement and dosage for optimal results. In the meantime, clinicians using acupuncture to relieve cancer pain should pay particular attention to safety and the available guidance on aspects such as dose and treatment techniques.

References

AACP. (2007). *AACP guidelines for safe practice*. AACP Ltd.

Aghabati, N., Mohammadi, E., Pour Esmaiel, Z. (2010). The effect of therapeutic touch on pain and fatigue of cancer patients undergoing chemotherapy. *Evidence Based Complementary and Alternative Medicine, 7*, 375–381.

Alimi, D., Rubino, C., Pichard-Leandri, E., Fermand-Brule, S., Dubreuil-Lemaire, M., Hill, C. (2003). Analgesic effect of auricular acupuncture for cancer pain: A randomized, blinded, controlled trial. *Journal of Clinical Oncology, 21*, 4120–4126.

Bardia, A., Barton, D. L., Prokop, L. J., Bauer, B. A., Moynihan, T. J. (2006). Efficacy of complementary and alternative medicine therapies in relieving cancer pain: A systematic review. *Journal of Clinical Oncology, 24*, 5457–5464.

Benham, A., Johnson, M. I. (2009). Could acupuncture needle sensation be a predictor of analgesic response? *Acupuncture in Medicine, 27*, 65–67.

Bing, Z., Villanueva, L., Le Bars, D. (1990). Acupuncture and diffuse noxious inhibitory controls: Naloxone-reversible depression of activities of trigeminal convergent neurons. *Neuroscience, 37*, 809–818.

Breivik, H., Cherny, N., Collett, B., de Conno, F., Filbet, M., Foubert, A. J., Cohen, R., Dow, L. (2009). Cancer-related pain: A pan-European survey of prevalence, treatment, and patient attitudes. *Annals of Oncology, 20*, 1420–1433.

Campbell, A. (1999). The limbic system and emotion in relation to acupuncture. *Acupuncture in Medicine, 17*, 124–130.

Campbell, A. (2006a). Point specificity of acupuncture in the light of recent clinical and imaging studies. *Acupuncture in Medicine, 24*, 118–122.

Campbell, A. (2006b). Role of C tactile fibres in touch and emotion—clinical and research relevance to acupuncture. *Acupuncture in Medicine, 24*, 169–171.

Caraceni, A., Portenoy, R. K. (1999). An international survey of cancer pain characteristics and syndromes. *Pain, 82*, 263–274.

Carlsson, C. (2002). Acupuncture mechanisms for clinically relevant long-term effects-reconsideration and a hypothesis. *Acupuncture in Medicine, 20*, 82–99.

Ceccherelli, F., Gagliardi, G., Ruzzante, L., Giron, G. (2002). Acupuncture modulation of capsaicin-induced inflammation: Effect of intraperitoneal and local administration of naloxone in rats. A blinded controlled study. *Journal of Alternative Complement Medicine, 8*, 341–349.

Chang, K., Brodie, R., Choong, M., Sweeney, K., Kerin, M. (2011). Complementary and alternative medicine use in oncology: A questionnaire survey of patients and health care professionals. *BMC Cancer, 11*, 196.

Chen, Z. J., Guo, Y. P., Wu, Z. C. (2008). Observation on the therapeutic effect of acupuncture at pain points on cancer pain. *Chinese Acupuncture Moxibustion, 28*, 251–253.

Cleeland, C. S. (2006). The measurement of pain from metastatic bone disease: Capturing the patient's experience. *Clinical Cancer Research, 12*, 6236–6241.

Clement-Jones, V., McLoughlin, L., Tomlin, S., Besser, G. M., Rees, L. H., Wen, H. L. (1980). Increased beta-endorphon but not metenkephalin levels in human cerebrospinal fluid after acupuncture for recurrent pain. *Lancet, 2*, 946–949.

Clohisy, D. R., Mantyh, P. W. (2003). Bone cancer pain. *Cancer, 97*, 866–873.

Cummings, M. (2011). Safety aspects of electroacupuncture. *Acupuncture in Medicine, 29*, 83–85.

Cummings, M., Baldry, P. (2007). Regional myofascial pain: Diagnosis and management. *Best Practice and Research Clinical Rheumatology, 21*, 367–387.

Dang, W., Yang, J. (1998). Clinical study on acupuncture treatment of stomach carcinoma pain. *Journal of Traditional Chinese Medicine, 18*, 31–38.

Diel, I. J. (2006). What do patients with metastatic bone pain need? *European Journal of Cancer Supplements, 4*, 1–3.

Dillon, M., Lucas, C. (1999). Auricular stud acupuncture in palliative care patients. *Journal of Palliative Medicine, 13*, 253–254.

Donovan-Rodriguez, T., Dickenson, A. H., Urch, C. E. (2005). Gabapentin normalizes spinal neuronal responses that correlate with behavior in a rat model of cancer-induced bone pain. *Anesthesiology, 102*, 132–140.

Ernst, E. (2003). The current position of complementary/alternative medicine in cancer. *European Journal of Cancer, 39*, 2273–2277.

Ernst, E. (2006). Acupuncture-a critical analysis. *Journal of International Medicine, 259*, 125–137.

Ernst, E., Lee, M. S. (2010). Acupuncture for palliative and supportive cancer care: A systematic review of systematic reviews. *Journal of Pain and Symptoms in Man, 40*, e3–e5.

Ernst, E., Lee, M. S., Choi, T. Y. (2011). Acupuncture: Does it alleviate pain and are there serious risks? A review of reviews. *Pain, 152*, 755–764.

Ernst, E., Pittler, M. H., Wider, B., Boddy, K. (2007). Complementary/alternative medicine for supportive cancer care: Development of the evidence-base. *Supplements in Care Cancer, 15*, 565–568.

Eustachi, A., Pajtler, H., Linde, K., Melchart, D., Weidenhammer, W. (2009). Patients of an interdisciplinary cancer treatment center: Use of, knowledge about, and demand for CAM treatment options. *Integrated Cancer Therapy, 8*, 56–62.

Ezzo, J., Berman, B., Hadhazy, V. A., Jadad, A. R., Lao, L., Singh, B. B. (2000). Is acupuncture effective for the treatment of chronic pain? A systematic review. *Pain, 86*, 217–225.

Fang, J., Jin, Z., Wang, Y., Li, K., Kong, J., Nixon, E. E., Zeng, Y., Ren, Y., Tong, H., Wang, Y., Wang, P., Hui, K. K.-S. (2009). The salient characteristics of the central effects of acupuncture needling: Limbic-paralimbic-neocortical network modulation. *Human Brain Mapping, 30*, 1196–1206.

Filshie, J. (1990). Acupuncture for malignant pain. *Acupuncture in Medicine, 8*, 38–39.

Filshie, J. (2005). Complementary medicine (CM) for cancer pain control. *European Journal of Cancer, 3*, 107–116.

Filshie, J., Bolton, T., Browne, D., Ashley, S. (2005). Acupuncture and self acupuncture for long term treatment of vasomotor symptoms in cancer patients—audit and treatment algorithm. *Acupuncture in Medicine, 23*, 171–180.

Filshie, J., Hester, J. (2006). Guidelines for providing acupuncture treatment for cancer patients—a peer-reviewed sample policy document. *Acupuncture in Medicine*, 24, 172–182.

Filshie, J., Penn, J., Ashley, S., Davies, C. L. (1996). Acupuncture for the relief of cancer-related breathlessness. *Journal of Palliative Medicine, 10*, 145–150.

Filshie, J., Rubens, C. (2011). Acupuncture in palliative care. *Acupuncture in Medicine, 29*, 166–167.

Freeman, M. D., Nystrom, A., Centeno, C. (2009). Chronic whiplash and central sensitization; an evaluation of the role of a myofascial trigger points in pain modulation. *Journal of Brachial Plexus and Peripheral Nerve Injury, 4*, 1–8.

Gao, X.-Y., Zhang, S.-P., Zhu, B., Zhang, H.-Q. (2008). Investigation of specificity of auricular acupuncture points in regulation of autonomic function in anesthetized rats. *Autonomic Neuroscience, 138*, 50–56.

Goblirsch, M. J., Zwolak, P., Clohisy, D. R. (2005). Advances in understanding bone cancer pain. *Journal of Cellular Biochemistry, 96*, 682–688.

Gori, L., Firenzuoli, F. (2007). Ear acupuncture in european traditional medicine. *eCAM, 4*, 13–16.

Gunn, C. (1989). Neuropathic pain: A new theory for chronic pain of intrinsic origin. *Acupuncture in Medicine, 6*, 50–53.

Guo, H. F., Tian, J., Wang, X., Fang, Y., Hou, Y., Han, J. (1996). Brain substrates activated by electroacupuncture of different frequencies (I): Comparative study on the expression of oncogene, c-fos and genes coding for three opioid peptides. *Brain Research. Molecular Brain Research, 43*, 157–166.

Haker, E., Egekvist, H., Bjerring, P. (2000). Effect of sensory stimulation (acupuncture) on sympathetic and parasympathetic activities in healthy subjects. *Journal of Autonomic Nervous System, 79*, 52–59.

Han, J.-S. (2003). Acupuncture: Neuropeptide release produced by electrical stimulation of different frequencies. *Trends in Neurosciences, 26*, 17–22.

Han, J.-S. (2004). Acupuncture and endorphins. *Neuroscience Letters, 361*, 258–261.
Han, J., Terenius, L. (1982). Neurochemical basis of acupuncture analgesia. *Annual Review of Pharmacology and Toxicology, 22*, 193–220.
Han, J. S., Yu, L. C., Shi, T. S. (1986). A mesolimbic loop of analgesia. III. A neuronal pathway from nucleus accumbens to periaqueductal grey. *Asian Pacific Journal of Pharmacology, 1*, 7–22.
Harding, C., Harris, A., Chadwick, D. (2009). Auricular acupuncture: A novel treatment for vasomotor symptoms associated with luteinizing-hormone releasing hormone agonist treatment for prostate cancer. *BJU International, 103*, 186–190.
Hopwood, V. (2004). Possible Acupuncture Mechanisms. In Acupuncture in Physiotherapy (Chapter 9, pp. 198–219). Oxford: Butterworth-Heinemann.
Hui, K. K., Liu, J., Makris, N., Gollub, R. L., Chen, A. J., Moore, C. I., Kennedy, D. N., Rosen, B. R., Kwong, K. K. (2000). Acupuncture modulates the limbic system and subcortical gray structures of the human brain: Evidence from fMRI studies in normal subjects. *Human Brain Mapping, 9*, 13–25.
Hui, K. K. S., Liu, J., Marina, O., Napadow, V., Haselgrove, C., Kwong, K. K., Kennedy, D. N., Makris, N. (2005). The integrated response of the human cerebro-cerebellar and limbic systems to acupuncture stimulation at ST 36 as evidenced by fMRI. *Neuroimage, 27*, 479–496.
Jadad, A. R., Moore, R. A., Carroll, D., Jenkinson, C., Reynolds, D. J. M., Gavaghan, G. J., McQuay, H. J. (1996). Assessing the quality of reports of randomized clinical trials: Is blinding necessary? *Controlled Clinical Trials, 17*, 1–12.
Laird, B., Colvin, M. F. (2008). Management of cancer pain: Basic principles and neuropathic cancer pain. *European Journal of Cancer, 44*, 1078–1082.
Langevin, H. M., Bouffard, N. A., Churchill, D. L., Badger, G. J. (2007). Connective tissue fibroblast response to acupuncture: Dose-dependent effect of bidirectional needle rotation. *Journal of Alternative Complement Medicine, 13*, 355–360.
Langevin, H. M., Storch, K. N., Cipolla, M. J., White, S. L., Buttolph, T. R., Taatjes, D. J. (2006). Fibroblast spreading induced by connective tissue stretch involves intracellular redistribution of alpha- and beta-actin. *Histochemistry and Cell Biology, 125*, 487–495.
Le Bars, D., Villanueva, L., Willer, J. C., Bouhassira, D. (1991). Diffuse noxious inhibitory controls (DNIC) in animals and in man. *Acupuncture in Medicine, 9*, 47–56.
Lee, H., Schmidt, K., Ernst, E. (2005). Acupuncture for the relief of cancer-related pain—A systematic review. *European Journal of Pain, 9*, 437–444.
Leng, G. (1999). A year of acupuncture in palliative care. *Journal of Palliative Medicine, 13*, 163–164.
Lipton, A. (2004). Pathophysiology of bone metastases: How this knowledge may lead to therapeutic intervention. *Supplements of Oncology, 2*, 205–213.
Lund, I., Lundeberg, T. (2006). Are minimal, superficial or sham acupuncture procedures acceptable as inert placebo controls? *Acupuncture in Medicine, 24*, 13–15.
Lund, I., Yu, L.-C., Uvnas-Moberg, K., Wang, J., Yu, C., Kurosawa, M., Agren, G., Rosén, A., Lekman, M., Lundeberg, T. (2002). Repeated massage-like stimulation induces long-term effects on nociception: Contribution of oxytocinergic mechanisms. *European Journal of Neuroscience, 16*, 330–338.
MacPherson, H., Green, G., Nevado, A., Lythgoe, M. F., Lewith, G., Devlin, R., Haselfoot, R., Aziz, A. (2008). Brain imaging of acupuncture: Comparing superficial with deep needling. *Neuroscience Letters, 434*, 144–149.
MacPherson, H., Thomas, K., Walters, S., Fitter, M. (2001). A prospective survey of adverse events and treatment reactions following 34,000 consultations with professional acupuncturists. *Acupuncture in Medicine, 19*, 93–102.
Mao-Ying, Q. L., Cui, K. M., Liu, Q., Dong, Z. Q., Wang, W., Wang, J., Sha, H., Wu, G. C., Wang, Y. Q. (2006). Stage-dependent analgesia of electro-acupuncture in a mouse model of cutaneous cancer pain. *European Journal of Pain, 10*, 689–694.

Mao-Ying, Q. L., Ren, D. H., Mi, W. L., Liu, Q., Wang, Y. Q. (2008). Analgesic effects of electroacupuncture combined with Celebrex on rats with tibial cancer pain. *Journal of Chinese Integrated Medicine*, *6*, 830–835.
Mayer, D. J., Price, D. D., Rafii, A. (1977). Antagonism of acupuncture analgesia in man by narcotic-antagonist naxalone. *Brain Research*, *121*, 368–372.
Mehling, W. E., Jacobs, B., Acree, M., Wilson, L., Bostrom, A., West, J., Acquah, J., Burns, B., Chapman, J., Hecht, F. M. (2007). Symptom management with massage and acupuncture in postoperative cancer patients: A randomized controlled trial. *Journal of Pain and Symptoms in Man*, *33*, 258–266.
Minton, O., Higginson, I. J. (2007). Electroacupuncture as an adjunctive treatment to control neuropathic pain in patients with cancer. *Journal of Pain and Symptoms in Man*, *33*, 115–117.
Paley, C., Johnson, M., Tashani, O., Bagnall, A.-M. (2011a). Acupuncture for cancer pain in adults. Cochrane Database of Systematic Reviews.
Paley, C. A., Tashani, O. A., Bagnall, A.-M., Johnson, M. I. (2011b). A Cochrane systematic review of acupuncture for cancer pain in adults. *BMJ Supplements of Palliative Care*, *1*, 51–55.
Peng, H., Peng, H., Xu, L., Lao, L. (2010). Efficacy of acupuncture in treatment of cancer pain: a systematic review. *Journal of Chinese Integrated Medicine*, *8*, 501–509.
Portenoy, R. K., Lesage, P. (1999). Management of cancer pain. *Lancet*, *353*, 1695–1700.
Qi-Liang, M.-Y., Ke-Mi, C., Qiong, L., Zhi-Qiang, D., Wei, W., Jun, W., Hong, S., Gen-Cheng, W., Yan-Qing, W. (2006). Stage-dependent analgesia of electro-acupuncture in a mouse model of cutaneous cancer pain. *European Journal of Pain 10*, 689–694.
Rui-Xin, Z., Aihui, L., Bing, L., Linbo, W., Jiajia, X., Ke, R., Jian-Tian, Q., Brian, M.B., Lixing, L. (2008). Electroacupuncture attenuates bone cancer-induced hyperalgesia and inhibits spinal preprodynorphin expression in a rat model. *European Journal of Pain*, *12*, 870–878.
Sandkühler, J. (2000). Learning and memory in pain pathways. *Pain*, *88*, 113–118.
Sandkühler, J., Chen, J. G., Cheng, G. (1997). Low-frequency stimulation of afferent adelta-fibers induces long-term depression at primary afferent synapses with substantia gelatinosa neurons in the rat. *Journal of Neuroscience*, *17*, 6483–6491.
Sevcik, M. A., Ghilardi, J. R., Peters, C. M., Lindsay, T. H., Halvorson, K. G., Jonas, B. M., Kubota, K., Kuskowski, M. A., Boustany, L., Shelton, D. L., Mantyh, P. W. (2005). Anti-NGF therapy profoundly reduces bone cancer pain and the accompanying increase in markers of peripheral and central sensitization. *Pain*, *115*, 128–141.
Theobald, D. E. (2004). Cancer pain, fatigue, distress, and insomnia in cancer patients. *Clinical Cornerstone*, *6*, S15–S21.
Thompson, J. W., Filshie J. (2005). Transcutaneous electrocal nerve stimulation (TENS) and acupuncture. In D. Doyle, G. Hanks, N. Cherny, K. Calman (Eds.), *Oxford Textbook of Palliative Medicine* (3rd edn., pp 421–436). Oxford: Oxford University Press.
Twycross, R. G. (1995). Management of pain in skeletal metastases. *Clinical Orthopaedics and Related Research*, *312*, 187–196.
Urch, C. E., Donovan-Rodriguez, T., Dickenson, A. H. (2003). Alterations in dorsal horn neurones in a rat model of cancer-induced bone pain. *Pain*, *106*, 347–356.
Urch, C. E., Donovan-Rodriguez, T., Gordon-Williams, R., Bee, L. A., Dickenson, A. H. (2005). Efficacy of chronic morphine in a rat model of cancer-induced bone pain: Behavior and in dorsal horn pathophysiology. *Journal of Pain*, *6*, 837–845.
Usichenko, T. I., Lehmann, C., Ernst, E. (2008). Auricular acupuncture for postoperative pain control: A systematic review of randomised clinical trials. *Anaesthesia*, *63*, 1343–1348.
Vallerand, A. H., Templin, T., Hasenau, S. M., Riley-Doucet, C. (2007). Factors that affect functional status in patients with cancer-related pain. *Pain*, *132*, 82–90.
Van Den Beuken-van Everdingen, M. H. J., de Rijke, J. M., Kessels, A. G., Schouten, H. C., van Kleef, M., Patijn, J. (2007a). High prevalence of pain in patients with cancer in a large population-based study in The Netherlands. *Pain*, *132*, 312–320.

Van Den Beuken-van Everdingen, M. H. J., de Rijke, J. M., Kessels, A. G., Schouten, H. C., van Kleef, M., Patijn, J. (2007b). Prevalence of pain in patients with cancer: A systematic review of the past 40 years. *Annals of Oncology, 18*, 1437–1449.

Wang, S.-M., Kain, Z. N., White, P. (2008). Acupuncture analgesia: I. The scientific basis. *Anesthesia and Analgesia, 106*, 602–610.

White, A., Cummings, M., Barlas, P., Cardini, F., Filshie, J., Foster, N. E., Lundeberg, T., Stener-Victorin, E., Witt, C. (2008a). Defining an adequate dose of acupuncture using a neurophysiological approach—a narrative review of the literature. *Acupuncture in Medicine, 26*, 111–120.

White, A., Cummings, M., Filshie, J. (2008b). *An Introduction to Western Medical Acupuncture*. London: Churchill Livingstone Elsevier.

White, A., Cummings, M., Filshie, J. (2008c). Neurological Mechanisms IV: Central regulatory effects. In A. White, M. Cummings, J. Filshie (Eds.), *An Introduction to Western Medical Acupuncture*, (Chapter 6, pp. 51–58). London: Churchill Livingstone Elsevier.

White, A., Foster, N. E., Cummings, M., Barlas, P. (2007). Acupuncture treatment for chronic knee pain: A systematic review. *Rheumatology, 46*, 384–390.

White, A., Hayhoe, S., Hart, A., Ernst, E., BMAS, AACP. (2001). Survey of adverse events following acupuncture (SAFA): A prospective study of 32,000 consultations. *Acupuncture in Medicine, 19*, 84–92.

Willer, J. C., De Broucker, T., Le Bars, D. (1989). Encoding of nociceptive thermal stimuli by diffuse noxious inhibitors controls (DNIC) in man. *Journal of Neurophysiology, 62*, 1028–1038.

Wong, R., Sagar, S. (2006). Acupuncture treatment for chemotherapy-induced peripheral neuropathy—a case series. *Acupuncture in Medicine, 24*, 87–91.

Wu, M. T., Hsieh, J. C., Xiong, J., Yang, C. F., Pan, H. B., Chen, Y. C., Tsai, G., Rosen, B. R., Kwong, K. K. (1999). Central nervous pathway for acupuncture stimulation: Localization of processing with functional MR imaging of the brain-preliminary experience. *Radiology, 212*, 133–141.

Zhang, R.-X., Li, A., Liu, B., Wang, L., Ren, K., Qiao, J.-T., Berman, B. M., Lao, L. (2007). Electroacupuncture attenuates bone cancer pain and inhibits spinal interleukin-1 beta expression in a rat model. *Anesthesia and Analgesia, 105*, 1482–1488.

Zhang, R.-X., Li, A., Liu, B., Wang, L., Xin, J., Ren, K., Qiao, J.-T., Berman, B. M., Lao, L. (2008). Electroacupuncture attenuates bone-cancer-induced hyperalgesia and inhibits spinal preprodynorphin expression in a rat model. *European Journal of Pain, 12*, 870–878.

Zhou, Z. F., Du, M. Y., Wu, W. Y., Jiang, Y., Han, J. S. (1981). Effect of intracerebral microinjection of naloxone on acupuncture- and morphine-analgesia in the rabbit. *Scientia Sinica, 24*, 1166–1178.

Chapter 4
Acupuncture for the Treatment of Hot Flashes in Cancer Patients

Francesco C. Peluso, Paul R. Graves and Hani Ashamalla

Abstract Hot flashes, a phenomenon characterized by an intense feeling of heat and visible reddening in the upper body, have frequently been described in cancer patients undergoing hormonal deprivation or hormonal ablation therapy. The occurrence of hot flashes can substantially affect the quality of life in such patients. Though several treatments are available to reduce hot flashes, many have significant side effects of their own. Acupuncture has emerged as a promising treatment modality to alleviate hot flashes in cancer patients. In prostate cancer patients, six different studies concluded that acupuncture reduces the incidence and severity of hot flashes well beyond the estimated placebo effect and the effects of alternative treatments such as venlafaxine with minimal side effects. In breast cancer patients, acupuncture trials have yielded similar results. However, there are more conflicting results among randomized clinical trials which use sham acupuncture as a control; with one study concluding that actual acupuncture is no better than sham acupuncture in reducing hot flash incidence. In fact, two systematic reviews concluded that current evidence did not suggest that acupuncture was an effective treatment for hot flashes in breast cancer and prostate cancer patients due to the paucity and poor quality of the primary data (Lee et al., Breast Cancer Research Treatments, 115:497–503, 2009; Supportive Care Cancer, 17:763–770, 2009). These conclusions are at least partly due to the inherent difficulties involved in the proper blinding of acupuncture practitioners and the development of an adequate placebo to mimic the therapeutic experience of acupuncture. Because the overall evidence from well-controlled, randomized clinical trials is currently limited, it is not possible to unequivocally state that acupuncture is more effective than venlafaxine for hot flashes – the medication that has yielded the most impressive benefits in treating hot flashes. However, since the majority of acupuncture trials have provided very encouraging results with minimal side effects, future studies are warranted to further investigate and assess the potential role of acupuncture in the treatment of hot flashes in cancer patients.

H. Ashamalla (✉) · P. R. Graves
Radiation Oncology Department, New York Methodist Hospital and Weill Medical College of Cornell University, Brooklyn, NY 11215, USA
e-mail: hashamalla@gmail.com

F. C. Peluso
State University of New York Downstate Medical Center, Brooklyn, NY, USA

W. C. S. Cho (ed.), *Acupuncture and Moxibustion as an Evidence-based Therapy for Cancer*, Evidence-based Anticancer Complementary and Alternative Medicine 3,
DOI 10.1007/978-94-007-4833-0_4, © Springer Science+Business Media Dordrecht 2012

4.1 Introduction

Prostate and breast cancer are two of the most common types of cancer. Treatment of these cancers frequently involves hormonal reduction and/or ablation. One consequence of the sudden deprivation of sex hormones is the ensuing predisposition for hot flashes or vasomotor instability.

A significant number of cancer patients undergoing hormonal deprivation therapy experience hot flashes. Androgen deprivation therapy (ADT) is now considered the gold standard treatment for metastatic cancer of the prostate (Spetz et al. 2003). Men with prostatic cancer can undergo either surgical or medical castration (treatment with GnRH analogues) castration coupled with anti-androgens for total androgen ablation. A systematic review (Spetz et al. 2003) of 143 randomized, prospective studies has shown that hot flash incidence is 45% in men receiving GnRH analogue coupled with anti-androgens; whereas individual studies report hot flash incidence ranging between 14–74.3%. One Scandinavian group (Spetz et al. 2001) reported a 74.3% incidence of hot flashes in 452 men undergoing complete androgen ablation.

Premenopausal women undergoing treatment for breast cancer can experience more frequent and severe hot flashes than women in the menopausal population (Carpenter et al. 1998). Overall, hot flashes occur in >65% of all breast cancer survivors and one study reported that 72% of women taking tamoxifen experienced hot flashes (Carpenter et al. 1998).

The occurrence of hot flashes is often associated with insomnia, fatigue, and irritability—with great detriment to the quality of life of the patients who incur them (Casper and Yen 1985). As a result, various pharmacologic interventions to reduce hot flash frequency and severity have been tested. However, many of these have the potential for significant adverse side effects (Sicat and Brokaw 2004). Consequently, a great deal of research has gone into evaluating the effectiveness of alternative treatment options, such as acupuncture.

Acupuncture, a 25-century-old treatment modality developed in China, has emerged as one strategy for the treatment of hot flashes in cancer patients. If practiced correctly, acupuncture is regarded as safe and has minimal side effects. This chapter will review the potential role of acupuncture as a method to reduce hot flashes in cancer patients.

4.2 Treatment Modalities of Acupuncture

Acupuncture is a technique in which very thin needles of varying lengths are inserted through the skin to treat a variety of conditions. This ancient form of traditional Chinese medicine has been used to treat myriad conditions. It has been used to reduce pain, combat addictive behaviors, and promote rehabilitation from strokes or other injuries (Lin and Chen 2008). With regard to cancer, acupuncture has been most widely applied to reduce the untoward effects of cancer treatments. Examples include the application of acupuncture to reduce nausea and vomiting from chemotherapy

(Collins and Thomas 2004) and to provide pain relief and improve movement (He et al. 1999; Deng et al. 2004; Capodice 2010; Morrow et al. 2011).

In traditional acupuncture, needles are inserted at specific locations termed acupoints, as defined by traditional Chinese medicine. Needles are inserted at acupoints just deep enough into the skin to keep them from falling out. They are usually left in place for less than half an hour. Skilled acupuncturists cause virtually no pain. The acupuncturist may twirl the needles, apply heat or a weak electrical current to enhance the effects of the therapy. Modern acupuncture needles are made of very thin stainless steel and are disposable. In 1996, the FDA approved the use of acupuncture by licensed practitioners (Lanfrey et al. 1996). By law, needles must be labeled for one-time use only.

4.3 Clinical Trials

To date, the most significant studies done to assess the efficacy of acupuncture in cancer patients have been conducted in the form of clinical trials. Quality systematic reviews have been published evaluating trials in both prostate cancer patients and breast cancer patients, both concluding that the limited evidence does not suggest that acupuncture is an effective treatment for hot flashes in cancer patients (Lee et al. 2009a,b). We have focused our discussion on the published studies contained in these reviews. The observational studies by Ashamalla et al. and Beer et al. discussed below, are articles published after the 2009 systematic review of acupuncture for prostate cancer patients. These studies were only available in abstract form at the time of Lee's systematic review but are provided here for completeness. Here we provide a review of these clinical trials that have been published as journal articles separated according to the type of cancer being treated and discussed in chronological order.

4.3.1 Acupuncture Trials in Prostate Cancer Patients

At the time of this writing, a total of six clinical studies have addressed the efficacy of acupuncture for the treatment of hot flashes in prostate cancer patients (Lee et al. 2009b). These studies, including their study designs, results and conclusions are summarized in Table 4.1.

The first clinical trial to suggest that acupuncture may reduce the incidence of hot flashes in men undergoing prostate cancer therapy was conducted by Hammar and colleagues (1999). In this pilot study, a total of seven men with vasomotor symptoms due to castration therapy underwent acupuncture therapy and the frequency of hot flashes was recorded in personal logbooks. Of the seven men, six completed a 10-week course of acupuncture. The frequency of hot flashes was reduced by 50–70% at various points with no adverse effect reported. This study did not include a placebo control group.

Table 4.1 Acupuncture trials for hot flashes in prostate cancer

Author	Therapy	Duration	No. of patients	HF measurement used	Acupuncture points	Percent reduction from baseline (%)	Control	Side effects
Hammar et al. (1999)	TA + electro-acupuncture	Weeks 1–2: twice weekly Weeks 3–12: once weekly	6	HF Frequency	B/L: BL15, BL23[a], BL32[a] U/L: GV20, HT7, PC6, LR3, SP6, SP9	70	None	NS
Hayes et al. (2005)	TA + electro-acupuncture	Weeks 1–2: twice weekly Weeks 3–12: once weekly	10	Mean HFS	B/L: GB34, BL15, BL23[a], BL32[a] U/L: GV20, HT7, PC6, LR2, SP6	43	None	NS
Harding et al. (2009)	AA	AA once weekly for 10 weeks	60	Daily record (at 0, 4 and 10 weeks). Frequency of HF during night and day	B/L: Auricular: autonomic, kidney, Shenmen, lung and liver	58	None	None
Frisk et al. (2009)	Electro-acupuncture	Weeks 1–2: twice weekly Weeks 3–12: once weekly	14	Mean HFS	B/L: BL15, BL23[a], BL32[a] U/L: GV20, HT7, PC6, LR3, SP6, SP9	78	None	[b]
	TA	Same as electroacupuncture arm	15	Mean HFS	Same as above but without electroacupuncture	73		
Beer et al. (2010)	TA + electro-acupuncture	Weeks 1–4: twice weekly Weeks 5–10: once weekly	22	Mean HFS	B/L: GB34, BL15, BL23[a], BL32[a] U/L: GV20, HT7, PC6, LR2, SP6	>50	None	Mild or grade 1 adverse events
Ashmalla et al. (2011)	TA + electro-acupuncture	Twice weekly for 4 weeks	14	Mean HFS	B/L: GB34, SP6[a], KI3, ST36[a], BL15[a] BL23[a], Taiyang, HT7, PC6, LI11	89.2	None	None

All acupuncture studies used 30 min sessions (except for Harding et al.'s study which used 40 min sessions). *AA* auricular acupuncture, *B/L* bilateral, *BL* bladder, *GB* gall bladder, *HFS* hot flash score, *HT* heart, *KI* kidney, *NS* not stated, *PC* pericardium, *SP* spleen, *ST* stomach, *TA* traditional acupuncture, *U/L* unilateral[a]Acupuncture point that received 2 Hz electrostimulation

[b]One patient felt that treatment caused distress, another reported fatigue on the day of treatment, and a third reported a centimeter sided hematoma at the insertion site of an acupuncture needles

In the clinical trial conducted by Hayes and colleagues that was published in abstract form only, ten patients were enrolled and treated with acupuncture twice weekly for 4 weeks. A 43% reduction in mean hot flash score—number of daily hot flashes multiplied by severity on a scale of 1 (mild) to 4 (very severe)—was reported with seven of the ten men experiencing at least a 50% reduction in hot flash score (HFS) at any time during a 16-week evaluation. No significant side effects were reported. This study did not include a placebo control group.

A study by Frisk and colleagues (2009) evaluated the ability of acupuncture to reduce hot flashes in prostate cancer patients. In this study, 31 men with hot flashes were recruited and randomized into two groups: one that received electroacupuncture (EA) and another that received traditional acupuncture (TA) weekly for 12 weeks. Of the 29 men that completed the treatment, the HFS decreased by 78% and 73% in the EA and TA groups respectively. Only a few minor side effects were reported including one local centimeter-sized hematoma, one episode of distress and one episode of fatigue among three separate patients. This study did not have a placebo control. Instead, a small group of patients were asked to record their HFS 6 weeks prior to treatment. The efficacies of EA and TA were evaluated by comparing the HFS before and after the respective treatments.

A larger study conducted by Harding and colleagues (2009) analyzed 60 patients for reduction of hot flashes after treatment with auriculo-acupuncture (AA). The study selected patients receiving luteinizing-hormone releasing hormone (LHRH) analogues for carcinoma of the prostate. Patients underwent weekly AA for a period of 10 weeks and consented to a questionnaire to assess their sense of well-being both before and after treatment. All men completed the treatment without any adverse effects and 95% of patients reported a significant decrease in the severity of symptoms. The mean reduction of hot flashes in this group was 58%. This study also did not have a placebo control.

Beer and colleagues' study (2010) analyzed the effect of acupuncture on HFS, quality of life, and sleep quality in patients undergoing hormonal therapy for prostate cancer. Patients were treated with TA and EA biweekly for 4 weeks then weekly for 6 weeks. Patients recorded their response during the course of treatment and hot flash scores were calculated from the patient's daily diaries. Of the patients in the study, 44% reported a 50% reduction in HFS by week 4 and 55% reported a 50% reduction in HFS upon completing 10 weeks of therapy.

Ashamalla and colleagues' study (2011) included 14 men treated with TA plus electrostimulation of select acupoints twice weekly for 4 weeks. The study recorded the mean HFS at 2 weeks, 6 weeks, and 8 months from the initiation of treatment. The mean percent HFS reduction at weeks 2 and 6 were 68.4% and 89.2%, respectively. In patients with adequate follow-up at 8-months, significant improvement of the HFS was still evident as there was a continued 80.3% reduction from mean baseline HFS. This study, like all those listed above, did not employ placebo control.

4.3.2 Acupuncture Trials in Breast Cancer Patients

A significant number of studies have been conducted addressing the efficacy of acupuncture in the treatment of hot flashes in breast cancer patients. Among these, there are a relatively small number of randomized, placebo-controlled, clinical trials (Lee et al. 2009a) using sham acupuncture. These studies, including their study designs, results and conclusions are summarized in Table 4.2.

In the study by Nedstrand and colleagues (2005), a total of 38 post-menopausal women with breast cancer were randomized into two groups. One received EA and the other received applied relaxation therapy for 12 weeks. The number of hot flashes was recorded daily in personal logbooks before and during treatment and at 3 and 6 months post-treatment. Of the 19 women in the acupuncture group, it was reported that hot flashes were reduced by 52% after 12 weeks of acupuncture, and by 58% after 6 months of follow up. Applied relaxation techniques also reduced hot flashes by 51% after 12 weeks and by 58% at 6-months follow-up.

In the prospective, randomized, controlled trial conducted by Deng and colleagues (2007), a total of 72 women with breast cancer were randomly assigned to obtain either sham acupuncture with retractable needles or true acupuncture. Treatment was given twice weekly for a period of 4 consecutive weeks. The frequency of hot flashes was evaluated at baseline, at 6 weeks and at 6 months after initiation of treatment. The mean number of hot flashes was reported to decrease from 8.7 to 6.2 (29%) in the true acupuncture group and from 10 to 7.6 in the sham group (24%). Although there were fewer hot flashes in the true acupuncture group (0.8 per day), it did not reach statistical significance. In this study the effectiveness of acupuncture was not significantly better than sham treatment but the authors suggested that longer and more intense acupuncture might produce a larger reduction of hot flashes.

Frisk and colleagues (2008) conducted a randomized, controlled study to compare acupuncture to hormonal therapy in reducing hot flashes in patients with a history of breast cancer. This study was part of an international multicenter study from three centers in Sweden. Forty-five women were randomized to receive either EA for 12 weeks or hormone therapy (HT) for 24 months. The number and severity of hot flash episodes were registered daily before, during, and up to 24 months after the initiation of treatment. For the 19 women that completed the EA treatment for 12 weeks, the median number of daily hot flashes decreased from 9.6 (baseline) to 4.3 at 12 weeks. Long-term follow-up also demonstrated a continued benefit for patients after EA therapy. Twelve months after the start of treatment, 14 women had a median of 4.9 daily hot flashes. At 24 months follow-up, seven women had a median of 2.1 daily hot flashes. The 18 women who received HT had the number of daily hot flashes reduced from a baseline of 6.6 to 0 at 12 weeks after initiation of HT. Therefore, acupuncture was shown to have a beneficial long-term effect in reducing hot flashes but was not as effective as hormone therapy. Nevertheless, hormone therapy is contraindicated in women with hormone receptor-positve breast cancer and has well-documented adverse cardiovascular effects in post-menopausal women.

In the prospective, randomized, controlled trial conducted by Hervik and Mjaland (2009), acupuncture was shown to provide effective relief from hot flashes in women

Table 4.2 Acupuncture trials for hot flashes in breast cancer

Author	Therapy	Treatment and Duration	No. of patients	HF measurement used in study	Acupoints	Percent reduction from baseline	Control	Side effects
Nedstrand et al. (2005)	electro-acupuncture	Weeks 1–2: twice weekly Weeks 3–12: once weekly	38	Mean HF frequency	B/L: BL15, BL23[a], BL32[a] U/L: GV20, HT7, PC6, LR3, SP6, SP9	50%	Applied relaxation (60 min, once weekly for 12 weeks)	NS
Deng et al. (2007)	TA	Twice weekly for 4 weeks	72	Mean HF frequency	B/L: GB20, BL13, PC7, HT6, KI7, ST36, SP6, ear Shenmen, ear sympathetic point U/L: GV14	29%	Sham TA (non-penetrating, non-acupoint)	Minor adverse effects. Slight bleeding at needle site
Frisk et al. (2008)	TA + electro-acupuncture	Weeks 1–2: twice weekly Weeks 3–10: once weekly	45	Median HF frequency	B/L: BL15, BL23[a], BL32[a] U/L: GV20, HT7, PC6, LR3, SP6, SP9	55%	Hormone therapy	NS
Hervik and Mjaland et al. (2009)	TA	Weeks 1–5: twice weekly Weeks 6–10: once weekly	59	Mean HF frequency	U/L: GB20, LU7, KI3, SP6, CV4, PC7, LR4, LR8	50% day, 60% night	Sham TA (2–3 mm penetration at non-acu points)	NS
Walker et al. (2010)	TA	12 weeks	47	Mean HFS	NS	50%	Venlafaxine (12 weeks course)	None

All acupuncture studies used 30 min sessions (except for Deng et al.'s study which used 20 min sessions) *B/L* bilateral, *BL* bladder, *GB* gall bladder, *GV* governor vessel, *HFS* hot flash score, *HT* heart, *KI* kidney, *LI* large Intestine, *LR* liver, *LU* lung, *NS* not stated, *PC* pericardium, *SP* spleen, *ST* stomach, *TA* traditional acupuncture, *U/L* unilateral

[a] Acupuncture point that received 2 Hz electrostimulation

following surgical intervention and treated with tamoxifen. In this study, 59 women were randomized into two groups: those receiving traditional acupuncture or those receiving sham acupuncture. Sham acupuncture for this study was defined as the insertion of needles superficially (2–3 mm deep) at non-acupoints: 5, 10 and 15 cm proximal to the upper border of the patella and over the highest point of the trapezius muscle. Women were treated for a period of 10 weeks. The mean number of hot flashes was recorded both before the treatment, during treatment, and 12 weeks post-treatment. The mean number of daytime and nighttime hot flashes was reported to decrease by 50% and 60% respectively, in the acupuncture group. The women in the sham acupuncture group experienced a 25% decrease in daily hot flashes during treatment, which reversed during the following 12 weeks. The Kupperman index, a validated health score, was reduced by 44% in the acupuncture group at the end of treatment while no changes were observed in the sham acupuncture group.

In the study conducted by Walker and colleagues (2010), 50 hormone receptor-positive breast cancer patients were randomly assigned to two groups, one that received 12 weeks of acupuncture ($n = 25$) and one that received venlafaxine (Effexor), ($n = 25$) treatment. Outcomes, including hot flash score, depression and other quality of life symptoms were measured for up to 1 year post treatment. It was reported that both treatment groups experienced significant decreases in hot flashes, depression, and had improvement in quality of life symptoms including mental health. Although acupuncture was found to be equally effective as venlafaxine in reducing hot flashes, the acupuncture group experienced significantly fewer side effects than the venlafaxine group. Whereas 18 of the 25 patients in the venlafaxine group experienced nausea, dry mouth, dizziness and anxiety, the acupuncture group experienced no significant adverse effects.

4.4 Review and Evaluation of Results

4.4.1 Review of Acupuncture Trials in Prostate Cancer Patients

All of the six clinical trials mentioned above demonstrated a significant reduction in hot flashes among prostate cancer patients compared to their occurrence prior to treatment. Most of these studies used the HFS as a tool to measure the efficacy of acupuncture treatment. The HFS is a nationally accredited system that has been used in numerous studies and has been proven to be reliable in estimating the quality and quantity of hot flashes experienced by cancer patients (Sloan et al. 2001).

The reported reduction in hot flashes from baseline in all of these studies approach or exceed the efficacy of SNRIs (namely venlafaxine) which have proven to be very effective in the alleviation of hot flashes in both men and women undergoing hormonal deprivation therapy for cancer. Studies of the efficacy of venlafaxine for alleviation of hot flashes have demonstrated decreases in median HFS of 54% and 45.5% among men and women respectively (Quella et al. 1999; Loprinzi et al.

2009a,b). In addition, acupuncture treatment was reported to be very well tolerated in the prostate cancer studies in Table 4.1, whereas venlafaxine treatment has been associated with a number of undesirable side effects including nausea, altered sexual drive, and sleeplessness (Quella et al. 1999; Nelson et al. 2006).

Acupuncture may have long-lasting effects on hot flashes in ADT patients which last well beyond treatment duration. This has been evidenced by follow-up studies conducted by Hammar et al. (1999), Frisk et al. (2009) and Ashamalla et al. (2011). Hammar et al. (1999) reported that at 6-month follow-up, the mean number of hot flashes per day was 50% lower than before therapy while 33% of patients still experienced greater than a 50% reduction. Frisk et al. (2009) reported that at 6-month follow-up, 33% of EA patients and 43% of TA patients experienced >50% reduction in the mean number of hot flashes per day. At 12-month follow-up, 18% of the available EA patients and 46% of the available TA patients still experienced a 50% decrease from their baseline. Ashamalla et al. (2011) reported that at 8-month follow-up, there was still an 80.3% decrease in HFS among patients and 91% of the men continued to experience a greater than 50% improvement.

4.4.2 *Review of Acupuncture Trials in Breast Cancer Patients*

The results of the acupuncture trials listed above for the treatment of hot flashes in breast cancer patients generally show significant reductions in hot flashes approaching that of venlafaxine treatment (50–60%). These acupuncture trials report minimal adverse side effects compared with both venlafaxine and hormonal therapies (Table 4.2).

The randomized, controlled study by Deng et al. (2007) stands out in concluding that there is no statistically significant difference between the effects of actual acupuncture and sham acupuncture. Deng's trial employed the use of retractable needles, which never pierce the skin while the device itself is kept upright by a tiny adhesive ring at its base. These sham devices were placed several centimeters away from the proper acupoints. Patients in the true acupuncture group had a mean daily hot flash decrease of 33% while those in the sham group experienced a decrease of 24%. When those who initially received the sham treatment were crossed over to true acupuncture at 7 weeks, they experienced another 9% decrease resulting in a 33% decrease overall. These results were not deemed statistically significant because they are within the range of placebo effect observed for hot flash treatment that ranges from 20–35% with 4 weeks of placebo treatment.

Another approach to conducting sham acupuncture has been to needle the skin at non-acupoints, such as the trial conducted by Vincent et al. (2007). This trial studied the efficacy of acupuncture on hot flashes in postmenopausal women. This randomized, sham-controlled clinical study also concluded that there is no difference between acupuncture and sham acupuncture for hot flashes. Of note, the study of Vincent et al. (2007) used different definitions for sham acupuncture. Their trial defined sham acupuncture as needling administered in non-acupuncture, non-meridian areas, whenever possible 5 cm or more away from the actual acupuncture point. 103

participants were randomized to either true or sham acupuncture for biweekly treatments for 5 weeks with another 7 weeks of follow-up for each arm of the study. At week 6, patients receiving true acupuncture experienced a 40% decrease in hot flashes while those receiving sham acupuncture experienced a 38% decrease in hot flashes. At week 12, the true acupuncture group had 13% more hot flashes than they did at week 6; those in the sham group continued to experience a decrease of another 5%. Therefore, at the end of 12 weeks, those who received true acupuncture only experienced a net decrease in hot flashes of 27% from baseline, while those who received sham had 45% decrease from baseline. The authors concluded that the results of the study suggest medical acupuncture was not any more effective for reducing hot flashes than was the chosen sham acupuncture.

The study by Vincent's group is intriguing because the placebo still involves piercing of the skin and although the areas were deemed non-acupuncture and non-meridian according to traditional Chinese medicine, they could still affect afferent nerve fibers in the skin. By stimulating afferent nerve fibers, there is potential release of β-endorphins which may contribute to the alleviation of hot flashes according to the current pathophysiologic model of hot flashes discussed later in this chapter (Zhao 2008). Furthermore, although this method of placebo was defined as a needling in non-meridian points, there was no mention of whether manual stimulation was used to achieve the Deqi sensation—the characteristic numbness or soreness experienced by the patient during true acupuncture (Vincent et al. 2007). If Deqi was induced, then the same physiological mechanism which is produced by manual acupuncture at normal acupoints may have been activated, and could explain why placebo patients in this trial still experienced a 45% reduction in hot flashes. If this was the case, the statistical differences observed in the reduction of hot flashes between the true acupuncture group and the sham acupuncture group may simply reflect different efficacy in placement of acupuncture needles rather than a difference between a true acupuncture treatment and a feigned one. Lastly, the 45% reduction experienced by the sham group is quite comparable to the effects of venlafaxine and suggests that acupuncture, regardless of acupoint placement, may still be clinically useful.

The sham retractable needle acupuncture device used in Deng's trial (2007) is a good placebo in the sense that it does not pierce the skin and thus there is no potential for inadvertent afferent nerve stimulation. However, it does not allow for adequate blinding. While neither the patient nor the doctor may know if the patient actually received true acupuncture or placebo, the acupuncturist cannot be effectively blinded as he/she will obviously be aware of the fact that the needles are authentic or sham devices. Although a single acupuncturist coached all acupuncturists conducting the sham acupuncture and also observed treatments periodically for integrity, this obviously leaves the study results vulnerable to bias (Ernst 2006). This problem is simply inherent in acupuncture research and there may be no way to provide a better placebo than the device used by Deng's group. However, the fact that Deng's trial is deemed placebo-controlled should not lend it any more authority than other non-controlled trials in light of this essential flaw in methodology.

4.5 Safety and Adverse Effects

As of 1996, acupuncture needles are deemed Class II medical devices by the FDA—permitting their use by licensed, registered, or certified practitioners. Needles are required by the FDA to have proper labeling and manufacturers must follow strict practices in their production. About 7–11% of patients may experience needling pain or bleeding at the site of needling. Major complications such as pneumothorax, cardiac tamponade, human immunodeficiency virus and hepatitis C infection are exceedingly rare especially if the procedure is performed by a well-trained acupuncturist with sterile, one-time use needles (Ernst 2006). Most of the serious side effects documented are the result of poor training and the large number of paramedics practicing non-sterile techniques. When considering acupuncture therapy for their patients, it is essential that physicians confirm that the licensed acupuncturist has adequate accreditation in accordance with the appropriate state legislature.

4.6 The Theoretical Pathophysiologic Model of Hot Flashes and the Biochemical Action of Acupuncture

Studies of the hot flash mechanism have been limited to postmenopausal women but it has been suggested that an analogous mechanism applies for the triggering of hot flashes in men and women receiving hormonal deprivation therapy. This is because hot flashes in both menopausal women and cancer patients are subjectively and objectively similar and are associated with the sudden withdrawal of sex hormones (Spetz et al. 2001). Estrogen and testosterone stimulate the production of endorphins, which modulate norepinephrine—a neurotransmitter thought to play a key role in the hot flash mechanism of Shanafelt and colleagues (Shanafelt et al. 2002).

Shanafelt et al. (2002) have presented a theoretical model for the hot flash mechanism that incorporates the findings and theories published by experts on the subject through 2002. Hot flashes are the result of dysfunction of the thermoregulatory nucleus located in the medial preoptic area of the hypothalamus. This nucleus is responsible for maintaining body temperature within a normal range termed the thermoregulatory zone. If body temperature increases, the nucleus initiates heat loss mechanisms such as peripheral vasodilation—occasionally resulting in a hot flash.

Shanafelt et al. (2002) proposes that norepinephrine is the primary neurotransmitter for lowering the thermoregulatory set point, citing that plasma levels of norepinephrine metabolites are increased before and during hot flashes, and intrahypothalamic injection of norepinephrine can induce a heat loss response. Following sex hormone withdrawal, the level of endorphins will decrease and may no longer be sufficient to effectively modulate hypothalamic norepinephrine. This relative excess of norepinephrine in the thermoregulatory nucleus triggers hot flashes when minor stimuli (emotional stress, caffeine, alcohol, etc.) are present.

Serotonin (5-HT) also plays a significant role in Shanafelt's model—explained in more detail in a work by Berendsen (2000). Both Shanafelt and Berendsen cite a number of studies demonstrating that blood serotonin levels are drastically lowered in women who experience menopause and return to normal with the injection of an estrogen (Berendsen 2000). This low blood serotonin level leads to the increase of 5-HT_{2A} receptors on blood platelets—possibly reflecting an increase of hypothalamic 5-HT_{2A} receptors. This is significant because 5-HT_{2A} receptors have been shown to mediate heat loss and an increased number of these receptors in the hypothalamus render it hypersensitive to serotonin (Berendsen 2000). This predisposes the hypothalamus to trigger autonomic heat loss mechanisms in response to relatively small increases of serotonin. In addition, mild stressors such as emotional stress, alcohol, and caffeine release 5-HT modulin, which by blocking 5-HT_{1B} auto-receptors, perpetuate a further release of serotonin (Shanafelt et al. 2002).

In summary, sex hormone withdrawal causes dysfunction in the thermoregulatory nucleus by two proposed mechanisms. Firstly, through decreased production of endorphins, increasing norepinephrine and decreasing the hypothalamic thermoregulatory set point. Secondly, through upregulation of 5HT_{2A} receptors that leads to the hypersensivity of the thermoregulatory nucleus towards serotonin (Berendsen 2000; Shanafelt et al. 2002).

A review by Lin and Chen (2008) of mechanisms of acupuncture analgesia provides a thorough overview of the evidence supporting the theory that the release of endorphins and serotonin are induced by acupuncture. Lin and Chen cite studies in the mid to late 1970s conducted by Pomeranz (Pomeranz and Cheng 1979; Pomeranz and Paley 1979) which suggest that EA causes the pituitary to release endogenous opioids into the plasma and exerts an analgesic effect on the central nervous system. Following Pomeranz's suggestion that different frequencies applied to acupuncture needles may release different endogenous opioids such as β-endorphin, enkephalin, endomorphin and dynorphin, research began to focus on establishing the relationship between specific endogenous opioids with specific EA frequencies.

Han's review (2004) of the results of studies attempting to link the release of opioid peptides to specific electrical frequencies concludes that EA at 2 Hz stimulates a strong release of enkephalin, beta-endorphin, and endomorphin but no release of dynorphin while EA at 100 Hz stimulates a strong release of dynorphin but not the release of any of the other three substances. It was also discovered that alternating between frequencies of 2 Hz and 100 Hz using a pulse generator significantly increases acupuncture's analgesic effect compared to the use of 2 Hz or 100 Hz exclusively. The relationship between different frequencies of EA and endogenous opiates produced suggests that different frequencies of electroacupuncture used for hot flash treatment may have varying efficacy depending on which opioid is most effective in suppressing norepinephrine.

Two hertz EA is the modality most utilized in hot flash acupuncture trials and may be preferable for its ability to stimulate the release a variety of endogenous opioids. Furthermore, studies by Tsai et al. have suggested that the analgesic effect of EA at 2 Hz is also mediated by serotonin, since the effect diminished after a serotonin synthesis inhibitor injection—suggesting that serotonin may also be released as a result of EA at 2 Hz (Lin and Chen 2008). This conclusion is further evidenced by the increase of serotonin in the spinal cord following 2 Hz EA and that serotonin's precursor responds to enhanced analgesia at 2 Hz EA (Lin and Chen 2008).

Among the trials listed in Tables 4.1 and 4.2, those that implemented 2 Hz EA tended to report greater reductions in hot flashes than those using manual stimulation exclusively—with the exception of Frisk's prostate cancer study (2009) which showed a slightly higher decrease in mean hot flash score among men receiving TA than EA. If these mechanisms for acupuncture analgesia are accurate, acupuncture may have the potential to alleviate hot flashes by two possible mechanisms: by increasing centrally acting endorphins which modulate norepinephrine and by increasing circulating 5-HT which decreases central 5-HT_{2A} receptor hypersensitivity and hyperdensity (Fig. 4.1).

4.7 Conclusion and Future Prospectives

In conclusion, to design a randomized, well-controlled study of acupuncture for the alleviation of hot flashes in cancer patients is a particularly challenging enterprise. The mechanisms for both hot flashes and the physiologic effects of acupuncture are not entirely known. There are inherent problems in developing an ideal placebo device for acupuncture—one that effectively blinds the acupuncturist as well as the patient and prescribing physician. This prevents effective double-blind studies in clinical trials for hot flash treatment. Loose definitions given to acupuncture and sham acupuncture may cause confusion when comparing various studies because different acupuncture techniques may have varying physiological effects on the body. In addition, chosen sham placebos which needle the skin may still stimulate affect afferent nerves—making it difficult to determine whether hot flash improvement is due to placebo effect or something more. Methods for blinding and controlling acupuncture studies must be further improved in the future to allow for more objective meta-analysis of acupuncture trials.

The measured outcomes of hot flashes should be standardized as well in order to more objectively compare the efficacy of different treatment modalities. Several studies found in both Tables 4.1 and 4.2 measure reduction in hot flash frequency, which does not take into account the severity of each hot flash. HFS is preferable as it gives a more comprehensive picture of the morbidity of hot flashes in cancer patients. It also provides more insight into the utility of a given treatment modality—as the ability to reduce the severity of a patient's hot flashes can be just as clinically meaningful as decreasing the frequency of his/her hot flashes alone.

The many variables in acupuncture studies including differing acupuncture protocols and measured study outcomes may undermine the credibility of study results and prevent researchers from coming to a consensus on the value of acupuncture in treating hot flashes. Future studies must seek to standardize the acupuncture protocol to the finest detail in order to allow their results to be interpreted more objectively and compared to those of other studies. The studies in Tables 4.1 and 4.2 suggest that the most promising protocol for hot flash acupuncture treatment should employ

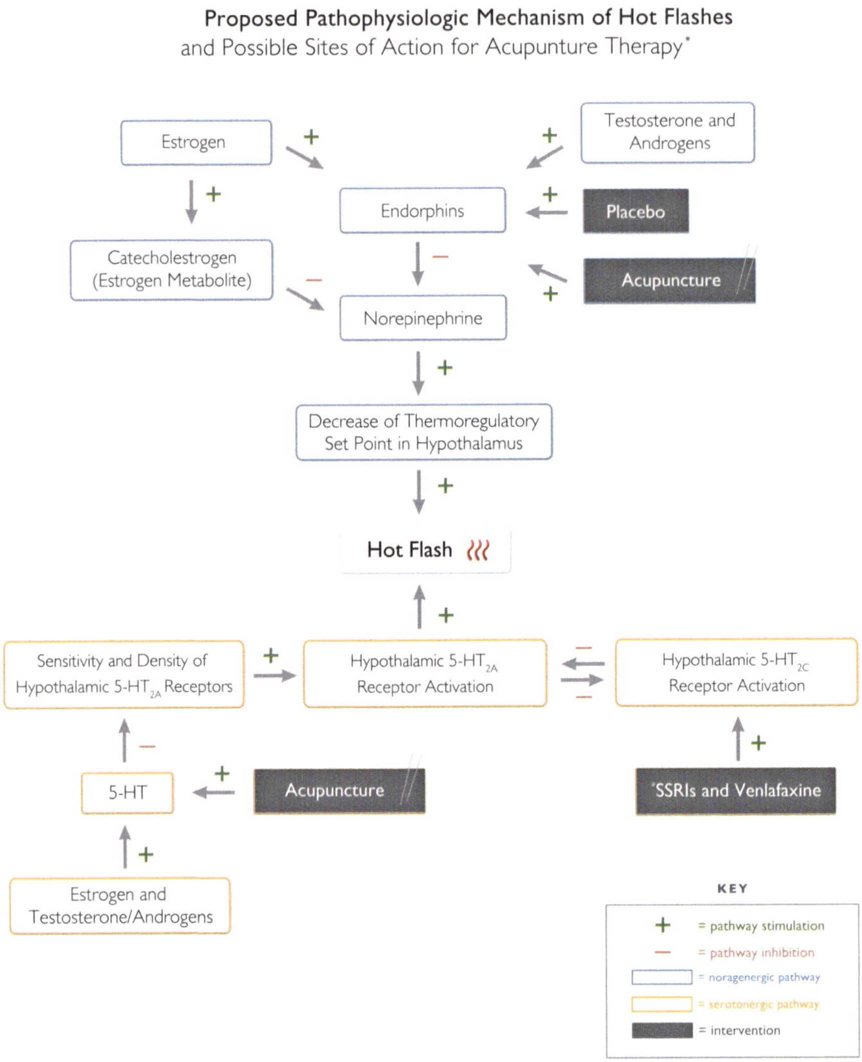

Fig. 4.1 Sex hormone withdrawal causes dysfunction in the thermoregulatory nucleus by two proposed mechanisms. Firstly, through decreased production of endorphins, increasing norepinephrine and decreasing the hypothalamic thermoregulatory set point. Secondly, through upregulation of 5-HT_{2A} receptors that leads to the hypersensivity of the thermoregulatory nucleus towards serotonin. Acupuncture may have the potential to alleviate hot flashes by two possible mechanisms: by increasing centrally acting endorphins which modulate norepinephrine and by increasing circulating 5-HT which decreases central 5-HT_{2A} receptor hypersensitivity and hyperdensity

2 Hz electrostimulation at multiple acupoints during biweekly sessions for at least 4 weeks to achieve the maximum anticipated effect that acupuncture therapy may provide. Attempts at standardizing acupuncture research methodology and developing improved placebo devices will help to advance our knowledge of the potential that

acupuncture may have in improving the quality of life for cancer patients suffering from hot flashes.

References

Ashamalla, H., Jiang, M. L., Guirguis, A., Peluso, F., Ashamalla, M. (2011). Acupuncture for the alleviation of hot flashes in men treated with androgen ablation therapy. *International Journal of Radiation Oncology, Biology, Physics*, *79*, 1358–1363.

Beer, T. M., Benavides, M., Emmons, S. L., Hayes, M., Liu, G., Garzotto, M., et al. (2010). Acupuncture for hot flashes in patients with prostate cancer. *Urology*, *76*, 1182–1188.

Berendsen, H. H. (2000). The role of serotonin in hot flushes. *Maturitas*, *36*, 155–164.

Capodice, J. L. (2010). Acupuncture in the oncology setting: clinical trial update. *Current Treatment Options of Oncology*, *11*, 87–94.

Carpenter, J. S., Andrykowski, M. A., Cordova, M., Cunningham, L., Studts, J., McGrath, P., et al. (1998). Hot flashes in postmenopausal women treated for breast carcinoma: prevalence, severity, correlates, management, and relation to quality of life. *Cancer*, *82*, 1682–1691.

Casper, R. F., & Yen, S. S. (1985). Neuroendocrinology of menopausal flushes: an hypothesis of flush mechanism. *Clinical Endocrinology (Oxf)*, *22*, 293–312.

Collins, K. B., & Thomas, D. J. (2004). Acupuncture and acupressure for the management of chemotherapy-induced nausea and vomiting. *Journal of American Academic Nurse Practise*, *16*, 76–80.

Deng, G., Cassileth, B. R., & Yeung, K. S. (2004). Complementary therapies for cancer-related symptoms. *Journal of Supportive Oncology*, *2*, 419–426; discussion 427–429.

Deng, G., Vickers, A., Yeung, S., D'Andrea, G. M., Xiao, H., Heerdt, A. S., et al. (2007). Randomized, controlled trial of acupuncture for the treatment of hot flashes in breast cancer patients. *Journal of Clinical Oncology*, *25*, 5584–5590.

Ernst, E. (2006). Acupuncture—a critical analysis. *Journal of International Medicine*, *259*, 125–137.

Frisk, J., Carlhall, S., Kallstrom, A. C., Lindh-Astrand, L., Malmstrom, A., & Hammar, M. (2008). Long-term follow-up of acupuncture and hormone therapy on hot flushes in women with breast cancer: a prospective, randomized, controlled multicenter trial. *Climacteric*, *11*, 166–174.

Frisk, J., Spetz, A. C., Hjertberg, H., Petersson, B., & Hammar, M. (2009). Two modes of acupuncture as a treatment for hot flushes in men with prostate cancer—a prospective multicenter study with long-term follow-up. *European Journal of Urology*, *55*, 156–163.

Hammar, M., Frisk, J., Grimas, O., Hook, M., Spetz, A. C., & Wyon, Y. (1999). Acupuncture treatment of vasomotor symptoms in men with prostatic carcinoma: a pilot study. *Journal of Urology*, *161*, 853–856.

Han, S. J. (2004). Acupuncture and endorphins. *Neuroscience Letters*, *361*, 258–261.

Harding, C., Harris, A., & Chadwick, D. (2009). Auricular acupuncture: a novel treatment for vasomotor symptoms associated with luteinizing-hormone releasing hormone agonist treatment for prostate cancer. *BJU International*, *103*, 186–190.

Hayes, M., Katovic, N. M., Donovan D., Emmons S., Benavides M., Montalto M., et al. (2005). Acupuncture for hot flashes in prostate cancer patients. *Journal of Clinical Oncology*, *23*, 8160.

He, J. P., Friedrich, M., Ertan, A. K., Muller, K., & Schmidt, W. (1999), Pain-relief and movement improvement by acupuncture after ablation and axillary lymphadenectomy in patients with mammary cancer. *Clinical and Experimental Obstetrics Gynecology*, *26*, 81–84

Hervik, J., & Mjaland, O. (2009). Acupuncture for the treatment of hot flashes in breast cancer patients, a randomized, controlled trial. *Breast Cancer Research Treatments*, *116*, 311–316.

Lanfrey, P., Mottet, N., Dagues, F., Bennaoum, K., Costa, P., Louis, J. F., et al. (1996). Hot flashes and hormonal treatment of prostate cancer. *Progrès en Urologie*, *6*, 17–22.

Lee, M. S., Kim, K. H., Choi, S. M., & Ernst, E. (2009a). Acupuncture for treating hot flashes in breast cancer patients: a systematic review. *Breast Cancer Research Treatments*, *115*, 497–503.

Lee, M. S., Kim, K. H., Shin, B. C., Choi, S. M., & Ernst, E. (2009b). Acupuncture for treating hot flushes in men with prostate cancer: a systematic review. *Supportive Care Cancer*, *17*, 763–770.

Lin, J. G., & Chen, W. L. (2008). Acupuncture analgesia: a review of its mechanisms of actions. *American Journal of Chinese Medicine*, *36*, 635–645.

Loprinzi, C. L., Dueck, A. C., Khoyratty, B. S., Barton, D. L., Jafar, S., Rowland, K. M. Jr., et al. (2009a). A Phase III randomized, double-blind, placebo-controlled trial of gabapentin in the management of hot flashes in men (N00CB). *Annals of Oncology*, *20*, 542–559.

Loprinzi, C. L., Sloan, J., Stearns, V., Slack, R., Iyengar, M., Diekmann, B., et al. (2009b). Newer antidepressants and gabapentin for hot flashes: an individual patient pooled analysis. *Journal of Clinical Oncology*, *27*, 2831–2837.

Morrow, P. K., Mattair, D. N., & Hortobagyi, G. N. (2011). Hot flashes: a review of pathophysiology and treatment modalities. *Oncologist*, *16*, 1658–1664.

Nedstrand, E., Wijma, K., Wyon, Y., & Hammar, M. (2005). Vasomotor symptoms decrease in women with breast cancer randomized to treatment with applied relaxation or electro-acupuncture: a preliminary study. *Climacteric*, *8*, 243–250.

Nelson, H. D., Vesco, K. K., Haney, E., Fu, R., Nedrow, A., Miller, J., et al. (2006). Nonhormonal therapies for menopausal hot flashes: systematic review and meta-analysis. *JAMA*, *295*, 2057–2071.

Pomeranz, B., & Cheng, R. (1979). Suppression of noxious responses in single neurons of cat spinal cord by electroacupuncture and its reversal by the opiate antagonist naloxone. *Experimental Neurology*, *64*, 327–341.

Pomeranz, B., & Paley, D. (1979). Electroacupuncture hypalgesia is mediated by afferent nerve impulses: an electrophysiological study in mice. *Experimental Neurology*, *66*, 398–402.

Quella, S. K., Loprinzi, C. L., Sloan, J., Novotny, P., Perez, E. A., Burch, P. A., et al. (1999). Pilot evaluation of venlafaxine for the treatment of hot flashes in men undergoing androgen ablation therapy for prostate cancer. *Journal of Urology*, *162*, 98–102.

Shanafelt, T. D., Barton, D. L., Adjei, A. A., & Loprinzi, C. L. (2002). Pathophysiology and treatment of hot flashes. *Mayo Clinic Proceeding*, *77*, 1207–1218.

Sicat, B. L., & Brokaw, D. K. (2004). Nonhormonal alternatives for the treatment of hot flashes. *Pharmacotherapy*, *24*, 79–93.

Sloan, J. A., Loprinzi, C. L., Novotny, P. J., Barton, D. L., Lavasseur, B. I., & Windschitl, H. (2001). Methodologic lessons learned from hot flash studies. *Journal of Clinical Oncology*, *19*, 4280–4290.

Spetz, A. C., Hammar, M., Lindberg, B., Spangberg, A., & Varenhorst, E. (2001). Prospective evaluation of hot flashes during treatment with parenteral estrogen or complete androgen ablation for metastatic carcinoma of the prostate. *Journal of Urology*, *166*, 517–520.

Spetz, A. C., Zetterlund, E. L., Varenhorst, E., & Hammar, M. (2003). Incidence and management of hot flashes in prostate cancer. *Journal of Supportive Oncology*, *1*, 263–6, 269–70, 272–3; discussion 267–8, 271–2.

Vincent, A., Barton, D. L., Mandrekar, J. N., Cha, S. S., Zais, T., Wahner-Roedler, D. L., et al. (2007). Acupuncture for hot flashes: a randomized, sham-controlled clinical study. *Menopause*, *14*, 45–52.

Walker, E. M., Rodriguez, A. I., Kohn, B., Ball, R. M., Pegg, J., Pocock, J. R., et al. (2010). Acupuncture versus venlafaxine for the management of vasomotor symptoms in patients with hormone receptor-positive breast cancer: a randomized controlled trial. *Journal of Clinical Oncology*, *28*, 634–640.

Zhao, Z. Q. (2008). Neural mechanism underlying acupuncture analgesia. *Progress in Neurobiology*, *85*, 355–375.

Chapter 5
Acupuncture and Moxibustion for Cancer-Related Symptoms

Raimond K. Wong and Stephen M. Sagar

Abstract Acupuncture and moxibustion is increasingly utilized in cancer management. Recent research has continued to provide new evidence to support the use of these complementary treatment modalities for the supportive care of cancer patients during and after conventional therapies. Apart from nausea and vomiting, for which the strongest evidence exists to support acupuncture treatment, there are multiple other symptoms that have been shown to benefit from acupuncture and moxibustion. These symptoms are commonly encountered by patients in their cancer journey and include the very debilitating cancer pain syndrome to the least apparent symptoms like anxiety, depression and cancer-related fatigue. The alleviation of these symptoms is essential to ensure better patients' quality of life. Adoption of these acupuncture-related treatment modalities into clinical practice should be based on best evidence that ideally derived from well designed randomized controlled clinical trials. Non-invasive form of acupuncture point stimulation using transcutaneous electrical stimulation is also being investigated and the results of recent studies are promising. This chapter reviewed the current evidence from published laboratory and clinical trials to inform proper recommendation, utilization and further research of acupuncture and moxibustion management for cancer-related symptoms.

5.1 Introduction

Recent advances in cancer treatment have improved treatment outcomes of cancer patients. However, cancer patients continue to experience a wide variety of symptoms related to the cancers and its treatments. More aggressive treatments lead to more severe acute toxicities and their effective managements becomes an important factor to ensure patients' treatment compliance that may indirectly affect treatment outcomes. Improved survival of cancer patients also increases the prevalence of patients with chronic toxicities. Effective managements of these chronic toxicities are thus also important to improve patients' quality of life. Conventional managements

R. K. Wong (✉) · S. M. Sagar
Departments of Oncology and Medicine, McMaster University;
Juravinski Cancer Centre, 699 Concession Street, Hamilton,
ON L8V 5C2, Canada
e-mail: wongrai@mcmaster.ca

W. C. S. Cho (ed.), *Acupuncture and Moxibustion as an Evidence-based Therapy for Cancer*, Evidence-based Anticancer Complementary and Alternative Medicine 3,
DOI 10.1007/978-94-007-4833-0_5,

of cancer-related symptoms may not be effective and research for effective treatment modalities continues. Acupuncture and its related techniques are one of the most common forms of complementary and alternative medicine that are widely accepted by the general public. Recent studies have shown that these interventions can provide effective relief for some cancer-related symptoms. This chapter reviews the current published evidence of the effectiveness of acupuncture and moxibustion in managing cancer-related symptoms.

5.2 Cancer Pain

Pain is common in patients with all types and all stages of cancer but particularly in advanced and terminal stages. In a recent systematic review, 33% of patient experienced pain after their curative treatments and 64% of patients with advanced stage disease have suffered from pain. In more than one third of patients who reported pain, the intensity of pain was noted to be moderate to severe (van den Beuken-van Everdingen et al. 2007).

Cancer pain can be broadly categorized into nociceptive, neuropathic or mixed according to mechanisms. Cancer itself and cancer treatments can damage organs and activate nociceptive receptors resulting in pain that is often localized (except from visceral origin where pain is often not well localized), constant and with an arching and throbbing quality. Direct nerve damages, however, typically result in burning and electric shock like quality pain that may radiate along the nerve innervation areas.

In conventional managements of cancer pain, clinical recognition of the pain mechanisms involved is important to direct management. For example, pain with a neuropathic component often needs medications such as anti-depressants and anti-convulsants to be effectively managed (Vorobeychik et al. 2011). In contrast, treatment of pain with acupuncture approaches requires the recognition of symptoms patterns. These patterns include the location and propagation pathway of pain in relationship to acupuncture meridian distributions or to the correspondence areas of established acupuncture "microsystems". In a "microsystem", the whole body is reflected in part of the body, such as the ear, the hand or the foot. Acupuncture points in a "microsystem" resemble the acupuncture points found in the whole body and can also be used to achieve treatment effects. Symptom patterns recognition also include the overall assessment of the body energetic status: an overall reduction of body energy often worsen pain experience and only by correcting this deficient status then pain can be effectively controlled.

5.2.1 *Acupuncture for Cancer Pain*

5.2.1.1 Mechanisms Exist to Suggest Acupuncture Can Be Effective for Pain

The mechanisms by which acupuncture treatments can relieve pain have been suggested in many laboratory and clinical studies. Opioid peptides have been shown to be released at various regions of the central nervous systems upon acupuncture stimulation (Ji-Sheng 2003). Levels of other neurotransmitters, such as substance P that is related to inflammation and pain, have been shown to be reduced by electroacupuncture compared to that of controls in animal studies (Lee et al. 2009a). Modulation of the threshold of neuronal discharge of spinal dorsal horn neurons by electroacupuncture was also demonstrated in animal studies (Rong et al. 2005). Functional MRI studies offered further insight into the yet unclear complexity of acupuncture effects on pain perception. In human studies, activities of various regions of the brain known to be involved in pain perception, including the sensory cortical areas and the limbic system, were shown to be modulated in acupuncture analgesia (Wu et al. 1999; Hui et al. 2000). The frequencies of stimulation utilized in electroacupuncture were also shown to exert different modulation effects on the dynamic nociceptive neural network: high frequency stimulation induced analgesic effect on broader areas of the body while low frequency stimulation was more effective for adjacent painful areas.

5.2.1.2 Clinical Evidence Supporting Acupuncture Effectiveness

Acupuncture has been used for non-cancer and cancer-related pain, in fact, for many non-pain clinical conditions in China. In the west, acupuncture has also been widely utilized for pain management. A recent study showed that over 80% of chronic pain clinics offer acupuncture as an option for pain control (Woollam and Jackson 1998). Although there is plenty of anecdotal evidence to suggest acupuncture is effective in managing cancer-related pain, the acceptable gold standard remains in evidence provided through randomized controlled trials. There were, however, only few randomized trials examining acupuncture for cancer-related pain conducted to date and all showed positive results.

In one of these trials, Alimi et al. (2003) randomized 90 patients who attained a pain clinic for cancer-related pain with neuropathic nature into three groups. One group received true auricular acupuncture, another group received placebo auricular acupuncture and the last group had placebo auricular seeds. Eleven patients were excluded from the study analysis because of refusal to continue and violation of protocol for change in analgesics. Intensities of pain, measured using a visual analogue scale were assessed at baseline, 1 and 2 months from randomization. Patients in the true acupuncture group reported lower pain scores at 2 months compared to baseline than the other two placebo groups ($p < 0.001$). While the result of this trial was conclusive, the trial also highlighted common issues in conducting placebo trials with acupuncture. Acupuncturists who performed the assigned treatments were not blinded since it would have been difficult to be 'blinded' to putting needles and seeds. Unlike most randomized trial designs, acupuncture points formulas were not used since it is considered inappropriate in acupuncture practice that advocates individualized treatment approach that is believed to be more clinically effective. This trial also demonstrated the usefulness and convenience of using a 'microsystem' acupuncture technique alone for cancer-related pain.

In a prospective, open label, randomized controlled trial, Pfister et al. (2010) demonstrated that acupuncture may effectively reduce the moderate or severe pain in patients after neck dissection and radiotherapy. Seventy patients were randomized into acupuncture plus usual care and usual care alone. Hegu (LI4), Sanyinjiao (SP6), Baihui (GV20), Luozhen and auricular Shenman were used in all patients and were chosen based on classical functions. Local Ashi points and distal 'zone' points were also used on an individual basis. At 6 weeks after acupuncture, Constant-Murley Scores that measure pain, pain free range of motion and level of daily activities were significantly higher by 11.3 points in the acupuncture group compared to control ($p = 0.008$).

Crew et al. (2010) reported on a randomized controlled trial that compared acupuncture *vs* sham acupuncture in breast cancer patients with arthralgia and joint stiffness due to aromatase inhibitors. A total of 43 patients were recruited into the trial. The acupuncture treatments were delivered according to standard protocols. Individualized points for specific painful joint areas were allowed. Mean pain scores were decreased significantly in the acupuncture group compared to that of control (3.0 *vs* 5.5; $p < 0.001$).

Another randomized and again unblinded trial conducted by Dang and Yang (1998) focused on patients with stomach cancer who presented with cancer-related pain. Forty-eight patients were randomized into three groups: acupuncture with filiform needles alone, acupuncture with filiform needles plus point injections and control. Compared to the control group, the authors concluded that acupuncture treatments decreased pain significantly in the short-term after treatments. However, there was no significant difference in pain control in the long-term. There was also significant difference in the enkephalin plasma level before and after acupuncture treatments between the treatment group and the control group, supporting the observed effectiveness of these acupuncture treatment approaches.

In another randomized unblinded study (Xia et al. 1986), 76 patients with either lung, esophageal or stomach cancer-related chest pain were randomized equally into acupuncture treatment or control group. An energetic point, Zusanli (ST36) and a parasympathetic point, Neiguan (PC6) were used in all patients in combination with body points selected according to symptom patterns. The chest pain in all patients in the treatment group but not in the control group was alleviated or disappeared.

Given the lower methodological qualities of randomized controlled trials conducted, several research groups have utilized systematic review to explore the efficacy of acupuncture treatments in reducing cancer-related pain (Lee et al. 2005; Peng et al. 2010; Paley et al. 2011). The Cochrane review conducted by Paley et al. (2011) was the most recent updated attempt to review this efficacy issue. This review concluded that there was a lack of high quality studies to provide strong evidence to support the positive efficacy of acupuncture in cancer-related pain reduction. More appropriate designed randomized studies are needed to clarify this efficacy question. However it is likely that a long period will be needed for these randomized studies to be designed, conducted and analyzed. Given that there are so many different acupuncture approaches that can be effective to manage cancer-related pain, the complexity and the practicality in examining all available approaches can be a major barrier in generating scientifically sound evidence to support acupuncture as an evidence-based option of cancer pain control.

In the meantime, well conducted prospective cohort and case controlled studies involving smaller number of patients such as those performed by Wong and Sagar (2006), Filshie and Redman (1985), as well as Paley and Johnson (2011) in examining acupuncture approaches for cancer pain will continue to offer insight and guidance in using acupuncture for cancer-related pain.

Continuous research in the efficacy of various acupuncture approaches for controlling cancer-related pain should be advocated. Acupuncture practitioners should keep themselves aware of the evidence that is based on well designed research results and continue to offer acupuncture as an option for cancer pain management. Convenience in treatment delivery, proven efficacy and practitioners training should be the basis in considering the types of acupuncture approach to be used for patients with cancer pain. When particular symptom pattern is recognized, selection of appropriate acupuncture points such as Qihai (CV6), ST36 can be used first, to improve deficient energy status. Points, preferably distal rather than close to the area of pain, selected from the involved meridian(s) can then be utilized to improve the 'energy flow' of the affected meridian(s). The addition of stimulating points, for example, LI4, sympathetic point and PC6, parasympathetic point, that are known to have analgesic effects can enhance the overall treatment results. A review of the recent Chinese publications regarding the usage of acupuncture and moxibustion in cancer pain provides an overview of the current pattern of practice (Huang 2011a).

5.2.2 Moxibustion for Cancer Pain

Moxibustion is a traditional Chinese medicine treatment modality that uses the heat produced by the burning of herbal preparations containing *Artemisia vulgaris*, instead of using needles, to stimulate acupuncture points (WHO Regional Office for the Western Pacific 2007). The herbal preparation is either formed into a small cone called moxa cone or into a cylinder shape called moxa stick. Moxibustion treatment is carried out either by directly burning moxa cone on the skin, or indirectly by burning moxa cone on a skin barrier made of various materials (for example, ginger and salt), or by burning a moxa stick to apply heat to acupuncture points without direct skin contact. Moxibustion is viewed to be important in traditional Chinese medicine practice in managing conditions that are diagnosed to have 'cold' or 'dampness' symptom pattern components or when sluggish or blockage of energy is perceived in a meridian. It is also utilized frequently for tonification of energy for weak patients. Since, the presence of pain represents a blockage of energy in the painful area, moxibustion has been advocated to treat cancer-related pain. Heat generated by moxa combustion helps to improve circulation of blood and energy in the body and *Artemisia vulgaris* that makes up the moxa cone itself has energy and blood motivating properties. Energetic points such as ST36, CV6 and Shenque (CV8) are common points for moxa treatment (Cheng 1987).

5.2.2.1 Mechanisms Also Exist to Support Moxibustion for Pain

Moxibustion, performed in various forms, has been shown to affect physiological functions. Microcirculatory changes with increase in local and whole body capillary blood flow were observed with moxibustion (Huang et al. 2011b). This increase in blood flow may help to alleviate inflammation that commonly occurs in cancer bearing areas (Laird et al. 2011). Autonomic nervous system activities were also influenced by moxibustion treatment with relative increase in parasympathetic activities (Litscher et al. 2009). Moxibustion may work through a correction of the autonomic nervous system activities by reducing the influence of the sympathetic nervous system, the chronic activation of which has been suggested to perpetuate pain and worsening pain experiences (Cho et al. 2011). Like acupuncture, moxibustion alone was shown to induce an increase secretion of endogenous morphine-like substances: endomorphin and dynorphin (Liu et al. 2010; Ma et al. 2010).

5.2.2.2 Some Clinical Evidence Suggests Moxibustion Is Effective

It is not surprising to find that there was no randomized placebo controlled trial conducted to provide good evidence that moxibustion can improve pain compared to placebo since it is not possible to generate acceptable placebo for a treatment involving heat sensation of a certain temperature range. In the few trials examining moxibustion in managing benign painful conditions reported in the literature, all adopted a comparison of moxibustion *vs* other interventions instead of a placebo (Chen et al. 2008; Su et al. 2009; Sun et al. 2009; Xu et al. 2009; Ma et al. 2010). Results of all these trials have suggested that moxibustion is effective in managing pain, but because of the poor study design of most trials, a recent systematic review still failed to provide concrete evidence of this treatment approach in managing benign painful conditions (Lee et al. 2010a).

In regards to the use of moxibustion in cancer-related pain, there was no clinical trial using moxibustion as a single treatment modality reported in the English literature. In the three published trials identified, all utilized moxibustion in combination with another active intervention in the treatment arms, Bian et al. (2004) examined the effectiveness of moxibustion and acupuncture and morphine injections compared to conventional morphine injections alone for cancer-related pain in 44 patients using a randomized trial design. The moxibustion combination group was shown to have better quality of life and better pain control. In another randomized study (Zhang (2007), 72 patients suffering from herpes zoster, a not uncommon condition experienced by cancer patients, were divided into two groups. The treatment group received acupuncture plus moxibustion and a control group received no active interventions. The herpes lesions were resolved within 3 days after treatments in 97% of patients and related symptoms including pain were demonstrated to be significantly better in the treatment group.

In a recent reported multicenter trial, 120 patients with herpes zoster infection were randomized equally into two groups. The treatment group was treated with plum blossom needles to the lesions and selected acupuncture points followed by cotton sheet moxibustion, while the controlled group was treated with antiviral treatment using acyclovir cream on the affected areas and oral valaciclovir hydrochloride and vitamin B1. At 7 days post treatment, 80% of patients in the treatment group was reported cured of their herpes lesions compared to 45% in the controlled group. Pain, duration of blister and scarring and the overall duration for healing were all significantly shorter in the treatment group. However, the technique of cotton sheet moxibustion that aims to apply heat directly to the herpes lesions instead of acupuncture points may suggest the positive results of this trial attritbuted to some form of hyperthermia treatment and not traditional moxibustion (Yang et al. 2012).

To date there was no good evidence to show moxibustion alone improves cancer-related pain management. The use of moxibustion should be used as an adjunct treatment to other interventions with proven efficacy. Moxibustion should also be used according to the traditional guidelines within the scope of Chinese medicine practice. Again prospective cohort data should be systematically obtained for continuous analysis and to further provide evidence and guidance in utilizing this treatment modality for cancer-related painful conditions.

5.2.3 Acupuncture-Like Transcutaneous Nerve Stimulation May Be an Option for Some Patients

Non-invasive approach using transcutaneous nerve stimulator (TENS) has the advantage of easy treatment delivery by staffs or by patients themselves after minimal training. Using low frequencies (< 10 Hz) and high intensity stimulation over acupuncture points, acupuncture-like TENS (ALTENS), was found to mimic acupuncture treatment in that the Deqi sensation in real needle acupuncture can be elicited at the acupuncture points. It is known that ALTENS mainly stimulates α-delta and C fibres and is believed to achieve pain control by activating the descending pain suppression system and by the release of endorphins. In chronic pain conditions, ALTENS has been suggested to provide more effective pain control than placebo, and improves function more than standard TENS, though a meta-analysis failed to show conclusive evidence (Gadsby and Flowerdew 2000; Carroll et al. 2001). In a recent Cochrane review that only include three small randomized studies with two using conventional TENS and not ALTENS (Hurlow et al. 2012). The other study compared ALTENS and sham ALTENS for cancer pain or nausea and vomiting. There were only 15 patients included. The conclusion of this review indicated that there is insufficient evidence to support, (or refute) the effectiveness of TENS in cancer pain management.

At the Juravinski Cancer Centre (Hamilton, Canada), ALTENS (with a random electrode stimulation set up for minimizing brain habituation) is being offered as one of the options for patients with cancer-related pain that is not controlled by optimal analgesics or radiation therapy. Unpublished data suggested positive benefit for ALTENS as an adjunctive treatment for cancer pain control.

5.3 Nausea and Vomiting

One of the commonest symptoms cancer patients often experience is nausea and vomiting. The presence of this symptom not only affects patient's quality of life but also can be a limiting factor for cancer treatments. Multiple causes have been shown to contribute to the occurrence of nausea and vomiting in cancer patients. These include pharmacological, visceral, intestinal, central nervous system and vestibular causes (Fessele 1996). Although, pharmacological causes, mainly related to chemotherapies and narcotics, account for most incidence of nausea and vomiting, a throughout assessment to exclude possible causes, other than pharmacological ones, is important to ensure appropriate management is initiated. It is obvious that nausea and vomiting that is caused by mechanical intestinal obstruction or intracranial space occupying lesion is not expected to be relieved by pharmacological or acupuncture techniques. Delay in initiating appropriate treatments can lead to undesirable consequences.

5.3.1 Acupuncture

5.3.1.1 Mechanisms Exist Showing Acupuncture May Work for Nausea and Vomiting

Vomiting centre situated in an area in the medulla, integrates afferent stimuli from various sources, creates nausea sensation and initiates the vomiting reflex. These afferent stimuli include nervous signals from a special chemoreceptor trigger area, situated on the floor of the fourth ventricle, which responds to chemicals like chemotherapy agents or opioid-like substances, serotonin and histamine. Stimuli from cerebral cortex, cerebellar and vestibular nuclei also influence this centre (Streitberger et al. 2006).

Mechanisms by which acupuncture can lessen nausea and vomiting have been suggested by several clinical studies. In a study using acupuncture on PC6, a common acupuncture treatment point for nausea and vomiting, has shown that vagal activities that may suppress the vomiting centre, are significantly enhanced in the treatment group when compared to a sham acupuncture group (Huang et al. 2005). Modulation of serotonin and endogenous opiod systems through acupuncture activation of the serotonergic and noradrenergic fibers has also been observed (Mao et al. 1980; Han and Terenius 1982). Direct and indirect influence of stomach and gut smooth muscle activities with facilitated gastric emptying, gastric relaxation and suppression of retrograde peristalsis have also been suggested (Shiotani et al. 2004; Tatewaki et al. 2005). Functional magnetic resonance study showed that the cerebellar vestibular system activities are influenced by PC6 acupuncture but not by sham acupuncture (Yoo et al. 2004) (Fig. 5.1).

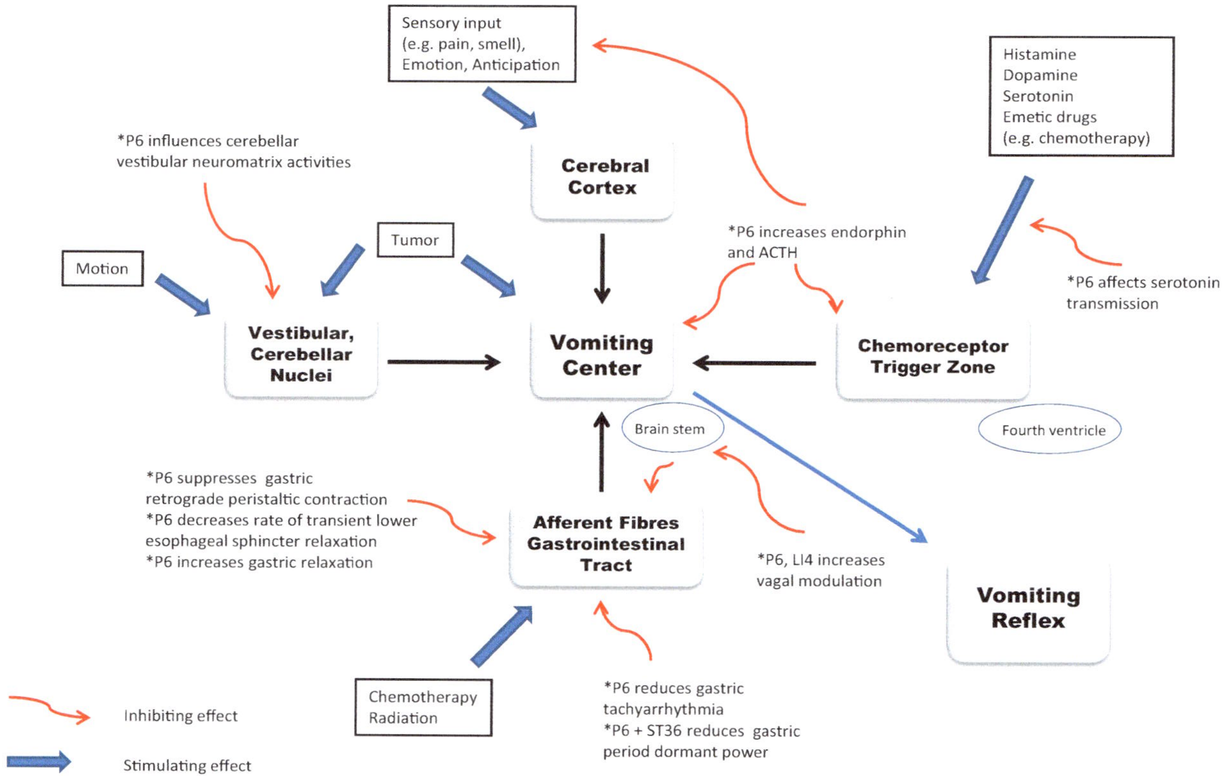

Fig. 5.1 Proposed mechanisms of action of acupuncture for nausea and vomiting. *ACTH* adrenocorticotropic hormone

5.3.1.2 Extensive Evidence Supports Acupuncture for Nausea and Vomiting

Extensive studies have been conducted and most reported positive effects of acupuncture for nausea and vomiting due to various causes. Over the last two decades, several meta-analysis and systematic reviews of randomized controlled trials were reported and continue to show acupuncture given alone or in combination with anti-emetic medications can provide better nausea control compared to control or anti-emetic medications (Vickers 1996; Lee and Done 2004; Ezzo et al. 2006; Lee and Fan 2009). These results have also led to the 1998 NIH (US) consensus statement that, "acupuncture is a proven effective treatment modality for nausea and vomiting".

The effect of PC6 acupuncture in managing nausea and vomiting has been mostly studied. Dundee et al. was the first group to show the use of PC6 alone increases the anti-emetic effect of drugs for peri-operative and chemotherapy-induced nausea and vomiting (Dundee et al. 1991). In a more recent meta-analysis of 26 randomized controlled trials examining acupuncture for postoperative nausea and vomiting, PC6 stimulation with acupuncture, acupressure or electrical stimulation was concluded to be effective in preventing postoperative nausea (RR 0.71, 95% CI of 0.61 to 0.83). PC6 stimulation when used with anti-emetic drugs was also found to reduce the risk of nausea, but not vomiting, when compared to anti-emetic drugs alone. There was no difference in the risk of postoperative nausea and vomiting between acupuncture and anti-emetic drugs. Side effects were minimal (Lee and Fan 2009). Invasive and non-invasive acupuncture on PC6 should be considered as an option for reducing the risk of postoperative nausea and vomiting (Gan et al. 2003).

In chemotherapy-induced nausea and vomiting, similar effectiveness of acupuncture point stimulation was identified in a systematic review of eleven randomized trials (Ezzo et al. 2006). However, the review suggested that electroacupuncture effectively reduced acute chemotherapy-induced nausea and vomiting but non-invasive electroacupuncture is not effective. Acupressure may be able to prevent acute nausea. This review also questioned the clinical relevance of acupuncture approaches when state-of-the-art anti-emetic medications are used. In a more recent randomized trial of acupuncture in a small pediatric cancer population, requirement for rescue anti-emetic medications was reduced in the acupuncture and anti-emetics group compared to anti-emetics alone group. The number of vomiting episodes was also shown to be reduced significantly in the treatment group (Gottschling et al. 2008).

Based on the available evidence, acupuncture should be considered as an option for managing postoperative and chemotherapy-induced nausea and vomiting, and should be used in combination with state-of-the-art anti-emetic medications. Electroacupuncture on PC6 should be recommended, however, acupressure on PC6 is still advisable if electroacupuncture is not practical. ST36 acupuncture point can be utilized in combination with PC6 to potentially improve treatment results (Ma 2009). ST36 should also be considered in patients considered to have 'low energy' since stimulation of this point has been considered to improve overall energy of a patient. According to acupuncture practice, overall energy should first be improved before direct symptoms management; otherwise, acupuncture treatment may not be as effective.

Various acupuncture points alternatives other than PC6 have also been suggested to be effective in managing nausea and vomiting according to some published reports (Shen et al. 2000; Somri et al. 2001; Ming et al. 2002; Gottschling et al. 2008). Korean hand acupuncture points K-K9 and K-D2 have also been shown to be viable alternatives (Schlager et al. 2000; Boehler et al. 2002).

5.3.2 Moxibustion for Nausea and Vomiting

5.3.2.1 Proposed Mechanisms by Which Moxibustion May Work for Nausea and Vomiting

Possible mechanisms by which moxibustion may exert beneficial effects in nausea and vomiting managements have been proposed. However, research in this area is still very limited. Moxibustion provides heat stimulation on acupuncture points in addition to the possible absorption of herbal extract through the skin. Treatment effects are likely mediated through mechanisms similar to that of acupuncture. Like acupuncture, moxibustion may modulate the activities of cortical and subcortical regions of the brain, brain stem areas and autonomic nervous system (Hui et al. 2000; Huang et al. 2005; Napadow et al. 2008).

5.3.2.2 Limited Evidence to Suggest Moxibustion for Nausea and Vomiting

Moxibustion as a single modality in managing nausea and vomiting has not been well studied. In a meta-analysis of moxibustion in cancer care (Lee 2010b), two small randomized studies have examined indirect moxibustion on CV8 in reducing chemotherapy-induced treatment toxicities in patients with nasopharyngeal cancers and gastric cancers as one of the study endpoints. In both studies, toxicities included nausea and vomiting were found to be significantly reduced with a combined risk ratio of 0.38 (95% CI of 0.22 to 0.65) (Cao et al. 1997; Chen et al. 2000). CV8 is the acupuncture point right on the umbilicus and needling is not advised for the fear of easy infection. This point is used in Chinese medicine to aim at treating abdominal, gynaecological and urinary symptoms, particularly in patients who present with 'cold' pattern (Wang, 2008).

Given the limited clinical evidence today, it is inconclusive in regards to the effectiveness of moxibustion alone for chemotherapy-induced nausea and vomiting. Adoption of this treatment modality should be used for selected patients according to traditional Chinese medicine practice and with appropriate precautions.

5.4 Postoperative Urinary Dysfunction

Patient underwent pelvic surgery for cancer commonly experience with urinary retention during the postoperative period as a result of bladder detrusor muscle dysfunction and reduced bladder sensation. This may lengthen hospital stay and increase the chance of urinary infection due to prolonged urinary catheter insertion (Chen et al. 2010).

Two publications have shown electroacupuncture on body acupuncture points including Guilai (ST29), ST36, Tiaokou (ST38), SP6 and Waiguan (TE5), was able to improve urinary flow rate, reduced residual bladder volume and shorten postoperative hospital stay compared to controls (Shi et al. 2008; Yi et al. 2011). A third study in patients who suffered from acute urinary retention after rectal cancer surgery, also showed acupuncture on body points that affect energy flow of the bladder meridian improves urinary flow and relieve retention symptoms in over 90% of patients (Dong et al. 2003).

In another randomized trial in patients who developed urinary retention after radical hysterectomy, patients who were randomized to receive acupuncture on Shuidao (ST28), ST36, SP6, scalp reproduction area plus moxibustion on CV8 showed significant improvement in bladder function ($p < 0.05$) after one and two courses of treatments, compared to acupuncture point injection on ST36 and SP6 (Yi et al. 2011). Unfortunate, the study did not have a control group. This latter study, however, provide insight in the usage of moxibustion in combination with acupuncture may enhance clinical effectiveness. Addition evidence to further support the effectiveness of indirect moxibustion on CV8 in managing urinary dysfunction was provided in another study. Stroked patients with urinary dysfunction were randomized to ginger-salt indirect moxibustion on CV8 and acupuncture. Urinary function in patients of the moxibustion group, including a reduction in urinary incontinence, was found to be significantly better than that of acupuncture group (Liu and Wang 2006).

5.5 Radiation-Induced Xerostomia (RIX)

Xerostomia, or dry mouth, remains a common complication of radiation treatment for head and neck cancers. Despite the use of more advanced radiation techniques that are able to reduce radiation dose to major salivary glands while delivering a radical dose to the cancer areas, up to 30% of patients still suffer from xerostomia and its associated symptoms that include loss of taste, difficulty in speech and swallowing. Current treatments mainly rely on symptomatic relief with saliva substitutes and pharmaceutical salivary stimulants with no long lasting effect. Recent studies have demonstrated acupuncture approaches may be viable treatment modalities for this condition with sustained benefit.

5.5.1 Acupuncture

5.5.1.1 Mechanisms of Acupuncture for RIX

Acupuncture has long been used for dry mouth symptom in traditional Chinese medicine. Recent advances in research have shed lights on the possible mechanisms by which acupuncture can have an effect on salivary production. Acupuncture has been shown to differentially affecting the autonomic nervous system activities with activation of the parasympathetic component that increases overall salivary production and deactivation of the sympathetic component that reduces salivary viscosity (Proctor and Carpenter 2007; Sakatani et al. 2010). Increase in blood flow to parotid glands and stimulation of glandular tissue regeneration of salivary glands have also been shown (Blom et al. 1992; Blom et al. 1993; Schneyer et al. 1993). The latter finding may explain the long-term benefits of acupuncture approaches in treating xerostomia as demonstrated in several clinical studies (Blom and Lundeberg 2000; Johnstone et al. 2002; Wong et al. 2003). In a fMRI study, stimulation of Erjian (LI2), a frequently utilized acupuncture point for xerostomia, has also been found to activate the insula region of the brain, the area associated with gustatory function, suggesting that acupuncture may act *via* the central nervous system resulting in a cascade of physiological events that lead to an improvement of salivary flow (Deng et al. 2008) (Fig. 5.2).

5.5.1.2 More Supportive Clinical Evidence of Acupuncture for RIX

After Blom et al. (1992) published the first report suggesting a positive effect of acupuncture for xerostomia, there has been a growing interest of research in evaluating different acupuncture approaches for this condition, particularly related to patients with RIX. The first randomized controlled trial of 38 patients with RIX divided into two groups: deep or superficial acupuncture treatments (Blom et al. 1996). Superficial acupuncture group was chosen to be the control despite previous evidence that superficial acupuncture may have certain degree of effectiveness and that should not be used as control for acupuncture study. Individualized body acupuncture points were utilized for the study. In this study, both groups showed a more than 20% increase in salivary flow rate in over 50% of patients after acupuncture treatments. In the treatment group, 68% of patients showed an increase in salivary flow rate compared to 50% of patients in the control group at one year. Moreover, the treatment group reported significantly greater improvement in symptoms with less dryness, less hoarseness and improved taste.

In another randomized controlled trial aimed to study the usefulness of acupuncture for pain and dysfunction in patients after neck dissection for cancers (Pfister et al. 2010). Over 80% of 58 patients recruited received radiation as a component of their treatments. Xerostomia inventory was set as a secondary endpoint of the study. Limbs acupuncture points were used including LI2 for xerostomia in the treatment group. Symptoms of xerostomia in the treatment group were found to be significantly reduced compared to that of the control ($p = 0.02$). Other prospective cohort studies are confirming the clinical usefulness of acupuncture for the relief of RIX (Rydholm and Strang 1999; Blom and Lundeberg 2000; Johnstone et al. 2001; Braga et al. 2008; Cho et al. 2008).

Interestingly, results from a few studies have suggested that acupuncture treatments may provide long-term improvement in symptoms related to RIX. In Blom

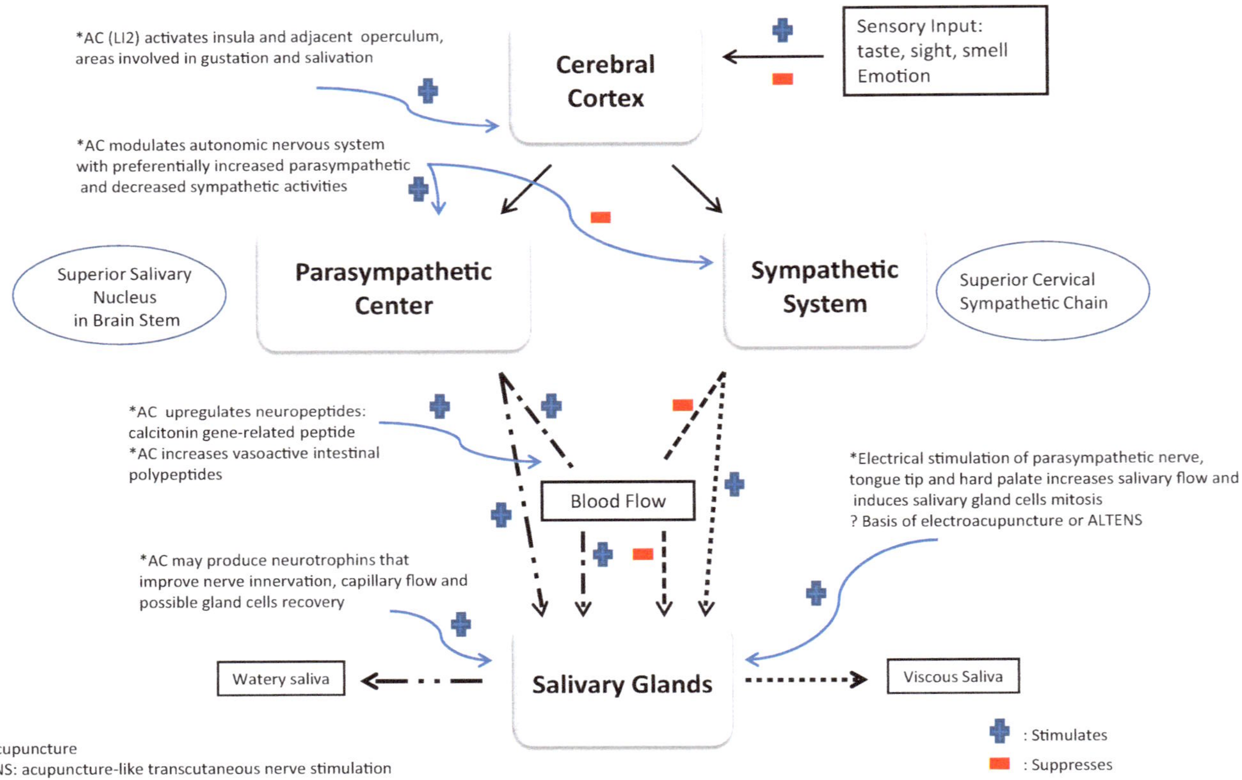

Fig. 5.2 Proposed mechanisms of action of acupuncture for xerostomia

et al's study of 70 patients with xerostomia due to either Sjögren's syndrome or radiotherapy treated with acupuncture, not only was there an increase in salivary flow rates observed immediately after acupuncture treatment, this increase were sustained up to 6 months follow up. At 3 years, patients who chose to have additional acupuncture treatment had consistently higher median salivary flow rate than those who did not have additional acupuncture. In another study (Johnstone et al. 2002), patients received initial weekly acupuncture treatments with ear points and LI2 for 3–4 weeks followed by monthly to bimonthly maintaining treatments were found to have sustained benefit.

Results of attempts in using acupuncture to prevent RIX have suggested positive outcomes. In a small randomized study involving only 24 patients who had radiation dose of greater than 5,000 cGy to over 50% of the parotid glands, the treatment group received acupuncture during radiation treatment and the control group had radiation treatment alone. Individualized body and auricular acupuncture points were used according to traditional Chinese medicine practice. Although all patients showed worsening of salivary function after radiation, there was significant difference in the mean resting and post stimulating salivary flow rates in favor of the treatment group. Xerostomia-related symptoms scores were also better in the treatment group (Braga Fdo et al. 2011). The small sample size of the study, however, had raised doubt in the study conclusion. Another larger randomized trial involving 96 eligible patients, also showed that patients received acupuncture during radiation treatment had reduced severity of xerostomia and maintained salivary flow rate better than those who did not have acupuncture (Meng et al. 2012). The beneficial effects were shown to occur as early as the third week and at 1 and 6 months after the completion of radiation. Unfortunately, the inclusion of only Chinese patients with nasopharyngeal cancers without advanced organ sparing radiation techniques made the results less generalizable. Further research in this prevention approach will be needed.

5.5.1.3 ALTENS: A Different Acupuncture Approach

Recognizing the possibility of fear for needle therapy in some patients and the possible difficulties in offering acupuncture treatments in conventional cancer clinics, at the Juravinski Cancer Centre, a different acupuncture-related approach was explored to manage RIX. In a Phase I and II study, preselected acupuncture points chosen according to traditional Chinese medicine principles were stimulated using acupuncture-like transcutaneous nerve stimulation (ALTENS) (Wong et al. 2003). Instead of needles, electrode pads applied on the skin overlying the acupuncture points were used for stimulation. Low frequency, high current intensity and random stimulation were used and treatments were given twice weekly for a total of 12 weeks. Salivary production, both basal and citric-acid primed, and xerostomia symptoms scores were all significantly improved in patients at 3 and 6 months after treatment completion. There were also improvement in swallowing, speech and taste. Built on these positive study results, a Phase II and III multicenter randomized study comparing ALTENS to oral pilocarpine, the current standard management, in treating established RIX was initiated by the Radiation Therapy Oncology Group (Wong et al. 2012). Acupuncture points used were Chenjiang (CV24), ST36, SP6 and LI4 selected based on the results of previous mentioned Phase II trial. The study has completed the required accrual of 190 patients quickly with a rate of 6–8 patient recruited per month suggesting high acceptance of this treatment modality by both patients and care providers in conventional clinical settings. The results of the Phase II (non-randomized) component of this study were reported recently demonstrated a 94% compliance rate for ALTENS treatments. At 3 months after randomization, 84% of the evaluable 35 patients achieved a positive treatment response with an improvement of xerostomia specific quality of life scores of 35.9%.

The results of a trial to examine ALTENS in preventing RIX were disappointing. In a Phase II randomized trial involving 60 patients who were to have conventional radiation treatment for head and neck cancers, ALTENS were given concurrently during radiation in the treatment group while the control group only had standard mouth care (Wong et al. 2010). ALTENS failed to exert any detectable differences in the mean salivary flow rate or xerostomia symptoms scores in the treatment group when compared to the controls. It was postulated that the acupuncture points stimulation that may induce salivary gland tissue regeneration during radiation may, in theory, render the glandular cells more sensitive to radiation damage and negate the beneficial effect of improved salivary function. The small sample size of the study may also be a factor affecting the results and the interpretation of the study conclusion.

5.5.2 *Moxibustion Is Not Indicated*

In traditional Chinese medicine, moxibustion is mainly used for 'cold' patterns since the warmth of burning moxa and the 'warm' nature of the herb, *Artemisia vulgaris* can drive the 'cold' away and promote blood and energy flow. In fact, there is description that moxibustion can cause dry mouth and is not advisable to be given in patients with 'heat' symptoms. A search in the literature has failed to show any reported study to investigate the effect of moxibustion in xerostomia conditions (Gu 1996).

5.6 Radiation Proctitis

Radiation proctitis is an inflammatory condition of the rectal mucosa as a result of radiation damage. This condition is seen often in patients receiving radiation treatment for pelvic cancers, particularly for prostate and cervical cancers, since high radiation dose volume will likely include the anterior portion of the rectum. Acute proctitis will usually subside after a few months but up to 5% will become chronic. Only one study investigated acupuncture as a treatment modality for radiation proctitis has been published (Zhang 1987). Forty-four cervix cancer patients who received radiation treatment and developed radiation proctitis were treated with acupuncture. 73%

of patients had complete response and marked reduction in symptoms was seen in 9%. At the Juravinski Cancer Centre, weekly acupuncture treatment on GV20 during the third to fifth week of radiotherapy has been offered to patients with locally advanced rectal cancers undergoing chemoradiation treatment and who presented with severe symptoms of tenesmus, increased rectal mucous secretion and bleeding. Preliminary experience in 24 patients showed marked improvement in patients' reported symptoms after one to two treatments (unpublished data). A formal in-house study is being planned. GV20 is indicated in traditional Chinese medicine for treating organs prolapse and to reduce leakage symptoms.

5.7 Quality of Life in Lymphoedema

Lymphoedema is a debilitating and disfiguring condition as a result of damage to the lymphatic drainage of part of the body. It commonly occurs in the limbs of patients who have had cancer treatments that cause damage to the axilla or groins. In one study on breast cancer patients, a prevalence of 29% was reported (Moffatt et al. 2003). Acupuncture directly on the affected area should be avoided to prevent the introduction of infection that may result in serious consequences. However, there is no contraindication to acupuncture in patients who have lymphoedema (Filshie 2001).

Recent experience in using acupuncture and moxibustion in the management of lymphoedema was reported with promising results. Kanakura et al. (2002) reported that acupuncture and moxibustion applied right after surgery or after the occurrence of lymphoedema in 24 patients who underwent pelvic lymph node dissection can prevent and improve the condition. However, measurements of lymphoedema used in the study were largely subjective.

Using traditional Chinese medicine principles to develop a acupuncture treatment protocol, Alem and Gurgel (2008) conducted a study on 29 breast cancer patients who suffered from lymphoedema of the upper limbs. Eleven acupuncture points were needled, without electrical stimulation, from the upper limb down to the leg on the unaffected contra-lateral side of the body. Jianyu (LI15), Jianliao (TE14), Chize (LU5), TE5 and LI4 were used for pain, heaviness and restricted movement of the upper limb; Zhongwan (CV12), Zhongji (CV3) and Qugu (CV2) for improved energy and increase lymphatic drainage; ST36, Yinlingquan (SP9) and SP6 for reducing oedema and promote "blood" flow. Twenty-four treatments were given once a week and no other interventions were given. Compared to baseline assessments, there were significant improvements in shoulder range of motion, degree of lymphoedema and sense of heaviness and tightness at 6 months. Interestingly, the degree of lymphoedema that was based on the skin characteristics, limb consistency and visual inspection showed improvements, circumferential measurements of the lymphoedematous limbs were not found to be significant. Logically, one would not expect that acupuncture approaches can correct anatomical damage and mechanical obstruction of lymphatics. The common presence of fibrosis in the affected limb will further prevent limb volume reduction.

Further study has demonstrated the feasibility of using acupuncture and moxibustion to treat cancer patients with upper body lymphoedema. Thirty-five subjects including breast cancer patients and head and neck cancer patients were managed with individualized acupuncture and moxibustion. Overall well being status of the patients was assessed using Measure Yourself Medical Outcome Profile. There was no significant adverse effect reported. Significant better well-being profile was noted after treatments. The authors concluded that acupuncture and moxibustion can be safely delivered to patients with lymphoedema provided that needling is avoided in the affected area (de Valois et al. 2011).

5.8 Cancer-Related Fatigue

Fatigue is a very common problem experienced by cancer patients and very often patients continue to have this symptom for a long time beyond active treatments (Wagner and Cella 2004). The underlying mechanism by which cancer-related fatigue occurs is not fully known. Apart from some correctable causes, for example, anemia, there is no effective treatment. Acupuncture and moxibustion approaches have been investigated for managing this distressful condition.

5.8.1 Proposed Mechanisms

Since the mechanisms by which cancer-related fatigue occurs is still not clearly known, any proposed mechanisms that acupuncture and moxibustion may act through are only theoretical. Fatigue has been found to be associated with changes in cytokine and hormonal levels and through modulating cytokines and hormonal secretions, acupuncture can play a role in treating fatigue (Glaus 1998; Stone et al. 1998). Study on human subjects who were experiencing fatigue also showed that overactive sympathetic activities are common in fatigue state. Acupuncture can modulate autonomic nervous system activities with preferential suppression of sympathetic activities and may lead to improvement of fatigue (Li et al. 2005).

5.8.2 Evidence Is Still Limited

To date, several studies have investigated the usefulness of acupuncture and moxibustion in managing this distressful symptom with mixed results. A Phase II study examined acupuncture for post chemotherapy fatigue that had lasted on average of 2 years, showed a mean improvement of 30% on the Brief Fatigue Inventory assessment (Vickers et al. 2004). Twice per week acupuncture treatments for 4 weeks were given for one cohort. Points that are indicated for fatigue in traditional Chinese medicine were used. These included classical energy points: ST36, Guanyuan

(CV4), CV6 and also Diji (SP8), SP9 and Quchi (LI11). For a second cohort, once weekly treatment for 6 weeks were delivered. Points included CV4, CV6, ST36, Taixi (KI3), Shufu (KI27) and SP6. There was no apparent significant difference in treatment responses between the twice weekly or weekly treatment.

In a small randomized controlled trial comparing acupuncture, acupressure and sham acupuncture in treating post chemotherapy fatigue in 47 cancer patients (Molassiotis et al. 2007). Results demonstrated significant improvement of the severity of fatigue measured by Multidimensional Fatigue Inventory in both the acupuncture (36%) and acupressure group (19%) compared to the sham acupuncture group (0.6%). Acupuncture provided higher fatigue relief than acupressure. Again, like the previous study, similar acupuncture points were used: ST36, SP6 and LI4. Patients, however, were treated three times per week for 2 weeks. More treatments were found to provide more sustained fatigue improvements.

In another randomized, double-blinded, controlled trial, 27 patients undergoing radiation therapy for cancers were randomized into a acupuncture and a sham acupuncture group (Balk et al. 2009). Typical acupuncture points including ST36, SP6, LI4 and KI3 were used given once to twice a week for 6 weeks. Non-penetrating needles were used for sham treatments. Although in both sham and true acupuncture groups, there was improvement in fatigue, there was no significant difference between the responses of the two groups. The result of this trial again cast some doubt in the effectiveness of acupuncture treatments in cancer-related fatigue but the sample size of this trial is far too small to make the results conclusive.

Traditionally, moxibustion is indicated to 'tonify' or to improve energy level of an individual. Indirect moxibustion on 'energy' points, ST36, CV4, CV6 and KI3 is usually recommended (Gu 1996). Adding moxibustion to acupuncture seems to be a logical choice to increase the probability of treatment success in cancer-related fatigue. Experiences in treating chronic fatigue using this strategy have suggested greater than 80% effectiveness (Wang et al. 2008a). However, this experience may not be completely generalizable to cancer-related fatigue. There is still no reported clinical trial investigating moxibustion alone in managing cancer-related fatigue.

5.9 Chemotherapy-Induced Peripheral Neuropathy

Chemotherapy-induced peripheral neuropathy (CIPN) occurs in 10–20% of patients who received neurotoxic chemotherapies including platinum compounds, vinca alkaloids, taxols and suramin (Forman 1990). With increasing indications of these chemotherapies and better survivals of cancer patients, the prevalence of CIPN is likely on the increase. Different components of the peripheral nervous system can be affected, but axonal degeneration is the commonest. Sensory neuropathy is predominant, while sensory-motor and autonomic nervous system dysfunction is less common. Patients usually present with numbness, paraesthesia, pin and needle sensation, and pain that is hard to describe but usually described in terms of burning, shooting or electric in nature. Impaired vibrational sense is common. There can be associated ataxia, myalgia and muscle weakness. CIPN symptoms can appear during the later courses of chemotherapy and can occur weeks or months after completion of chemotherapy (Windebank and Grisold 2008). Although peripheral nerve damages can recover in most patients, the recovery is usually incomplete with persistent symptoms resulting in poorer quality of life. Treatments for CIPN are largely for symptomatic relief of pain and paraesthesia. Centrally acting drugs like tricyclic anti-depressant, ion channel blockers have been shown to be moderately effective but with significant side effects that may limit their practical usefulness. Moreover, the beneficial effects are not long lasting, symptoms reoccur once medications are discontinued.

5.9.1 Evidence from Clinical Trials Continue to Support Acupuncture Usefulness

Approach in treating syndrome pattern that includes paraesthesia, hyperalgia, pain, pin and needles in both feet and hands has been described in TCM. The symptoms presented by patients with CIPN can be considered as a state with deficiency in energy and blood, and that the body is unable to direct these essential components to the four limbs resulting in sensory and motor dysfunctions.

Acupuncture treatments that aim to improve total energy and blood in the body and direct them to the limbs have been shown to be clinically effective. In recent clinical trials, acupuncture has been shown to improve symptoms due to peripheral neuropathy in HIV and diabetic patients (Abuaisha et al. 1998; Phillips et al. 2004). The first reported study on acupuncture for CIPN was reported by Wong and Sagar (2006) at the Juravinski Cancer Centre. This prospective pilot study involved patients with CIPN after combined taxol and platinum chemotherapies for gynaecological cancers treated with a selected acupuncture protocol. Five consecutive patients with WHO grade II CIPN symptoms were recruited. Mean duration of symptoms was 18 months (ranged from 6–38 months). Pain, pin and needle sensation and numbness of the hands and feet were the main presenting symptoms. In three patients, imbalance in gait was also present. After acupuncture treatments, marked improvement in pain was noted with average pain score came down from 7.8/10–3/10. All patients had a reduction in analgesic dosage. Gait was improved in all the three patients. Numbness and pin and needle sensation were significantly better. At 6 months follow up, symptoms improvement was sustained in four patients. Although the number of patients in this study was small, the results suggested acupuncture can be useful in CIPN. A Phase II study at the Juravinski Cancer Centre examining the effectiveness of acupuncture alone or ALTENS alone in CIPN management has completed recruitment. Results of the preliminary analysis were presented at the International Scientific Acupuncture and Meridian Symposium and continued to show that acupuncture or ALTENS using a selected protocol acupuncture points improved symptoms of CIPN at three months follow-up. Complete analysis is pending to be completed in 2012.

Follow the reported study by Wong and Sagar (2006), a few other pilot studies were conducted with results supporting the effectiveness of acupuncture in CIPN. In one study (Donald et al. 2011), 18 patients were treated with individualized acupuncture treatments with core acupuncture points including SP6 and ST36 similar to Wong and Sagar's study (2006). Improvement in symptoms especially in pain, and analgesic dosage were noted in 14 patients. In another study (Schroeder et al. 2011), six patients received acupuncture and best medical care were compared to a control group of five patients who received best medical care alone. All patients had nerve conduction study prior to interventions. Five patients in the treatment group had improvement in CIPN symptoms after acupuncture and all had improved nerve conduction studies while one patient in the control group showed improvement in nerve conduction study but no improvement in symptoms. With these positive pilot studies, a well designed randomized controlled trial is justified to clarify the efficacy of acupuncture in CIPN.

5.10 Vasomotor Symptoms Reduction

Vasomotor symptoms with hot flashes and sweating are common complications as a result of hormonal ablative therapies for breast and prostate cancer. Frequent hot flashes with associated fatigue, insomnia and irritability, were shown to adversely affecting quality of life (Oldenhave et al. 1993). Management of vasomotor symptoms involves hormonal replacement therapy and non-hormonal centrally active drugs including gabapentin, venalfaxine and anti-depressants (Bordeleau et al. 2007). However, their usage are often limited by associated side effects. Treatment of vasomotor symptoms in cancer patients remains a challenge and research for optimal non-hormonal approaches is continuously advocated.

5.10.1 Acupuncture Can Be Useful in Women Suffered from Vasomotor Symptoms

Acupuncture has been found to increase secretion of central β-endorphins, thereby potentially stabilizing thermoregulation and decreasing vasomotor symptoms (Filshie et al. 2005; Mayor 2008; Lee et al. 2009b). Sense of well-being was found to increase in women who underwent acupuncture as a result of enhanced brain serotonin, norepinephrine, and oxytocin activities (Nedstrand et al. 2006).

Uncontrolled small clinical studies have demonstrated improvement in vasomotor symptoms in breast cancer women; however, results are inconsistent (Borud et al. 2009a, 2010; de Valois et al. 2010). A retrospective audit of acupuncture and self acupuncture in 194 patients with breast or prostrate cancers showed up to a 50% reduction of hot flashes in some patients who successfully continued acupuncture for up to 6 years later (Filshie et al. 2005). A systematic review, conducted in 2008, of six randomized controlled trials of acupuncture compared with sham, hormonal replacement therapy, or Effexor XR failed to show statistical significant difference, however reported decreases of hot flashes with the use of both true acupuncture and sham acupuncture (Lee et al. 2009b).

Results from newer randomized trials continued to support the effectiveness of acupuncture in vasomotor symptoms management. In a more recent reported randomized trial comparing acupuncture plus self-care to self-care alone in postmenopausal women suffering from hot flashes, hot flashes frequencies and intensities were found to be improved significantly in the acupuncture plus self-care group. The vasomotor, sleep and somatic dimensions of the Women's Health Questionnaires were also improved (Borud et al. 2009b). In another study with similar design for perimenopausal and postmenopausal women with hot flashes, acupuncture plus usual care was also found to significantly improve hot flashes and related symptoms compared to usual care alone (Kim et al. 2010).

Frisk et al. (2012) randomized 45 breast cancer patients suffering from vasomotor symptoms to electroacupuncture for 12 weeks or hormonal therapy for 2 years. Scores in Health-related Quality of Life and Women's Health Questionnaire were improved significantly from baseline in both groups. Numbers of hot flashes per day were reduced and all sleep parameters were enhanced. The authors suggested that electroacupuncture can be considered as an alternative treatment to hormonal therapy for hot flashed in this group of patients.

Acupuncture has been suggested to be an alternative treatment for vasomotor symptoms in women with breast cancers who were refractory to, or unable to tolerate other treatments (Deng et al. 2007; Walker et al. 2010).The Society of Integrative Oncology's evidence-based clinical practice guidelines indicated that although there is no strong evidence to support the use of acupuncture for treatment of hot flashes, it is, however, a safe, tolerable treatment and could be used to treat hot flashes failing conventional treatments (Deng et al. 2009).

To answer the question regarding what are the acupuncture points and approached that should be recommended in managing vasomotor symptoms, a recent consensus building conference was held involving ten acupuncture experts. Consensus was made for eight syndromes and about five indicative symptoms for each syndrome. The choices of acupuncture points used, however, were quite different and probably reflecting the different in approaches by different acupuncture schools for the same clinical problem (Alraek et al. 2011).

5.10.2 Acupuncture Usefulness for Man with Vasomotor Symptoms Is Less Conclusive

A systematic review of acupuncture for vasomotor symptoms in prostate cancer patients has failed to show supportive evidence that acupuncture can exert a positive effect in reducing vasomotor symptoms (Lee et al. 2009c). However, this systematic review only included one randomized study and five uncontrolled studies reported prior to 2009 and that meet the study criteria. More studies, unfortunately, all uncontrolled, have been reported and suggested that acupuncture can provide relief in vasomotor symptoms in patients who underwent androgen ablative therapies for prostate cancers (Harding et al. 2009; Beer et al. 2010; Ashamalla et al. 2011). Further well designed trials are needed to clarify acupuncture usefulness in this condition.

5.10.3 *Moxibustion Can Be Useful*

To date, there is only one randomized trial conducted to examine the effect of moxibustion alone in vasomotor symptoms in post menopausal women. In this trial, 51 patients were randomized into three groups: Group A in which moxibustion was based on clinical expert opinion. In this group, CV12, CV4, bilateral ST36 and SP6 were used. These points were indicated for improving physical function and to treat gynecological diseases. Group B in which moxibustion was based on published literature. In this group, Mingmen (GV4), CV4, CV6 and bilateral Shenshu (UB23) points were used. Group C was the control waiting list. Treatment groups A and B were found to have significant reduction in the frequency (60% reduction *vs* increased frequency in the control group) and severity (40–50% reduction) of hot flashes. Group B also had significant better scores on the Menopausal-Specific Quality of Life Scale compared to the other two groups (Park et al. 2009).

5.10.4 *ALTENS Is Being Examined*

At the Juravinski Cancer Centre, non-invasive acupuncture approach using ALTENS is being examined in treating vasomotor symptoms of breast cancer patients as a result of hormonal ablation therapies. Apart from working through mechanisms by which acupuncture may improve vasomotor symptoms, recent evidence has also suggested that ALTENS can stimulate a neuroreflex network involving the autonomic nervous system that participates in body temperature regulation (Haker et al. 2000). This Phase II randomized study will compare ALTENS plus standardized life-style interventions to standardized life-style interventions alone. Sixty-eight eligible patients with a Hot Flashes Score of > 15 will be randomized. Hot Flashes Scores, heart rate variability and quality of life will be assessed. The choice of acupuncture points to treat vasomotor syndrome was based on the traditional Chinese medicine (TCM) concept. This concept explains the occurrence of vasomotor syndrome according to its meridian and Zhangfu (organs) models. It conceptualizes that Zhangfu functions and overall meridian energy decline with increasing age. At around age 50, "kidney" function and its meridian energy start to become deficient. As "kidney" is the foundation that supports and interacts with other Zhangfus and meridians to work properly, its deficiency cascades into multiple dysfunctions and imbalances of bodily functions, particularly involving the "liver", "heart" and "spleen". In women present with vasomotor syndrome, the "liver" tends to become overactive causing symptoms of hot flashes, sweating, irritability, mood swings, headache, dizziness, irregular menstrual flow, back discomfort and feeling of weakness in the knees. The "heart" also becomes overactive manifesting with palpitation, chest tightness, insomnia, and feeling of heat in the face, palms and soles. On the other hand, the "spleen" like the "kidney" becomes deficient resulting in decreased appetite, loose stool, cold hands and feet, fluid retention with swollen face and limbs, and generalized fatigue. The lack of "blood" during this period has also been viewed as a contributing factor to multiple symptoms.

TCM acupuncture treatment approach for vasomotor syndrome thus aims to improve "kidney" and "spleen" deficiencies and, at the same time, suppress "heart" and "liver" overactivities. The promotion of "blood" is also utilized to achieve symptom control. Selection of acupuncture points was based on a review of the published clinical studies identified through PubMed, non-PubMed and acupuncture texts describing experiences in treating vasomotor syndrome using body acupuncture points (Cheng 1987; Wyon et al. 2004; Huang et al. 2006; Zhou et al. 2006; Nir et al. 2007; Vincent et al. 2007; Avis et al. 2008; Kim et al. 2010). Shenshu (BL23), SP6, Xuehai (SP10), Taichong (LR3), Shenmen (HT7) and KI3 were selected and will be treated using ALTENS two times a week for 12 weeks. If this study results were positive, this may provide yet another approach utilizing acupuncture principles and may provide more options for patient care and further research.

5.11 Chemotherapy-induced Cognitive Dysfunction

Sixteen to fifth percent of cancer patients who received chemotherapy may develop cognitive impairment that can be long lasting for up to 10 years after treatments were completed (Tannock et al. 2004). The role of acupuncture for chemotherapy-induced cognitive impairment is not clear. In an animal study, acupuncture was shown to improve cognitive impairment caused by multi-infarcts of the brain (Yu et al. 2005). Johnston et al. (2007) has proposed that evidence exists to suggest acupuncture may be effective in managing this condition since it has been shown to provide benefit to a range of psychoneurological symptoms that are similar to those experienced by patients with chemotherapy-induced dysfunction. There was no reported study of moxibustion in this condition. Obviously, with the increasing prevalence of cancer patients who underwent successful chemotherapies, investigations for effective treatment options for this condition are increasingly necessary.

5.12 Myelosuppression

Myelosuppression is a common complication of chemotherapy treatments. It also occurs when significant amount of bone marrow is radiated to a certain dose. Patients, especially elderly who develop myelosuppression have increased risk of infection, bleeding and anaemia that not only can limit chemotherapy dosage but also can lead to significant treatment-related morbidities, mortalities and poor quality of life. Moreover, the lowering in immunological function can adversely affect cancer treatment outcomes. Current treatment has to rely on the use of expensive recombinant human granulocyte-colony stimulating factor (G-CSF) and transfusion of blood components, all with associated side effects.

Traditional Chinese medicine views the depressed immunity and susceptibility to infection and cancer progression as the weakening of the body healthy energy or Qi and that the "kidney" function is declined leading to an inability to maintain blood elements. Multiple traditional Chinese medicine treatment approaches aim to improve body Qi and to strengthen "kidney" function has been developed including the use of herbs, acupuncture and moxibustion.

In animal studies, acupuncture and moxibustion have been shown to promote the repair of damage done to bone marrow cells by chemotherapies through the upregulation of DNA excision repair-related proteins (Lu et al. 2009a). Acupuncture and moxibustion have also been shown to improve cell cycle regulator protein, cyclin D1 resulting in shortening of the cell cycles of hematopoietic cells and increased DNA synthesis with quicker repopulation of hematopoietic cells (Lu et al. 2011).

In an interesting case report (Grass 2003) of a patient who suffered from sustained myelosuppression requiring regular blood transfusions after chemotherapy treatments for chronic lymphocytic leukaemia, the patient received electroacupuncture to Jingming (BL1), point associated with sea of blood; Geshu (BL17), influential point of "blood"; LR3, point associated with nourishment of "liver" blood and SP6 weekly for 8 treatments. After the start of treatments, all peripheral blood parameters continued to be improved and no further transfusions were required. This case demonstrated the temporal changes in blood parameters in response to electroacupuncture.

A number of clinical trials have been conducted showing promising results in using acupuncture and or moxibustion in managing chemotherapy-induced myelosuppression. A meta-analysis reported by Lu et al. (2007) reviewed 11 randomized controlled trials published from 1979–2004 that meet the study criteria. Only studies that use manual acupuncture or electroacupuncture or warm needling were included. Daily treatments were commonly employed. Effective rates of leukopenia recovery from 50–90% were reported in all studies. Electroacupuncture appeared to be more effective than manual acupuncture. Though the positive results of this meta-analysis was encouraging, the authors noted that publication bias, poor quality of study methodologies, short follow-up periods and incomplete chemotherapy deliveries in some studies seriously affect the interpretation of the results.

In a recent, though small but well designed trial (Lu et al. 2009b), 17 patients were divided into a real acupuncture group and a sham acupuncture group. In the active treatment group, acupuncture points were selected based on practitioners' experience and from literature. These points include LR3, KI3, SP6, ST36, SP10, LI4, PC6, LI11 and GV20. TDP infra-red heating to the feet were applied in place of moxibustion. Superficial needling at non-acupuncture points were used as sham control. The incidence of grade 2 or greater leukopenia in the acupuncture group (30%) was significantly less than that in the control group (90%). The adjusted absolute neutrophil counts and plasma G-CSF, however, did not show significant different between the two groups. Larger trial is necessary to confirm the observed effectiveness.

In other controlled but non-randomized studies, acupuncture plus or minus moxibustion were all reported positive in correcting chemotherapy-induced leukopenia compared to controls that included G-CSF like drugs or no active treatment (Chen and Chen 2001; Ye et al. 2007). ST36 were used in all studies and SP6 was used in two. Daily treatments for 3–4 weeks were employed.

Indirect moxibustion alone may also be effective for chemotherapy-induced leukopenia. In a randomized trial that compared ginger indirect moxibustion to a Chinese patent medicine in 221 patients, the effective rates were improved by two folds in the moxibustion group compared to the control group after ten daily treatments. The effectiveness seemed to sustain after 15 days follow-up (Zhao et al. 2007).

It is still unclear as to when the acupuncture or moxibustion should be commenced in order to reduce the severity of chemotherapy-induced leukopenia. While in the meta-analysis mentioned above, the timing in starting the acupuncture was found to be not significant for treatment effectiveness, in the two positive randomized trials, the treatments were started one to two weeks prior to chemotherapy.

5.13 Anxiety, Depression

Anxiety is a common reaction in cancer patients. The presence of anxiety can reduce pain threshold, causes insomnia, worsen quality of life and may affect cancer treatment outcome (Jones 2001). Relief of anxiety by acupuncture was found to associate with increase in pain threshold (Widerstrom-Noga et al. 1998). Depression, though less common, is also frequently encountered by cancer patients (Jones 2001). Recent laboratory evidence has shown that the presence of tumor alone can stimulate cytokines production in behaviour related brain regions and can alter the regulation of the hypothalamic-pituitary-adrenal axis resulting in a depression-like behaviour (Pyter et al. 2009).

Adequate management of anxiety and depression in cancer patients is important to ensure better quality of life and to ensure optimum treatment outcomes. Conventionally, depression and anxiety are managed with the use of oral medications, such as amitriptyline or serotonin reuptake inhibitor drugs and inevitably, with associated side effects. Clinical studies have shown acupuncture may be a viable alternative to drugs treatments for anxiety and depression. In a recent review of conducted animal and clinical studies published in the English literature from year 2000 onwards, despite some methological issues, acupuncture was shown to have sufficient evidence to support its effectiveness for anxiety disorders (Errington-Evans 2011). The most frequently use acupuncture points among all studies were PC6, HT7, LR3, GV20 and Yintang (EX-HN3). One or three treatments per week, half hour per treatment and a total of ten treatments were the most common regime utilized.

Although a Cochrane review conducted in year 2005 concluded that there was insufficient evidence to determine the efficacy of acupuncture compared to medication, or to wait list control, or sham acupuncture in the management of depression, a more recent extensive review done by the Department of Veteran Affairs (US) has a different conclusion (Smith et al. 2010; Williams et al. 2011). This review included all the relevant published literature from year 2006–2011 and found that acupuncture showed promise in treating depression. For major depressive disorder, acupuncture showed greater effect than sham control on depressive symptoms but did not improve response or remission rates. Moreover, it did not differ significantly from short-term use of anti-depressants. This conclusion was largely based on a meta-analysis of eight randomized controlled trial included in this review (Wang et al. 2008b).

In another randomized trial conducted in China, 80 patients with cancer-related depression and sleep disorders to an acupuncture group and a fluoxetione control group (Feng et al. 2011). The mean Self-rating Depression Scale and Hamilton Depression Rating Scale scores were decreased significantly in the treatment group (43.6 and 9.8) compared to that of control (50.7 and 13.7). Sleep disorder symptoms were also significantly improved similarly in the treatment group.

In a single-blinded placebo-controlled study comparing the addition of acupuncture to oral anti-depressant, mianserin, to mianserin alone, acupuncture was shown to improve the course of depression (Roschke et al. 2000). The benefit of acupuncture seemed to appear immediately after start of treatments and since pharmaceutical anti-depressants are not usually effective until 2 weeks after starting therapy, their combination with acupuncture may enable more rapid onset of treatment response.

5.14 Gastrointestinal Dysfunction Other Than Nausea and Vomiting

Apart from nausea and vomiting that is commonly experienced by most cancer patients, there are other gastrointestinal dysfunctions that may occur in some patients. Gastroparesis, dysfunctional gastric retention creating symptoms of postprandial fullness, bloating, nausea and vomiting, early satiety and epigastric discomfort, can be caused by cancer and non-cancer-related causes. It can present as a paraneoplastic disorders associated with breast, small-cell lung and pancreas cancers. Abdominal surgeries also precipitate gastroparesis. Current treatments mainly rely on dietary and lifestyle modification, and gastric prokinetic medications including metoclopramide and anti-emetics. Acupuncture has been shown to increase gastric emptying and reduce symptoms of gastroparesis in diabetic patients (Chang et al. 2001a, 2001b). In a recent randomized controlled trial in liver cancer patients who developed gastroparesis after abdominal surgery (Sun et al. 2010). A total of 63 eligible patients were randomized to receive acupuncture or intramuscular metoclopramide treatment. Complete recovery was defined as the absence of gastric juice drained from gastric tube, no vomiting after removal of gastric tube and patient was able to tolerate semi-liquid diet. CV12, ST36, SP6 and PC6 were needled once a day. After acupuncture treatments, 90% of patients in the acupuncture group achieved complete recovery and only 32% in the control group.

Dysphagia is another condition that many patients who received head and neck cancer radiation can experience as a result of mucosal damage of pharynx and direct radiation damage of the swallowing muscles. Chronic dysphagia can result from fibrosis of the damaged muscles. A significant number of patients with dysphagia are at risk of aspiration pneumonia and may rely on percutaneous endoscopic gastrostomy (PEG) for feeding during treatment and, sometimes for a sustained period. Many studies have investigated acupuncture as a treatment modality for cancer-related dysphagia and have suggested moderate symptom relief (Shen and Shen 1996; Zheng and Ruan 2002; Zhou and Zhang 2006). A more recent retrospective case report in head and neck patients with post radiation dysphagia demonstrated that acupuncture treatments were able to shorten the period needed for PEG feeding (Lu et al. 2010). Nine of the ten patients treated showed various degree of improvement in swallowing. 86% of PEG tube dependent patients were able to have PEG removed after acupuncture treatments.

5.15 Hiccups and Yawning

Persisting hiccups and yawning are rarely encountered in cancer patients. Persistent hiccups have been associated with drug treatments, particularly with some types of chemotherapy, steroid and analgesics and direct tumor involvement of the brain stem area (Amirjamshidi et al. 2007; Kang et al. 2011; Tazi et al. 2011). Acupuncture has been used successfully in treating hiccups in non-cancer patients (Yan 1988; Lin 2006; Chang et al. 2008). In a recent case study of 16 cancer patients with persistent hiccups, acupuncture was shown to be an effective treatment option (Ge et al. 2010). Acupuncture points: BL17, GV14, CV12, PC6, ST36, Pishu (BL20), Weishu (BL21) and Qimen (LR14) were used. The mean hiccups severity measured by Hiccups Assessment Instruments before treatment was 5.2/10. After treatments, 13 patients had complete remission and 8 of this 13 patients achieved remission after only one treatment session. The authors reviewed laboratory evidence that acupuncture stimulation of PC6, ST36 and CV12 can activate the nucleus tractus neurons and subncucleus reticularis doraslis neurons that are implicated to be involved in hiccups reflex arc (Sun et al., 2007; Ji et al., 2009).

Persistent yawning has been linked to drugs, for example, anti-depressants, opioid and dopaminergic medications, and direct tumor involvement of the brain stem (Patatanian and Williams 2011). Radiation treatments that include the brain stem area can also induce yawning (Wong et al. 1997; Wong and Sagar 2000). One case report has shown that acupuncture on PC6 was able to abort persistent yawning in a patient receiving radiation treatment that include the brain stem for brain cancer (Wong and Sagar 2000).

5.16 Conclusion

Cancer patients suffer from a variety of cancer-related symptoms during and after cancer therapies. With recent improvement in cancer survival, increasing number of patients will also be affected by long-term and often debilitating treatment toxicities leading to poorer quality of life. The search for effective management options for cancer-related symptoms has become more important. Among all complementary and alternative therapies, acupuncture and related techniques are increasing accepted by cancer patients and are more widely provided by health care providers. Results from recent research have suggested acupuncture and related techniques are effective options for treating both short-term and long-term cancer-related symptoms. Future effort with innovative research design involving multiple disciplines and collaborative systematic data collection will continue to provide evidence to guide optimal utilization of these treatment techniques in cancer care and to reveal the underlying mechanisms of treatment effects.

References

Abuaisha, B. B., Costanzi, J. B., Boulton, A. J. (1998). Acupuncture for the treatment of chronic painful peripheral diabetic neuropathy: A long-term study. *Diabetes Research and Clinical Practice*, *39*, 115–121.

Alem, M., & Gurgel, M. S. (2008). Acupuncture in the rehabilitation of women after breast cancer surgery—a case series. *Acupuncture in Medicine*, *26*, 87–93.

Alimi, D., Rubino, C., Pichard-Leandri, E., Fermand-Brule, S., Dubreuil-Lemaire, M. L., Hill, C. (2003). Analgesic effect of auricular acupuncture for cancer pain: A randomized, blinded, controlled trial. *Journal of Clinical Oncology*, *21*, 4120–4126.

Alraek, T., Borud, E., White, A. (2011). Selecting acupuncture treatment for hot flashes: A Delphi consensus compared with a clinical trial. *Journal of Alternative and Complementary Medicine*, *17*, 33–38.

Amirjamshidi, A., Abbassioun, K., Parsa, K. (2007). Hiccup and neurosurgeons: a report of 4 rare dorsal medullary compressive pathologies and review of the literature. *Surgical Neurology*, *67*, 395–402.

Ashamalla, H., Jiang, M. L., Guirguis, A., Peluso, F., Ashamalla, M. (2011). Acupuncture for the alleviation of hot flashes in men treated with androgen ablation therapy. *International Journal of Radiation Oncology, Biology, Physics*, *79*, 1358–1363.

Avis, N. E., Legault, C., Coeytaux, R. R., Pian-Smith, M., Shifren, J. L., Chen, W., et al. (2008). A randomized, controlled pilot study of acupuncture treatment for menopausal hot flashes. *Menopause*, *15*, 1070–1078.

Balk, J., Day, R., Rosenzweig, M., Beriwal, S. (2009). Pilot, randomized, modified, double-blind, placebo-controlled trial of acupuncture for cancer-related fatigue. *Journal of the Society for Integrative Oncology*, *7*, 4–11.

Beer, T. M., Benavides, M., Emmons, S. L., Hayes, M., Liu, G., Garzotto, M., et al. (2010). Acupuncture for hot flashes in patients with prostate cancer. *Urology*, *76*, 1182–1188.

Bian, D., Cheng, Z. D., Zhang, N. S., et al. (2004). Effects of Acupoint-injection plus moxibustion on IL-2/IL-2R expression in peripheral blood in the patient with carcinous pain. *Chinese Acupuncture Moxibustion*, *24*, 641–644.

Blom, M., & Lundeberg, T. (2000). Long-term follow-up of patients treated with acupuncture for xerostomia and the influence of additional treatment. *Oral Diseases*, *6*, 15–24.

Blom, M., Dawidson, I., Angmar-Mansson, B. (1992). The effect of acupuncture on salivary flow rates in patients with xerostomia. *Oral Surgery, Oral Medicine, Oral Pathology*, *73*, 293–298.

Blom, M., Lundeberg, T., Dawidson, I., Angmar-Mansson, B. (1993). Effects on local blood flux of acupuncture stimulation used to treat xerostomia in patients suffering from Sjogren's syndrome. *Journal of Oral Rehabilitation*, *20*, 541–548.

Blom, M., Dawidson, I., Fernberg, J. O., Johnson, G., Angmar-Mansson, B. (1996). Acupuncture treatment of patients with radiation-induced xerostomia. *European Journal of Cancer, Part B, Oral Oncology*, *32B*, 182–190.

Boehler, M., Mitterschiffthaler, G., Schlager, A. (2002). Korean hand acupressure reduces postoperative nausea and vomiting after gynecological laparoscopic surgery. *Anesthesia and Analgesia, 94*, 872–875.

Bordeleau, L., Pritchard, K., Goodwin, P., Loprinzi, C. (2007). Therapeutic options for the management of hot flashes in breast cancer survivors: An evidence-based review. *Clinical Therapeutics, 29*, 230–241.

Borud, E. K., Alraek, T., White, A., Fonnebo, V., Eggen, A. E., Hammar, M., et al. (2009a). The acupuncture on hot flushes among menopausal women (ACUFLASH) study, a randomized controlled trial. *Menopause, 16*, 484–493.

Borud, E. K., Alraek, T., White, A., Grimsgaard, S. (2009b). The acupuncture treatment for postmenopausal hot flushes (Acuflash) study: Traditional Chinese medicine diagnoses and acupuncture points used, and their relation to the treatment response. *Acupuncture in Medicine, 27*, 101–108.

Borud, E. K., Alraek, T., White, A., Grimsgaard, S. (2010). The Acupuncture on Hot Flashes Among Menopausal Women study: Observational follow-up results at 6 and 12 months. *Menopause, 17*, 262–268.

Braga, F. P., Sugaya, N. N., Hirota, S. K., Weinfeld, I., Magalhaes, M. H., Migliari, D. A. (2008). The effect of acupuncture on salivary flow rates in patients with radiation-induced xerostomia. *Minerva Stomatologica, 57*, 343–348.

Braga Fdo, P., Lemos, C. A. Jr., Alves, F. A., Migliari, D. A. (2011). Acupuncture for the prevention of radiation-induced xerostomia in patients with head and neck cancer. *Brazilian Oral Research, 25*, 180–185.

Cao, J. X., Xiao, X. H., Tang, X. Y. (1997). Elemene fluorouracil Moxibustion "Shenque" effect in the treatment of advanced gastric cancer observed. *Chinese Journal of Clinical Oncology, 24*, 549–550.

Carroll, D., Moore, R. A., McQuay, H. J., Fairman, F., Tramer, M., Leijon, G. (2001). Transcutaneous electrical nerve stimulation (TENS) for chronic pain. Cochrane Database System Review, *3*, CD003222.

Chang, C. C., Chang, Y. C., Chang, S. T., Chang, W. K., Chang, H. Y., Chen, L. C., et al. (2008). Efficacy of near-infrared irradiation on intractable hiccup in custom-set acupoints: Evidence-based analysis of treatment outcome and associated factors. *Scandinavian Journal of Gastroenterology, 43*, 538–544.

Chang, C. S., Ko, C. W., Wu, C. Y., Chen, G. H. (2001a). Effect of electrical stimulation on acupuncture points in diabetic patients with gastric dysrhythmia: A pilot study. *Digestion, 64*, 184–190.

Chang, X., Yan, J., Yi, S., Lin, Y., Yang, R. (2001b). The affects of acupuncture at sibai and neiting acupoints on gastric peristalsis. *Journal of Traditional Chinese Medicine, 21*, 286–288.

Cheng, X. (Ed.). (1987). *Chinese Acupuncture and Moxibustion*. Beijing: Foreign Languages.

Chen, S., & Chen, Y. (2001). Observation on the effect of electro-acupuncture therapy on T-cell subpopulation, NK cytoactive, leukocyte count, and humoral immunity of patients treated by chemotherapy. *International Journal of Clinical Acupunture, 12*, 91–95.

Chen, K., Jiang, Y., Wen, H. (2000). Clinical study on treatment of nasopharyngeal carcinoma by radio- and chemotherapy with supplementary moxibustion on Shenque point. *Zhongguo Zhong Xi Yi Jie He Za Zhi, 20*, 733–735.

Chen, R. X., Kang, M. F., He, W. L., Chen, S. Y., Zhang, B. (2008). Moxibustion on heat-sensitive acupoints for treatment of myofascial pain syndrome: A multi-central randomized controlled trial. *Zhongguo Zhen Jiu, 28*, 395–398.

Chen, X. J., Song, Y. Y., Cai, L. Z., Du, K. H., Lin, C. Q., Su, Y. Z., et al. (2010). Influence of urodynamic factors on urinary retention in patients with cervical carcinoma after radical hysterectomy. *Zhonghua Fu Chan Ke Za Zhi, 45*, 677–681.

Cho, J. H., Chung, W. K., Kang, W., Choi, S. M., Cho, C. K., Son, C. G. (2008). Manual acupuncture improved quality of life in cancer patients with radiation-induced xerostomia. *Journal of Alternative and Complementary Medicine, 14*, 523–526.

Cho, D. S., Choi, J. B., Kim, Y. S., Joo, K. J., Kim, S. H., Kim, J.C., et al. (2011). Heart rate variability in assessment of autonomic dysfunction in patients with chronic prostatitis/chronic pelvic pain syndrome. *Urology, 78*, 1369–1372.

Crew, K. D., Capodice, J. L., Greenlee, H., Brafman, L., Fuentes, D., Awad, D., et al. (2010). Randomized, blinded, sham-controlled trial of acupuncture for the management of aromatase inhibitor-associated joint symptoms in women with early-stage breast cancer. *Journal of Clinical Oncology, 28*, 1154–1160.

Dang, W., & Yang, J. (1998). Clinical study on acupuncture treatment of stomach carcinoma pain. *Journal of Traditional Chinese Medicine, 18*, 31–38.

de Valois, B. A., Young, T. E., Melsome, E. (2011). Assessing the feasibility of using acupuncture and moxibustion to improve quality of life for cancer survivors with upper body lymphoedema. *European Journal of Oncology Nursing, 16*, 301–9.

de Valois, B. A., Young, T. E., Robinson, N., McCourt, C., Maher, E. J. (2010). Using traditional acupuncture for breast cancer-related hot flashes and night sweats. *Journal of Alternative and Complementary Medicine, 16*, 1047–1057.

Deng, G., Vickers, A., Yeung, S., D'Andrea, G. M., Xiao, H., Heerdt, A. S., et al. (2007). Randomized, controlled trial of acupuncture for the treatment of hot flashes in breast cancer patients. *Journal of Clinical Oncology, 25*, 5584–5590.

Deng, G., Hou, B. L., Holodny, A. I., Cassileth, B. R. (2008). Functional magnetic resonance imaging (fMRI) changes and saliva production associated with acupuncture at LI-2 acupuncture point: A randomized controlled study. *BMC Complement Alternative Medicine, 8*, 37.

Deng, G. E., Frenkel, M., Cohen, L., Cassileth, B. R., Abrams, D. I., Capodice, J. L., et al. (2009). Evidence-based clinical practice guidelines for integrative oncology: Complementary therapies and botanicals. *Journal of the Society for Integrative Oncology, 7*, 85–120.

Donald, G. K., Tobin, I., Stringer, J. (2011). Evaluation of acupuncture in the management of chemotherapy-induced peripheral neuropathy. *Acupuncture in Medicine, 29*, 230–233.

Dong, W. H., Zhan, L. Y., Chen, F. (2003). The aetiology and management of acute urinary retention after rectal surgery. *Xian Dai Zhong Xi Yi Jie He Zha Zhi, 12*, 2082–2083.

Dundee, J. W., Yang, J., McMillan, C. (1991). Non-invasive stimulation of the P6 (Neiguan) antiemetic acupuncture point in cancer chemotherapy. *Journal of the Royal Society of Medicine, 84*, 210–212.

Errington-Evans, N. (2011). Acupuncture for Anxiety. *CNS Neuroscience Therapy, 18*, 227–284.

Ezzo, J. M., Richardson, M. A., Vickers, A., Allen, C., Dibble, S. L., Issell, B. F., et al. (2006). Acupuncture-point stimulation for chemotherapy-induced nausea or vomiting. Cochrane Database System Review, 2, CD002285.

Feng, Y., Wang, X. Y., Li, S. D., Zhang, Y., Wang, H. M., Li, M., et al. (2011). Clinical research of acupuncture on malignant tumor patients for improving depression and sleep quality. *Journal of Traditional Chinese Medicine, 31*, 199–202.

Fessele, K. S. (1996). Managing the multiple causes of nausea and vomiting in the patient with cancer. *Oncology Nursing Forum, 23*, 1409–1415; quiz 1416–1417.

Filshie, J. (2001). Safety aspects of acupuncture in palliative care. *Acupuncture in Medicine, 19*, 117–122.

Filshie, J., & Redman, D. (1985). Acupuncture and malignant pain problems. *European Journal of Surgical Oncology, 11*, 389–394.

Filshie, J., Bolton, T., Browne, D., Ashley, S. (2005). Acupuncture and self acupuncture for long-term treatment of vasomotor symptoms in cancer patients-audit and treatment algorithm. *Acupuncture in Medicine, 23*, 171–180.

Forman, A. (1990). Peripheral neuropathy in cancer patients: Incidence, features, and pathophysiology. *Oncology, 4*, 57–62.

Frisk, J., Källström, A. C., Wall, N., Fredrikson, M., Hammar, M. (2012). Acupuncture improves health-related quality-of-life (HRQoL) and sleep in women with breast cancer and hot flushes. *Supportive Care in Cancer, 20*, 715–724.

Gadsby, J. G., & Flowerdew, M. W. (2000). Transcutaneous electrical nerve stimulation and acupuncture-like transcutaneous electrical nerve stimulation for chronic low back pain. *Cochrane Database System Review, 2,* CD000210.

Gan, T. J., Meyer, T., Apfel, C. C., Chung, F., Davis, P. J., Eubanks, S., et al. (2003). Consensus guidelines for managing postoperative nausea and vomiting. *Anesthesia and Analgesia, 97,* 62–71.

Ge, A. X., Ryan, M. E., Giaccone, G., Hughes, M. S., Pavletic, S. Z. (2010). Acupuncture treatment for persistent hiccups in patients with cancer. *Journal of Alternative and Complementary Medicine, 16,* 811–816.

Glaus, A. (1998). Fatigue in patients with cancer. Analysis and assessment. *Recent Results Cancer Research, 145*(I-XI), 1–172.

Gottschling, S., Reindl, T. K., Meyer, S., Berrang, J., Henze, G., Graeber, S., et al. (2008). Acupuncture to alleviate chemotherapy-induced nausea and vomiting in pediatric oncology—a randomized multicenter crossover pilot trial. *Klinische Padiatrie, 220,* 365–370.

Grass, G. W. (2003). Reversal of chemotherapy-induced myelosuppression with electroacupuncture. *Medical Acupuncture, 15,* 35–39.

Gu, Y. Z. (Ed.). (1996). *Jiu Fa Yang Sheng.* Liaoning: Liaoning Scientific Technology.

Haker, E., Egekvist, H., Bjerring, P. (2000). Effect of sensory stimulation (acupuncture) on sympathetic and parasympathetic activities in healthy subjects. *Journal of Autonomous Nerveous System, 79,* 52–59.

Han, J. S., & Terenius, L. (1982). Neurochemical basis of acupuncture analgesia. *Annual Review of Pharmacology and Toxicology, 22,* 193–220.

Harding, C., Harris, A., Chadwick, D. (2009). Auricular acupuncture: A novel treatment for vasomotor symptoms associated with luteinizing-hormone releasing hormone agonist treatment for prostate cancer. *BJU International, 103,* 186–190.

Huang, S. T., Chen, G. Y., Lo, H. M., Lin, J. G., Lee, Y. S., Kuo, C. D. (2005). Increase in the vagal modulation by acupuncture at neiguan point in the healthy subjects. *The American Journal of Chinese Medicine, 33,* 157–164.

Huang, M. I., Nir, Y., Chen, B., Schnyer, R., Manber, R. (2006). A randomized controlled pilot study of acupuncture for postmenopausal hot flashes: Effect on nocturnal hot flashes and sleep quality. *Fertility and Sterility, 86,* 700–710.

Huang, Q. F. (2011a). Exploration of clinical regularities in acupuncture-moxibustion treatment for cancer pain. *Journal of Acupuncture Tuina Science, 9,* 346–350.

Huang, T., Wang, R. H., Huang, X., Tian, Y. Y., Zhang, W. B., Ayali, H., et al. (2011b). Comparison of the effects of traditional box-moxibustion and eletrothermal Bian-stone moxibustion on volume of blood flow in the skin. *Journal of Traditional Chinese Medicine, 31,* 44–45.

Hui, K. K., Liu, J., Makris, N., Gollub, R. L., Chen, A. J., Moore, C. I., et al. (2000). Acupuncture modulates the limbic system and subcortical gray structures of the human brain: Evidence from fMRI studies in normal subjects. *Human Brain Mapping, 9,* 13–25.

Hurlow, A., Bennett, M. I., Robb, K. A., Johnson, M. I., Simpson, K. H., Oxberry, S. G. (2012). Transcutaneous electric nerve stimulation (TENS) for cancer pain in adults. *Cochrane Database Systematic Reviews, 3,* CD006276.

Ji, L. X., Yan, L. P., Wang, H. J., Li, L., He, W., Ben, H., et al. (2009). Effects of electroacupuncture of "Neiguan" (PC 6), "Zhongwan" (CV 12) and "Zusanli" (ST 36) on electrical activities of neurons subnucleus reticularis dorsalis in rats. *Zhen Ci Yan Jiu, 34,* 27–30.

Ji-Sheng, H. (2003). Acupuncture: Neuropeptide release produced by electrical stimulation of different frequencies. *Trends in Neuroscience, 26,* 17–22.

Johnston, M. F., Yang, C., Hui, K. K., Xiao, B., Li, X. S., Rusiewicz, A. (2007). Acupuncture for chemotherapy-associated cognitive dysfunction: A hypothesis-generating literature review to inform clinical advice. *Integrative Cancer Therapies, 6,* 36–41.

Johnstone, P. A., Peng, Y. P., May, B. C., Inouye, W. S., Niemtzow, R. C. (2001). Acupuncture for pilocarpine-resistant xerostomia following radiotherapy for head and neck malignancies. *International Journal of Radiation Oncology, Biology, Physics, 50,* 353–357.

Johnstone, P. A., Niemtzow, R. C., Riffenburgh, R. H. (2002). Acupuncture for xerostomia: Clinical update. *Cancer, 94*, 1151–1156.

Jones, R. D. (2001). Depression and anxiety in oncology: The oncologist's perspective. *The Journal of Clinical Psychiatry, 8*(62 Suppl), 52–55; discussion 56–57.

Kanakura, Y., Niwa, K., Kometani, K., Nakazawa, K., Yamaguchi, Y., Ishikawa, H., et al. (2002). Effectiveness of acupuncture and moxibustion treatment for lymphedema following intrapelvic lymph node dissection: A preliminary report. *The American Journal of Chinese Medicine, 30*, 37–43.

Kang, J. H., Hui, D., Kim, M. J., Kim, H. G., Kang, M. H., Lee, G. W., et al. (2011). Corticosteroid rotation to alleviate dexamethasone-induced hiccup: A case series at a single institution. *Journal of Pain and Symptom Management 43*, 625–630.

Kim, K. H., Kang, K. W., Kim, D. I., Kim, H. J., Yoon, H. M., Lee, J. M., et al. (2010). Effects of acupuncture on hot flashes in perimenopausal and postmenopausal women—a multicenter randomized clinical trial. *Menopause, 17*, 269–280.

Laird, B. J., Scott, A. C., Colvin, L. A., McKeon, A. L., Murray, G. D., Fearon, K. C., et al. (2011). Cancer pain and its relationship to systemic inflammation: An exploratory study. *Pain 152*, 460–463.

Lee, A., & Done, M. L. (2004). Stimulation of the wrist acupuncture point P6 for preventing postoperative nausea and vomiting. Cochrane Database System Review, *3*, CD003281.

Lee, H., Schmidt, K., Ernst, E. (2005). Acupuncture for the relief of cancer-related pain—a systematic review. *European Journal of Pain, 9*, 437–444.

Lee, A., & Fan, L. T. (2009). Stimulation of the wrist acupuncture point P6 for preventing postoperative nausea and vomiting. Cochrane Database System Review 2, CD003281.

Lee, H. J., Lee, J. H., Lee, E. O., Lee, H. J., Kim, K. H., Lee, K. S., et al. (2009a). Substance P and beta endorphin mediate electroacupuncture induced analgesic activity in mouse cancer pain model. *Acupuncture and Electro-Therapeutics Research, 34*, 27–40.

Lee, M. S., Kim, K. H., Choi, S. M., Ernst, E. (2009b). Acupuncture for treating hot flashes in breast cancer patients: A systematic review. *Breast Cancer Research and Treatment, 115*, 497–503.

Lee, M. S., Kim, K. H., Shin, B. C., Choi, S. M., Ernst, E. (2009c). Acupuncture for treating hot flushes in men with prostate cancer: A systematic review. *Supportive Care Cancer, 17*, 763–770.

Lee, M. S., Choi, T. Y., Kang, J. W., Lee, B. J., Ernst, E. (2010a). Moxibustion for treating pain: A systematic review. *The American Journal of Chinese Medicine, 38*, 829–838.

Lee, M. S., Choi, T. Y., Park, J. E., Lee, S. S., Ernst, E. (2010b). Moxibustion for cancer care: A systematic review and meta-analysis. *BMC Cancer, 10*, 130.

Li, Z., Wang, C., Mak, A. F., Chow, D. H. (2005). Effects of acupuncture on heart rate variability in normal subjects under fatigue and non-fatigue state. *European Journal of Applied Physiology, 94*, 633–640.

Lin, Y. C. (2006). Acupuncture for persistent hiccups in a heart and lung transplant recipient. *The Journal of Heart and Lung Transplantation, 25*, 126–127.

Litscher, G., Zhang, W., Yi, S. H., Wang, L., Huang, T., Gaischek, I., et al. (2009). The future of acupuncture moxibustion—a transcontinental three-center pilot study using high-tech methods. *Evidence-Based Complementary and Alternative Medicine, 21*, 115–121.

Liu, H. L., & Wang, L. P. (2006). Randomized controlled study on ginger-salt-partitioned moxibustion at shenque (CV8) on urination disorders poststroke. *Zhongguo Zhen Jiu, 26*, 621–624.

Liu, H. R., Qi, L., Wu, L. Y., Ma, X. P., Qin, X. D., Huang, W. Y., et al. (2010). Effects of moxibustion on dynorphin and endomorphin in rats with chronic visceral hyperalgesia. *World Journal of Gastroenterology, 16*, 4079–4083.

Lu, W., Hu, D., Dean-Clower, E., Doherty-Gilman, A., Legedza, A. T., Lee, H., et al. (2007). Acupuncture for chemotherapy-induced leukopenia: Exploratory meta-analysis of randomized controlled trials. *Journal of the Society for Integrative Oncology, 5*, 1–10.

Lu, M., Cao, D. M., Li, D. M., Zhao, X. X., Li, J. W., Li, H. X., et al. (2009a). Effects of acupuncture and moxibustion on DNA excision repair-related proteins of bone marrow cell in cyclophosphamide-induced mice. *Zhongguo Zhen Jiu, 29*, 821–824.

Lu, W., Matulonis, U. A., Doherty-Gilman, A., Lee, H., Dean-Clower, E., Rosulek, A., et al. (2009b). Acupuncture for chemotherapy-induced neutropenia in patients with gynecologic malignancies: A pilot randomized, sham-controlled clinical trial. *Journal of Alternative and Complementary Medicine*, *15*, 745–753.

Lu, W., Posner, M. R., Wayne, P., Rosenthal, D. S., Haddad, R. I. (2010). Acupuncture for dysphagia after chemoradiation therapy in head and neck cancer: A case series report. *Integrative Cancer Therapies*, *9*, 284–290.

Lu, M., Cao, D. M., Zhao, X. X. (2011). Study on dynamic effect of acupuncture on marrow cell cycle regulatory protein cyclin D1 expression and cell cycle in mice with cyclophosphamide induced myelosuppression. *Zhongguo Zhong Xi Yi Jie He Za Zhi*, *31*, 238–243.

Ma, L. (2009). Acupuncture as a complementary therapy in chemotherapy-induced nausea and vomiting. *Proceedings (Baylor University Medical Center)*, *22*, 138–141.

Ma, S. X., Wu, F. W., Cui, J. M., Jin, Z. H., Kong, L. J. (2010). Effect on moxibustion at Sanyinjiao (SP6) for uterine contraction pain in labor: A randomized controlled trial. *Zhongguo Zhen Jiu*, *30*, 623–626.

Mao, W., Ghia, J. N., Scott, D. S., Duncan, G. H., Gregg, J. M. (1980). High versus low intensity acupuncture analgesia for treatment of chronic pain: Effects on platelet serotonin. *Pain*, *8*, 331–342.

Mayor, D. F. (2008). Electroacupuncture parameters and beta-endorphin revisited. *Acupuncture in Medicine*, *26*, 197–198.

Meng, Z., Garcia, M. K., Hu, C., Chiang, J., Chambers, M., Rosenthal, D. I., et al. (2012). Randomized controlled trial of acupuncture for prevention of radiation-induced xerostomia among patients with nasopharyngeal carcinoma. *Cancer*, *118*, 3337–3344.

Ming, J. L., Kuo, B. I., Lin, J. G., Lin, L. C. (2002). The efficacy of acupressure to prevent nausea and vomiting in post-operative patients. *Journal of Advanced Nursing*, *39*, 343–351.

Moffatt, C. J., Franks, P. J., Doherty, D. C., Williams, A. F., Badger, C., Jeffs, E., et al. (2003). Lymphoedema: An underestimated health problem. *Monthly Journal of the Association of Physicians*, *96*, 731–738.

Molassiotis, A., Sylt, P., Diggins, H. (2007). The management of cancer-related fatigue after chemotherapy with acupuncture and acupressure: A randomised controlled trial. *Complementary Therapies in Medicine*, *15*, 228–237.

Napadow, V., Ahn, A., Longhurst, J., Lao, L., Stener-Victorin, E., Harris, R., et al. (2008). The status and future of acupuncture mechanism research. *Journal of Alternative and Complementary Medicine*, *14*, 861–869.

Nedstrand, E., Wyon, Y., Hammar, M., Wijma, K. (2006). Psychological well-being improves in women with breast cancer after treatment with applied relaxation or electro-acupuncture for vasomotor symptom. *Journal of Psychosomatic Obstetrics and Gynaecology*, *27*, 193–199.

Nir, Y., Huang, M. I., Schnyer, R., Chen, B., Manber, R. (2007). Acupuncture for postmenopausal hot flashes. *Maturitas*, *56*, 383–395.

Oldenhave, A., Jaszmann, L. J., Haspels, A. A., Everaerd, W. T. (1993). Impact of climacteric on well-being. A survey based on 5,213 women 39–60 years old. *American Journal of Obstetrics and Gynecology*, *168*, 772–780.

Paley, C. A., & Johnson, M. I. (2011). Acupuncture for cancer-induced bone pain: A pilot study. *Acupuncture in Medicine*, *29*, 71–73.

Paley, C. A., Johnson, M. I., Tashani, O. A., Bagnall, A. M. (2011). Acupuncture for cancer pain in adults. Cochrane Database System Rev, *1*, CD007753.

Park, J. E., Lee, M. S., Jung, S., Kim, A., Kang, K., Choi, J., et al. (2009). Moxibustion for treating menopausal hot flashes: A randomized clinical trial. *Menopause*, *16*, 660–665.

Patatanian, E., & Williams, N. T. (2011). Drug-induced yawning—a review. *The Annals of Pharmacotherapy*, *45*, 1297–1301.

Peng, H., Peng, H. D., Xu, L., Lao, L. X. (2010). Efficacy of acupuncture in treatment of cancer pain: A systematic review. *Zhong Xi Yi Jie He Xue Bao*, *8*, 501–509.

Pfister, D. G., Cassileth, B. R., Deng, G. E., Yeung, K. S., Lee, J. S., Garrity, D., et al. (2010). Acupuncture for pain and dysfunction after neck dissection: Results of a randomized controlled trial. *Journal of Clinical Oncology*, *28*, 2565–2570.

Phillips, K. D., Skelton, W. D., Hand, G. A. (2004). Effect of acupuncture administered in a group setting on pain and subjective peripheral neuropathy in persons with human immunodeficiency virus disease. *Journal of Alternative and Complementary Medicine*, *10*, 449–455.

Proctor, G. B., & Carpenter, G. H. (2007). Regulation of salivary gland function by autonomic nerves. *Autonomic Neuroscience*, *133*, 3–18.

Pyter, L. M., Pineros, V., Galang, J. A., McClintock, M. K., Prendergast, B. J. (2009). Peripheral tumors induce depressive-like behaviors and cytokine production and alter hypothalamic-pituitary-adrenal axis regulation. *Proceedings of the National Academy of Sciences of the United States of America*, *106*, 9069–9074.

Rong, P. J., Zu, B., Huang, Q. F., Gao, X. Y., Ben, H., Li, Y. H. (2005). Acupuncture inhibition on neuronal activity of spinal dorsal horn induced by noxious colorectal distention in rat. *World Journal of Gastroenterology*, *11*, 1011–1017.

Roschke, J., Wolf, C., Muller, M. J., Wagner, P., Mann, K., Grozinger, M., et al. (2000). The benefit from whole body acupuncture in major depression. *Journal of Affective Disorders*, *57*, 73–81.

Rydholm, M., & Strang, P. (1999). Acupuncture for patients in hospital-based home care suffering from xerostomia. *Journal of Palliative Care*, *15*, 20–23.

Sakatani, K., Kitagawa, T., Aoyama, N., Sasaki, M. (2010). Effects of acupuncture on autonomic nervous function and prefrontal cortex activity. *Advances in Experimental Medicine and Biology*, *662*, 455–460.

Schlager, A., Boehler, M., Puhringer, F. (2000). Korean hand acupressure reduces postoperative vomiting in children after strabismus surgery. *British Journal of Anaesthesia*, *85*, 267–270.

Schneyer, C. A., Humphreys-Beher, M. G., Hall, H. D., Jirakulsomchok, D. (1993). Mitogenic activity of rat salivary glands after electrical stimulation of parasympathetic nerves. *American Journal of Physiology*, *264*, G935–938.

Schroeder, S., Meyer-Hamme, G., Epplee, S. (2011). Acupuncture for chemotherapy-induced peripheral neuropathy (CIPN): A pilot study using neurography. *Acupuncture in Medicine*, *30*, 4–7.

Shen, H., & Shen, C. X. (1996). Acupuncture treatment on "Tian Tu" (CV22) for dysphagia in advanced esophageal cancer; a 120 cases report. *Zhejiang Journal of Traditional Chinese Medicine*, *31*, 561.

Shen, J., Wenger, N., Glaspy, J., Hays, R. D., Albert, P. S., Choi, C., et al. (2000). Electroacupuncture for control of myeloablative chemotherapy-induced emesis: A randomized controlled trial. *JAMA*, *284*, 2755–2761.

Shi, J. L., Chen, Y. Q., Wen, L., et al. (2008). Electroacupuncture in the treatment of urinary retention in postoperative period of rectal cancer patients. *Zhongguo Zhong Xi Yi Jie He Za Zhi*, *28*, 158–159.

Shiotani, A, Tatewaki M, Hoshino E, Takahashi, T (2004) Effects of electroacupuncture on gastric myoelectrical activity in healthy humans. *Neurogastroenterol and Motility*, *16*, 293–298

Smith, C. A., Hay, P. P., Macpherson, H. (2010). Acupuncture for depression. Cochrane Database System Review, *1*, CD004046.

Somri, M., Vaida, S. J., Sabo, E., Yassain, G., Gankin, I., Gaitini, L. A. (2001). Acupuncture versus ondansetron in the prevention of postoperative vomiting. A study of children undergoing dental surgery. *Anaesthesia*, *56*, 927–932.

Stone, P., Richards, M., Hardy, J. (1998). Fatigue in patients with cancer. *European Journal of Cancer*, *34*, 1670–1676.

Streitberger, K., Ezzo, J., Schneider, A. (2006). Acupuncture for nausea and vomiting: An update of clinical and experimental studies. *Autonomic Neuroscience*, *129*, 107–117.

Su, J. C., Cao, L. H., Li, Z. D., Wang, S. C., Zhang, Q. J., Ma, Y. H., et al. (2009). Controlled clinical trials of initial observation on therapeutic effects of moxibustion for osteoarthritis of the knee: Multi-center clinical effect. *Zhongguo Gu Shang*, *22*, 914–916.

Sun, B. M., Luo, M., Wu, S. B., Chen, X. X., Wu, M. C. (2010). Acupuncture versus metoclopramide in treatment of postoperative gastroparesis syndrome in abdominal surgical patients: A randomized controlled trial. *Zhong Xi Yi Jie He Xue Bao, 8*, 641–644.

Sun, G. J., Wang, S. J., Du, Y. J., Hu, H. P., Wu, X. P., Kong, L. H. (2007). Study on dual-directional regulation induced by acupuncture at different acupoints in the rat with motility abnormality of the stomach. *Zhongguo Zhen Jiu, 27*, 839–842.

Sun, L. H., Ge, J. J., Yang, J. J., She, Y. F., Li, W. L., Li, X. H., et al. (2009). Randomized controlled clinical study on ginger-partitioned moxibustion for patients with cold-damp stagnation type primary dysmenorrhea. *Zhen Ci Yan Jiu, 34*, 398–402.

Tannock, I. F., Ahles, T. A., Ganz, P. A., Van Dam, F. S. (2004). Cognitive impairment associated with chemotherapy for cancer: Report of a workshop. *Journal Clinical Oncology, 22*, 2233–2239.

Tatewaki, M., Strickland, C., Fukuda, H., Tsuchida, D., Hoshino, E., Pappas, T. N., et al. (2005). Effects of acupuncture on vasopressin-induced emesis in conscious dogs. *American Journal of Physiology. Regulatory, Integrative and Comparative Physiology, 288*, R401–408.

Tazi, I., Zaoui, S., Nafil, H., Mahmal, L. (2011). Hiccups ad severe hyponatremia induced by low dose cyclophosphamide therapy for Burkitt lymphoma. *Annales de Biologie Clinique, 69*, 613–614.

van Den Beuken-van Everdingen, M. H., de Rijke, J. M., Kessels, A. G., Schouten, H. C., van Kleef, M., Patijn, J. (2007). Prevalence of pain in patients with cancer: A systematic review of the past 40 years. *Annals of Oncology, 18*, 1437–1449.

Vickers, A. J. (1996). Can acupuncture have specific effects on health? A systematic review of acupuncture antiemesis trials. *Journal of the Royal Society of Medicine, 89*, 303–311.

Vickers, A. J., Straus, D. J., Fearon, B., Cassileth, B. R. (2004). Acupuncture for postchemotherapy fatigue: A Phase II study. *Journal of Clinical Oncology, 22*, 1731–1735.

Vincent, A., Barton, D. L., Mandrekar, J. N., Cha, S. S., Zais, T., Wahner-Roedler, D. L., et al. (2007). Acupuncture for hot flashes: A randomized, sham-controlled clinical study. *Menopause, 14*, 45–52.

Vorobeychik, Y., Gordin, V., Mao, J., Chen, L. (2011). Combination therapy for neuropathic pain: A review of current evidence. *CNS Drugs, 25*, 1023–1034.

Wagner, L. I., & Cella, D. (2004). Fatigue and cancer: Causes, prevalence and treatment approaches. *British Journal of Cancer, 91*, 822–828.

Walker, E. M., Rodriguez, A. I., Kohn, B., Ball, R. M., Pegg, J., Pocock, J. R., et al. (2010). Acupuncture versus venlafaxine for the management of vasomotor symptoms in patients with hormone receptor-positive breast cancer: A randomized controlled trial. *Journal of Clinical Oncology, 28*, 634–640.

Wang, Q. C. (Ed.). (2008). *New Acupuncturiology*. Beijing: Zhong Yi Gu Ji.

Wang, T., Zhang, Q., Xue, X., Yeung, A. (2008a). A systematic review of acupuncture and moxibustion treatment for chronic fatigue syndrome in China. *The American Journal of Chinese Medicine, 36*, 1–24.

Wang, H., Qi, H., Wang, B. S., Cui, Y. Y., Zhu, L., Rong, Z. X., et al. (2008b). Is acupuncture beneficial in depression: A meta-analysis of 8 randomized controlled trials? *Journal of Affective Disorders, 111*, 125–134.

WHO Regional Office for the Western Pacific (2007) WHO international standard terminologies on traditional medicine in the Western Pacific Region.

Widerstrom-Noga, E., Dyrehag, L. E., Borglum-Jensen, L., Aslund, P. G., Wenneberg, B., Andersson, S. A. (1998). Pain threshold responses to two different modes of sensory stimulation in patients with orofacial muscular pain: Psychologic considerations. *Journal of Orofacial Pain, 12*, 27–34.

Williams, J. W., Gierisch, J. M., McDuffie, J., Strauss, J. L., & Nagi, A. (2011). An overview of complementary and alternative medicine therapies for anxiety and depressive disorders: Supplement to efficacy of complementary and alternative medicine therapies for posttraumatic stress disorder. Washington: Department of Veterans Affairs.

Windebank, A. J., & Grisold, W. (2008). Chemotherapy-induced neuropathy. *Journal of Peripheral Nervous System, 13*, 27–46.
Wong, R. K., & Sagar, S. M. (2000). The treatment of persistent yawning with acupuncture. *Acupuncture in Medicine, 18*, 124–126.
Wong, R., & Sagar, S. (2006). Acupuncture treatment for chemotherapy-induced peripheral neuropathy—a case series. *Acupuncture in Medicine, 24*, 87–91.
Wong, K. Y., Ngan, K. C., Sin, V. C., Lau, W. H. (1997). Sphenoidal sinus mucocoele and yawning after radiation treatment for nasopharyngeal carcinoma. *Clinical Oncology (Royal College of Radiologists), 9*, 415–417.
Wong, R. K., Jones, G. W., Sagar, S. M., Babjak, A. F., Whelan, T. (2003). A Phase I-II study in the use of acupuncture-like transcutaneous nerve stimulation in the treatment of radiation-induced xerostomia in head-and-neck cancer patients treated with radical radiotherapy. *International Journal of Radiation Oncology, Biology, Physics, 57*, 472–480.
Wong, R. K., Sagar, S. M., Chen, B. J., Yi, G. Y., Cook, R. (2010). Phase II randomized trial of acupuncture-like transcutaneous electrical nerve stimulation to prevent radiation-induced xerostomia in head and neck cancer patients. *Journal of the Society for Integrative Oncology, 8*, 35–42.
Wong, R. K., James, J. L., Sagar, S., Wyatt, G., Nguyen-Tan, P. F., Singh, A. K., et al. (2012). Phase 2 results from radiation therapy oncology group study 0537: A Phase 2/3 study comparing acupuncture-like transcutaneous electrical nerve stimulation versus pilocarpine in treating early radiation-induced xerostomia. *Cancer, 118*, 4244–4252.
Woollam, C. H., & Jackson, A. O. (1998). Acupuncture in the management of chronic pain. *Anaesthesia, 53*, 593–595.
Wu, M. T., Hsieh, J. C., Xiong, J., Yang, C. F., Pan, H. B., Chen, Y. C., et al. (1999). Central nervous pathway for acupuncture stimulation: Localization of processing with functional MR imaging of the brain-preliminary experience. *Radiology, 212*, 133–141.
Wyon, Y., Wijma, K., Nedstrand, E., Hammar, M. (2004). A comparison of acupuncture and oral estradiol treatment of vasomotor symptoms in postmenopausal women. *Climacteric, 7*, 153–164.
Xia, Y. Q., Zhang, D., Yang, C. X., Xu, H. L., Li, Y., Ma, L. T. (1986). An approach to the effect on tumors of acupuncture in combination with radiotherapy or chemotherapy. *Journal of Traditional Chinese Medicine, 6*, 23–26.
Xu, K. S., Huang, M. W., Yao, L. Y., Chen, J., Su, J., Zheng, J. Q. (2009). Clinically randomized controlled trials of moxibustion with salt in bamboo circle for treatment of periarthritis of shoulder. *Zhongguo Zhen Jiu, 29*, 77–80.
Yan, L. S. (1988). Treatment of persistent hiccupping with electro-acupuncture at "hiccup-relieving" point. *Journal of Traditional Chinese Medicine, 8*, 29–30.
Yang, J. X., Xiang, K. W., Zhang, Y. X. (2012) Treatment of herpes zoster with cotton sheet moxibustion: multicentre randomized controlled trial. *Zhongguo Zhen Jiu, 32*, 417–421.
Ye, F., Liu, D., Wang, S., Xu, L. (2007). Effects of electro-acupuncture on T cell subpopulations, NK activity, humoral immunity and leukocyte count in patients undergoing chemotherapy. *Journal of Traditional Chinese Medicine, 27*, 19–21.
Yi, W. M., Pan, A. Z., Li, J. J., Luo, D. F., Huang, Q. H. (2011). Clinical observation on the acupuncture treatment in patients with urinary retention after radical hysterectomy. *Chinese Journal of Integrative Medicine, 17*, 860–863.
Yoo, S. S., Teh, E. K., Blinder, R. A., Jolesz, F. A. (2004). Modulation of cerebellar activities by acupuncture stimulation: Evidence from fMRI study. *Neuroimage, 22*, 932–940.
Yu, J., Liu, C., Zhang, X., Han, J. (2005). Acupuncture improved cognitive impairment caused by multi-infarct dementia in rats. *Physiology and Behavior, 86*, 434–441.
Zhang, M., Qiu, L., Zhang, J. (2007). Observation on therapeutic effect of surround needling plus surround moxibustion on herpes zoster. *Zhongguo Zhen Jiu, 27*, 123–125.
Zhang, Z. H. (1987). Effect of acupuncture on 44 cases of radiation rectitis following radiation therapy for carcinoma of the cervix uteri. *Journal of Traditional Chinese Medicine, 7*, 139–140.

Zhao, X. X., Lu, M., Zhu, X., Gao, P., Li, Y. L., Wang, X. M., et al. (2007). Multi-central clinical evaluation of ginger-partitioned moxibustion for treatment of leukopenia induced by chemotherapy. *Zhongguo Zhen Jiu, 27*, 715–720.

Zheng, P., & Ruan, J. (2002). Effect of acupuncture combined with psychotherapy on quality of life in patients with nasopharyngeal cancer in post radiation therapy. *Chinese Journal of Information of Traditional Chinese Medicine, 9*, 63–64.

Zhou, H., & Zhang, P. (2006). Effect of swallowing training combined with acupuncture on dysphagia in nasopharyngeal carcinoma after radiotherapy. *Chinese Journal of Rehabilitation Theory Practice, 12*, 58–59.

Zhou, J., Qin, Z. Y., Li, W. L., Zhang, C. P., Tian, L. Y., Zhang, Y. J., et al. (2006). Clinical observation on therapeutic effect of electroacupuncture at Sanyinjiao (SP 6) on peri-menopausal syndrome. *Zhongguo Zhen Jiu, 26*, 617–620.

Chapter 6
Use of Acupuncture and Moxibustion in the Control of Anticancer Therapy-induced Nausea and Vomiting

Rie Konno and Aye A. Gyi

Abstract Anticancer-related adverse events, particularly chemotherapy-induced nausea and vomiting, are significant problems for both healthcare professionals and patients. The use of alternative medicine is receiving more recognition for control of such adverse events as an adjunct therapy along with administration of anti-emetics. This chapter examines the current available research evidence on the efficacy of acupuncture and moxibustion for reducing anticancer treatment-induced nausea and vomiting as well as safety of such treatments, searching the major databases resulted in four systematic reviews and three new trials being identified and reviewed. These evidence supports the use of acupoint-stimulation for reducing chemotherapy-induced nausea and vomiting in both adult and pediatric cancer patients with very low risk of serious adverse events. Concerning different stimulation methods, acupressure on pericardium meridian demonstrates reasonably strong evidence for reducing the severity of acute nausea. Electroacupuncture on pericardium meridian can alleviate acute vomiting. In contrast, manual acupuncture and non-invasive stimulation methods fail to provide strong evidence for such effect. A meta-analysis of two small-scale studies showed significant beneficial effects of moxibustion but further large-scale studies are needed to provide indisputable recommendations for practice. Overall, well-designed studies with a large sample size are needed for developing a solid evidence base that promotes acupuncture and moxibustion in cancer care.

6.1 Introduction

The practice of acupuncture originated in China over 3,500 years ago. Today, acupuncture is widely used throughout the world and is one of the main pillars of traditional Chinese medicine. Acupuncture has become increasingly popular in

---

R. Konno (✉)
Joanna Briggs Institute, Faculty of Health Sciences, The University of Adelaide, Adelaide, South Australia, Australia
e-mail: rie.konno@adelaide.edu.au

A. A. Gyi
Neurosurgery Department, School of Medical Science, Faculty of Health Sciences, The University of Adelaide, Adelaide, South Australia, Australia

W. C. S. Cho (ed.), *Acupuncture and Moxibustion as an Evidence-based Therapy for Cancer*, Evidence-based Anticancer Complementary and Alternative Medicine 3,
DOI 10.1007/978-94-007-4833-0_6, © Springer Science+Business Media Dordrecht 2012

Western world and is often referred to as medical acupuncture in that context. The general theory of acupuncture is based on the premise that there are patterns of energy flow (Qi) through the body that are essential for good health. Disruptions of this flow are believed to be responsible for disease. Acupuncture may correct imbalances of flow at identifiable points close to the skin (Ma 2009).

Acupuncture is a therapeutic technique that involves stimulation of anatomical locations on the skin by a variety of techniques. The most studied mechanism of stimulation of acupuncture points employs penetration of the skin by thin, solid, metallic needles, which are manipulated manually (manual acupuncture) or by electrical stimulation (electroacupuncture) (Ezzo et al. 2006; Urroz et al. 2012). Electrical stimulation can also be applied *via* electrodes on the skin surface or by a relief band, a wristwatch-like device (non-invasive electrostimulation). Pressure can be applied either by pressing on the point with the fingers or by wearing an elastic wristband with an embedded stud (acupressure) (Ezzo et al. 2006; Allais et al. 2012).

Several professional bodies have provided recommendations and guidelines for using acupuncture for several indications, including various types of pain and several kinds of nausea and vomiting (Cassileth et al. 2007; Deng et al. 2007, American Cancer Society (http://www.cancer.org/Treatment/TreatmentsandSideEffects/ComplementaryandAl lternativeMedicine/ManualHealingandPhysicalTouch/acupuncture?sitearea = ETO), World Health Organization (http://apps.who.int/medicinedocs/en/d/Js4926e/6.html)). They all recognize the beneficial effects of acupuncture for controlling anticancer treatment-induced nausea and vomiting and recommend its clinical use for managing such symptoms.

The acupuncture points that have been widely used for nausea control are Neiguan (PC6) and Zusanli (ST36) (World Health Organisation 2003). PC6 is located between the tendons of palmaris longus and flexor carpi radialis at 2 body-inches proximal to the wrist crease (1 body-inch is the greatest width of a patient's thumb at the distal phalanx). ST36 is located on the anterior lateral side of the leg, 1 body-inch from the anterior crest of the tibia (World Health Organisation 2003). PC6 is the most commonly used acupuncture point to control nausea and vomiting, and PC6 can be stimulated by various methods (Ezzo et al. 2006).

Stimulation of these areas by moxibustion—the use of a cone or cylinder of dried herbs burned on or near the skin at acupuncture points to strengthen blood, stimulate Qi and maintain general health—is most commonly practiced in conjunction with acupuncture (Manheimer et al. 2009). In traditional Chinese medicine moxibustion can be used on its own or to augment the effect of acupuncture needles.

A number of other indications have been investigated, but there is a lack of adequate evidence to recommend for or against use of these indications (Manheimer et al. 2009). In some cases, this is due to methodological challenges inherent in acupuncture trials, such as placebo control and blinding. Other challenges include the diversity of approaches, the practice of individualizing treatment for each patient, and practitioners' differing skill levels. However, the body of trial data for acupuncture continues to grow, with innovative approaches to these methodological quandaries being developed.

Many acupuncture-related adverse events, most of them owing to improper technique have been described (Zhang et al. 2010). Adverse effects due to improper sterilization and disposing of needles can lead to infection or cross-transmission of human immunodeficiency virus, hepatitis and other infectious diseases. Mild side effects, including bleeding or bruising at needles sites, fainting, and nausea, may also occur. Complications, including bent or broken needles, typically occur due to improper technique. Serious adverse effects, however, are few, and acupuncture can generally be considered inherently safe in the hands of well-trained practitioners (Zhang et al. 2010).

This book chapter is designed to provide an evidence-based guide on using acupuncture and/or moxibustion to control anticancer therapy-induced nausea and vomiting based on a thorough systematic review of the available scientific studies. Furthermore, this chapter contains a detailed methodology and practical processes for assessing, pooling, disseminating and using the best available international evidence concerning acupuncture. In all healthcare systems, there is a growing consensus that evidence-based practice offers the most responsible course of action for improving health outcomes. All clinicians and healthcare professionals want to provide the best possible care for patients, families and communities, and our aim in this chapter is to close the gap between evidence and action, and therefore make this possible.

6.2 SR Method

To identify existing evidence, the following major databases were searched: PubMed, CINAHL, EMBASE, TRIP, Cochrane Library, CCTR (Cochrane Controlled Trials Registry) and JBI Library. Regarding the use of acupuncture, a previous Cochrane systematic review (SR) (2006) examined studies published up to 2003. Therefore, this particular search was extended to identify new trials published from 2004 to the current date (October 2011) with specific reference to the use of acupuncture. Concerning trials that used moxibustion, one SR (2010) considered studies published until 2005 and this search for new trials aimed to identify relevant studies published from 2006 to the present (March 2012). The search aimed to identify randomised controlled trials (RCT) and SRs of RCTs published in any language. This resulted in the finding that the majority of studies were published in English and a few were published in Chinese.

6.3 Result for Acupuncture

The database search identified two SRs investigating the effectiveness or adverse events of acupuncture for chemotherapy-induced nausea and vomiting (CINV) in patients with mixed cancer type (Ezzo et al. 2006) and patients with only breast cancer (Chao et al. 2009). A third SR reported on adverse events caused by acupuncture

(Ladas et al. 2010). The details of the three SRs are presented in Table 6.1. The details of the primary studies from the three SRs are listed in Table 6.2.

Three new trials were also identified as reporting on the effects of acupuncture (Reindl et al. 2006; Gottschling et al. 2008) or a combination of acupressure and acustimulation (Melchart et al. 2006). These include one trial on adult patients (Melchart et al. 2006) and two trials on paediatric patients (Reindl et al. 2006; Gottschling et al. 2008). The study by Reindl et al. (2006) constituted a preliminary report of Gottschling et al. (2008). As such only the latest study (Gottschling et al. 2008) was reviewed in this chapter.

6.3.1 A Cochrane SR by Ezzo et al. (2006)

Ezzo et al. (2006) examined the evidence for the effectiveness of acupuncture-point stimulation therapies including manual acupuncture, electroacupuncture, acupressure and non-invasive electro stimulation for controlling CINV in patients of any age group and cancer type.

The databases searched were MEDLINE, EMBASE, PsychLIT, MANTIS, Science Citation Index, CCTR (Cochrane Controlled Trials Registry), Cochrane Complementary Medicine Field Trials Register, Cochrane Pain, Palliative Care and Supportive Care Specialized Register, Cochrane Cancer Specialized Register, and conference abstracts. The SR included studies published up to 2003. The inclusion criteria were any type of cancer, any stage of cancer and any age group as long as the outcomes of interest were related to chemotherapy-induced nausea and/or vomiting. The review identified 11 RCTs of moderate to high quality. The details of the primary studies consisting of SRs are provided in Table 6.2.

The review defined acute nausea and vomiting as being events occurring within 24 h following the initiation of chemotherapy, and delayed nausea and vomiting referred to such events occurring after 24 h to 5–8 days (Ezzo et al. 2006).

All studies administered standard anti-emetics for both experimental and control groups. Most included studies used an anti-emetic regimen following the American Society of Clinical Oncology (ASCO) guidelines using 5-HT_3 antagonist plus steroid prior to chemotherapy, and steroid plus either metoclopramide or a 5-HT_3 antagonist for delayed nausea. The results of the review will be presented in a later section.

6.3.2 A Systematic Review by Chao et al. (2009)

A more recently published SR by Chao et al. (2009) examined the effectiveness of acupoint-stimulation for chemotherapy-induced adverse events including CINV for patients with breast cancer.

This particular review searched studies published from 1999–2008 in the English and Chinese languages. Eleven studies discussed CINV but only following three

Table 6.1 Included systematic reviews: acupuncture point stimulation

Author(s) and year of publication	Included study design(s)	Number of included studies	Type of cancer	Intervention (s)	Outcome measures
Ezzo et al. (2006)	RCTs	11 RCTs	Any cancer type of any age group	Acupuncture (manual acupuncture, electroacupuncture, acupressure and non-invasive electrostimulation)	Chemotherapy-induced: acute nausea, acute vomiting, delayed nausea, delayed vomiting
Chao et al. (2009)	RCTs and before and after studies	In total 23 studies, of 11 studies reporting on nausea and vomiting, only 3 studies were deemed high quality	Breast cancer	Acupuncture (manual acupuncture, electroacupuncture and acupressure)	Anticancer therapy-related nausea and vomiting and other adverse events
Jindal et al. (2008)	RCTs and meta-analyses or SRs	For adverse events, 22 RCTs were reviewed For efficacy of acupuncture, the data from Cochrane SR by Ezzo et al. (2006) were used	Children with various diagnosis (not specific to cancer)	Acupuncture (manual acupuncture, electroacupuncture, acupressure and non-invasive electrostimulation)	Adverse events, nausea and vomiting, asthma, seasonal allergic rhinitis, neurologic disorder, gastrointestinal disorders, addiction

RCT randomized controlled trial, *SR* systematic review

Table 6.2 Primary studies from systematic reviews: effectiveness of acupuncture point stimulation

Authors (year)	Included SR	Study design	Sample size	Type of cancer	Intervention(s)	Control	Outcome measures
Dibble et al. (2000)	Ezzo et al. (2006); Chao et al. (2009)	RCT with parallel design	17	Breast cancer	Acupressure at Neiguan (PC6) and Zusanli (ST36) for up to 3 min every morning (and as required) Plus antiemetics	Antiemetics only	Acute and delayed nausea
Dundee et al. (1987)	Ezzo et al. (2006)	RCT with cross-over design	10	Testicular cancer patients with prior history of chemotherapy-induced emesis or nausea	Electroacupuncture to PC6 until Deqi elicited for five to six sessions per day for 3 days	Antiemetics plus sham point in right elbow for 3 days. Only one of the treatments was sham Antiemetics plus sham point in right elbow	Acute vomiting
Dundee et al. (1988)	Ezzo et al. (2006)	RCT with parallel design	20	Various cancer patients receiving chemotherapy for the first time	Low frequency electroacupuncture (10 Hz for 5 min before or at the start of chemotherapy) Deqi elicited Plus antiemetics	Antiemetics only	Acute vomiting

Table 6.2 (continued)

Authors (year)	Included SR	Study design	Sample size	Type of cancer	Intervention(s)	Control	Outcome measures
McMillan et al. (1991)	Ezzo et al. (2006)	RCT with cross-over design	16	Patients with any cancer receiving chemotherapy for five consecutive days with or without prior history of chemotherapy-induced emesis or nausea or both	TENS stimulation on PC6 point before the chemotherapy for 5 min and stimulation for further 5 min every 2 h if awake Plus antiemetics	Antiemetics only	Acute vomiting and acute nausea
Noga et al. (2002)	Ezzo et al. (2006)	RCT with parallel design	120 (110) evaluable	Hematologic cancer	Acupressure band (sea-band) for PC6 for 24 h after chemotherapy Plus antiemetics	Antiemetics plus SeaBand at sham point	Acute vomiting, Acute nausea, delayed vomiting and delayed nausea
Pearl et al. (1999)	Ezzo et al. (2006)	RCT with cross-over design	42 (32 evaluable)	Gynaecologic cancer patients receiving single infusion chemotherapy	TENS (relief-band) for PC6 point for 7 days from discharge from the hospital Plus antiemetics	Antiemetics plus sham relief band at P6 for the same period	Acute vomiting, acute nausea, delayed vomiting and nausea

Table 6.2 (continued)

Authors (year)	Included SR	Study design	Sample size	Type of cancer	Intervention(s)	Control	Outcome measures
Roscoe et al. (2002)	Ezzo et al. (2006)	RCT with cross-over design	42 (38 evaluable)	Breast, lung, ovarian, colorectal cancer patients who had moderate to greater level of chemotherapy-induced nausea after first course	TENS (relief-band) prior to chemotherapy and for as long as helpful Plus antiemetics	Antiemetics plus sham ReliefBand Antiemetics only	Acute nausea and delayed nausea
Roscoe et al. (2003)	Ezzo et al. (2006)	RCT with parallel design	747 (700 evaluable)	Any cancer patients receiving first doxorubicin or cisplatin therapy	Bilateral acupressure (sea-band) for 5 days Single acustimulation (relief-band) for 5 days Plus antiemetics	Antiemetics only	Acute and delayed vomiting Acute and delayed nausea
Shen et al. (2000)	Ezzo et al. (2006); Chao et al. (2009)	RCT with parallel design	104	Breast cancer patients receiving high-dose chemotherapy. Prior history of chemotherapy-induced nausea or vomiting or both	Low frequency of electroacupuncture (2–10 Hz) at PC6 and ST36 Deqi elicited for 20 min for 2 h before chemotherapy for 5 days Plus antiemetics	Sham acupuncture plus antiemetics	Acute vomiting

Table 6.2 (continued)

Authors (year)	Included SR	Study design	Sample size	Type of cancer	Intervention(s)	Control	Outcome measures
Streiberg et al. (2003)	Ezzo et al. (2006)	RCT with parallel design	80	Mixed cancers	Needle acupuncture at PC6 for 30 min Deqi elicited. Then remained in place for 20 min without additional stimulation. Before the first chemotherapy session and the day after (The use of antiemetics was not reported)	Non-invasive placebo acupuncture at P6.	Acute vomiting and acute nausea
Treish et al. (2003)	Ezzo et al. (2006)	RCT with parallel design	49 (37 evaluable)	Mixed cancers	ReliefBand for 5 days Plus antiemetics	Sham ReliefBand plus antiemetics	Acute vomiting, acute nausea, delayed vomiting and delayed nausea
Dibble et al. (2007)	Chao et al. (2009)	RCT with 3 arms	53 (47 evaluable)	Breast cancer	Self-acupressure at PC6 for 6 min in the morning and 3 min anytime of the day as required for 2 weeks	Acupressure at Houxi (SI3) No acupressure	Acute nausea and acute vomiting

Table 6.2 (continued)

Authors (year)	Included SR	Study design	Sample size	Type of cancer	Intervention(s)	Control	Outcome measures
Molassiotis et al. (2007)	Chao et al. (2009)	RCT	36	Breast cancer	Acupressure wristband for 5 days	No acupressure	Experience and intensity of emesis
Roscoe et al. (2005)	Chao et al. (2009)	RCT with 3 arms	63	Breast cancer	Electroacupuncture band for 5 days	Sham acupoint No electro-acupuncture	Daily emesis, episodes number, severity level
Gu et al. (2007)	Chao et al. (2009)	RCT with cross-over design	120	Breast cancer	Intravenously ondansetron 8 mg and dexamethasone 2.5 mg blocking both acupuncture points of ST36 once a day for 3 days	Intravenously both ondansetron 8 mg and dex-amethasone 5 mg 30 min before chemotherapy	Antiemetic rate
Ho (2006)	Chao et al. (2009)	RCT	60	Breast cancer	Self-digital acupressure plus mental support for 10 days	Mental support	Antiemetic rate
Xu et al. (2005)	Chao et al. (2009)	RCT	100	Breast cancer	Manual acupuncture injected drug ST36	Usual care (intramuscular injection)	Acute nausea and vomiting

Table 6.2 (continued)

Authors (year)	Included SR	Study design	Sample size	Type of cancer	Intervention(s)	Control	Outcome measures
Ning (2004)	Chao et al. (2009)	RCT	90	Breast cancer	Manual acupuncture therapy injected drug at ST36, ST6 and Hegu (LI4)	Manual acupuncture therapy injected in LI4, PC6	Antiemetic rating
Nystrom et al. (2008)	Chao et al. (2009)	Pre- and post-study	5	Breast cancer	Manual acupuncture therapy at PC6 for 10 times over 3 weeks	No acupuncture therapy	Nausea
Choo et al. (2006)	Chao et al. (2009)	Pre- and post-study	27	Breast cancer	Electroacupuncture 10 Hz at PC6 and ST36 for 10 min before chemotherapy and 20 min during chemotherapy	No control group	Acute nausea and vomiting

RCT randomized controlled trial

(Roscoe et al. 2005; Dibble et al. 2007; Molassiotis et al. 2007) were deemed to be of reasonably high quality, scoring three out of five using the modified Jade scale (Jadad et al. 1996). Consequently, this chapter discusses only the data from these three studies.

The SR analysed the data narratively without pooling. The detailed results of the SR are presented in a later section in this chapter.

6.3.3 New Trials

The details of the three newly identified trials are listed in Table 6.3.

6.3.4 Studies Examining Manual Acupuncture or Electroacupuncture

From the Cochrane SR, the following four studies assessed manual acupuncture and electroacupuncture. Manual acupuncture involves insertion and manual rotation of needles while electroacupuncture employs electrical stimulation *via* inserted needles.

Only one study used manual acupuncture and it failed to identify evidence that encouraged the use of manual acupuncture for treating CINV. Streitberger et al. (2003) examined whether manual acupuncture reduces chemotherapy-induced acute nausea and vomiting on 80 patients with various types of cancer. The acupuncture was applied at PC6 for 30 min both before the first chemotherapy session and the following day. Deqi sensation was elicited, which is a sensation that patients feel when the needle reaches the Qi level. The needle was left for 20 min without further manipulation. The control group received non-invasive placebo acupuncture at the same point. As for anti-emetics, all patients received 8 mg of 5-HT_3 without steroid. The result did not show a statistically significant benefit of acupuncture compared with the control ($p = 0.82$) concerning the occurrence of acute nausea and vomiting.

The following three studies assessed electroacupuncture but no indisputable evidence was found to promote the use of electroacupuncture for reducing CINV. In the three studies, all patients received anti-emetics following the ASCO guideline. A study by Shen et al. (2000) used three-armed parallel group design to compare: (1) low frequency (2–10 Hz) electroacupuncture at PC6 and ST36 points for 20 min, (2) acupuncture with fake electrostimulation, and (3) no acupuncture. One hundred and four females with breast cancer participated. The intervention was provided 2 h before chemotherapy every day over a 5-day period. A statistically significant reduction in the frequency of vomiting was found in the electroacupuncture group compared with the other two groups during the study period ($p < 0.001$). However, no significant difference was found in the follow-up period (6–9 days) regarding the number of vomiting episodes.

Table 6.3 Newly identified studies on acupoint stimulation

Author(s) and year of publication	Study design	Sample size	Type of patients	Intervention(s)	Control	Outcome measures
Melchart et al. (2006)	Randomized cross-over trial	28	Chemotherapy for stomach cancer, testicles cancer, esophagus cancer, lung cancer, and others	Acupuncture at PC6 once before chemotherapy for 20 min. Deqi was elicited Plus acupressure band at PC6 for 72 or 96 h Plus standard antiemetics	Sham point plus standard antiemetics	Nausea rate based on daily intensity rating
Gottschling et al. (2008)	Multicentre cross-over study	23	Children from 6 to 18 years of age with solid tumor who are going through chemotherapy	Acupuncture (or laser acupuncture) for 20 min on a first day preferably before chemotherapy started, and every day throughout the chemotherapy course Acupuncturists were allowed to tailor point combination Plus standard antiemetics	Antiemetics only	The average amount of 5-HT_3antagonists per day, number of vomiting, nausea score
Ladas et al. (2010)	Retrospective chart review	32	Patients with cancer treatment-related thrombocytopenia	Individualized acupuncture therapy based on traditional Chinese medicine treatment theory Used needles were 0.16 and 0.20 mm diameter (40 and 36 gauge) and 15, 30 or 40 mm length)	N/A	Adverse events

Dundee et al. (1987, 1988) reported two small studies with conflicting results. However, due to the small sample size in both studies, the results should be interpreted with caution. A first study by Dundee et al. (1987) examined acupressure at PC6. Deqi was elicited. Electroacupuncture was applied (10 Hz, pulse width 0–25 ms) using a DC stimulator. Ten patients with testicular cancer participated. The session was held for 5 to 6 times over 3 days. At least 8 h interval was maintained between each session. The control group received sham acupuncture in the right elbow. The result showed significant reduction of nausea in the group with acupuncture on PC6 over the acupuncture on sham point group ($p < 0.001$).

Another study by Dundee et al. (1988) used the same intervention involving 20 patients with various types of cancer. The session was held for 5 min prior to the chemotherapy or soon after the initiation of chemotherapy. The control group received only anti-emetics. There was no statistically significant group difference (risk ratio (RR) 0.50; 95% CI 0.17 to 1.46).

In the next section, the data are pooled, if appropriate, to determine the effectiveness of acupuncture and/or electroacupuncture according to acuity of nausea and vomiting. No other SRs or primary studies were identified from the search addressing the effectiveness of manual acupuncture or electroacupuncture for anticancer treatment-induced nausea and vomiting for all age groups.

6.3.4.1 Effects of Acupuncture or Electroacupuncture for Nausea and Vomiting Within 24 h

Since no new SRs or new primary studies were identified, the data presented by the Cochrane SR (2006) are deemed the most up-to-date evidence.

Only one study was identified that assessed manual acupuncture. The use of manual acupuncture (Streitberger et al. 2003) did not provide statistically significant effects on acute vomiting. Similarly, use of manual acupuncture did not provide significant reduction in severity of acute nausea (standard mean difference (SMD) 0.02; 95% CI −0.42 to 0.40; $p = 0.9$).

The Cochrane SR pooled the data from the three studies reporting on electroacupuncture. The electroacupuncture group indicated significantly fewer episodes of acute vomiting (57%) over the control group (80%) (RR 0.76; 95% CI 0.60 to 0.97; $p = 0.02$). The SR also pooled the data from all four studies to determine the overall effects of acupuncture involving insertion of needles (manual acupuncture and/or electroacupuncture) for CINV.

Acute vomiting occurred in 37% of the acupuncture group and 60% in the control group. The meta-analysis revealed that acupuncture alone or electroacupuncture can significantly reduce acute vomiting (RR 0.74; 95% CI 0.57 to 0.94; $p = 0.01$).

From these results, the following evidence is derived to guide practice:

- Electroacupuncture can be used to reduce chemotherapy-induced acute vomiting in conjunction with standardized anti-emetics.
- There is no reasonable evidence to encourage the use of manual acupuncture for reducing CINV. Further high quality studies are required.

- There is a lack of evidence supporting the use of electroacupuncture for reducing chemotherapy-induced acute nausea. More high quality studies are required.

6.3.4.2 Effects of Acupuncture or Electroacupuncture for Nausea and Vomiting after 24 h

Of the four acupuncture or electroacupuncture studies from the Cochrane SR, no studies reported on the outcomes concerning delayed nausea and vomiting that occurred 24 h or later after chemotherapy began. No new trial and no other SR was found that addressed delayed nausea and vomiting.

Judging by these results the following evidence statement can be drawn:

- No sufficient data were available to determine the effect of manual or electroacupuncture for reducing chemotherapy-induced delayed nausea and vomiting.

6.3.5 Studies Examining Acupressure

Acupressure involves pressure on the acupuncture point by finger or devices such as a small plastic button attached to a self-administering device. The Cochrane SR reviewed three studies reporting on the effects of acupressure for improving CINV and the SR by Chao et al. (2009) also reported a further two studies. Of five primary studies from the SRs, four reported favourable results for encouraging the use of acupressure while one study found a conflicting result.

Using a three-armed controlled trial design, Roscoe et al. (2003) compared bilateral acupressure band (SeaBand) on PC6 point, single acustimulation band (ReliefBand) and anti-emetics only (Roscoe et al. 2005). The study involved 747 patients who are receiving initial doxorubicin or cisplatin. The bilateral bands were worn on both wrists. The single acustimulation band was worn on one wrist but the patients were allowed to wear it on their wrist or alternated between wrists as desired. These patients were also allowed to the change level of stimulation between 10 to 35 mA as desired. Both bands were given to patients prior to the chemotherapy and they were worn for 5 days. All patients received anti-emetics as recommended in the ASCO guideline. The study indicated a favourable result for the acupressure group with significantly less acute nausea compared to the other two groups ($p<0.05$). For acute vomiting and delayed nausea or vomiting, no significant group differences were reported. Furthermore, acustimulation resulted in significantly less nausea and vomiting only in men ($p<0.05$) compared to the control group. Women showed less but not statistically significant acute nausea in the acupressure group compared to the control group ($p = 0.052$).

In a small study by Dibble et al. (2000), seventeen women with breast cancer were instructed to administer self-acupressure at PC6 and ST36 points for up to 3 min in the morning before chemotherapy and anytime throughout the day if required. The control group received only anti-emetics. Anti-emetics were administered following the ASCO guideline. The study highlighted significantly fewer episodes of nausea ($p < 0.01$) and nausea intensity ($p < 0.04$) in the acupressure group during the first 10 days of the chemotherapy cycle compared to the control group.

Another study by Dibble et al. (2007) was reviewed in the SR by Chao et al. (2009). The study involved in total 160 women with breast cancer receiving chemotherapy. The duration of follow-up was 21 days and it emerged that acupressure had a statistically significant effect in reducing the amount of delayed vomiting and delayed intensity of nausea. In contrast, no significant effects were demonstrated for acute nausea or vomiting compared with the sham point group and control group.

A study by Molassiotis et al. (2007) included in the SR by Chao et al. (2009) also reported favourable results supporting the use of acupressure. Thirty-six patients with breast cancer were allocated either to the SeaBand group or control group. SeaBand was worn for 5 days following chemotherapy. The result demonstrated acupressure provided beneficial effects by inducing fewer experiences of nausea and retching, and occurrence of nausea, vomiting and retching and distress were all significantly lower in the experimental group compared to the control group. The experience of vomiting was not statistically significant. Caution should be applied to these results due to the small sample size. The authors also noted that the use of standardized anti-emetics was not possible from day 2 to day 3 due to ethical considerations.

A study by Noga et al. (2002) from the Cochrane SR (Ezzo et al. 2006) reported a conflicting outcome. The study examined whether the use of an acupressure wrist band can reduce chemotherapy-induced acute nausea and vomiting and delayed nausea and vomiting. One hundred and twenty patients with hematologic cancer were involved. SeaBand was worn at PC6 for 24 h following chemotherapy. The control group received an acupressure band at a sham point. All patients received anti-emetics following the ASCO guideline. The result did not confirm beneficial effects that had been reported in other studies. The authors reported no significant group difference in patients' demographic data. No significant difference was found in the demographic data of patients in both groups. The authors called for further clinical trials with placebo-controlled design and investigation of the mechanism of acupressure on the human body.

6.3.5.1 Effects of Acupressure on Acute Nausea and Vomiting

The Cochrane SR conducted a meta-analysis using data from two studies (Dibble et al. 2000; Roscoe et al. 2005) that reported on the same outcome measures (mean severity of acute nausea). Other studies could not be pooled due to reported outcome measures at different time points. The pooled data showed that acupressure had a positive effect on reducing mean acute nausea severity over control within the first 24 h (SMD -0.19; 95% CI -0.37 to -0.01; $p = 0.04$).

Based on this result the following evidence statement can be made:

- The use of acupressure may reduce the severity of chemotherapy-induced acute nausea.

The data from three studies were combined to determine the effects on acute vomiting. Overall, 17% of patients in the acupressure group and 20% in control group had acute vomiting. However the difference was not statistically significant (RR 0.83; 95% CI 0.60 to 1.16; $p = 0.3$).

Based on this analysis, the following evidence statement can be elucidated:

- There is no strong evidence to support the use of acupressure band for reducing chemotherapy-induced acute vomiting.

6.3.5.2 Effects on Delayed Nausea and Vomiting

The following evidence statement can be drawn:

- No indisputable evidence was found to support or to discourage the use of acupressure for reducing chemotherapy-induced delayed nausea or vomiting.

In addition, Melchart et al. (2006) reported on the combination of acupuncture and acupressure for CINV but the study failed to demonstrate a beneficial effect of such a combination. Twenty-eight cancer patients were randomly allocated to the experimental group with a combination of acupuncture and acupressure at point PC6 while the control group used a close sham point. The study was conducted over one chemotherapy cycle. The study did not find any statistically significant difference between the experimental group and the control group at the sham point for the nausea score. The authors suggested that more large-scale studies are required.

6.3.6 Studies Examining Non-invasive Electrostimulation

Non-invasive electrostimulation provides electrostimulation on the surface of the skin without insertion of acupuncture needles or application of pressure on acupuncture point(s). The Cochrane SR reviewed five studies assessing non-invasive electrostimulation for reducing chemotherapy-induced nausea and/or vomiting. The SR by Chao et al. (2009) also reported on one new study. Overviews of all six studies are presented in the following section. These studies used transcutaneous electrical nerve stimulation (TENS) with wrist band on the PC6 point. Three studies reported some beneficial effects of non-invasive acustimulation for CINV, while two studies found no significant effects on nausea or vomiting at any time point during the study period.

A double-blind, placebo-controlled parallel-subjects trial with a follow-up crossover trial by Pearl et al. (1999) compared TENS with ReliefBand on PC6 and sham ReliefBand at the same point for managing chemotherapy-induced nausea and/or vomiting. Forty-two patients with gynaecologic cancer participated in the trial. All patients were given ReliefBand following their discharge from the hospital after chemotherapy and the band was worn for 7 days. All patients received anti-emetics as recommended in the ASCO guideline. Of these 42 patients, 32 were evaluable for the parallel-subjects component, 16 in each group. The percentage of patients with absent or minimal nausea was 59% overall, which was similar to that for both the active (56%) and placebo (62%) groups. The incidence and severity of nausea and vomiting was similar for each group. Eighteen patients completed two consecutive cycles and were evaluable for the cross-over component. The average age of the cross-over patients and their dose intensity were comparable with those of the overall study population (56.3 *vs* 58.6 years and 22.7 *vs* 22.7 mg/m^2/week, respectively). Overall, the percentage of cycles with absent or minimal nausea was 47%, which was similar to that of the active (50%) and placebo (44%) cycles. However, the severity of nausea was significantly less in the active cycles during days 2–4. Patients averaged less than one episode of vomiting daily in each cycle.

The study showed that the ReliefBand is an effective adjunct to standard anti-emetic agents for controlling nausea induced by cisplatin-based chemotherapy in gynecologic oncology patients.

Roscoe et al. (2002) reported that TENS had beneficial effects for delayed nausea and vomiting as well as less rescue anti-emetic pills being required. Their study compared the effects of TENS (ReliefBand) on the control group without any acu-stimulation. Forty-two patients with breast cancer, lung cancer, ovarian cancer or colorectal cancer were involved in this study. Patients in the experimental group wore the band before chemotherapy for as long as helpful. All patients received anti-emetics including ondansetron and granistron without dexamethasone. This was not consistent with the ASCO guideline. There was no statistically significant difference between the groups regarding the severity of nausea. The experimental group had less delayed nausea and vomiting compared with the control group ($p < 0.06$). The use of significantly less anti-emetic pills was reported in the experimental group ($p < 0.05$).

A study by Treish et al. (2003) also compared the effect of TENS using active ReliefBand and sham ReliefBand with 49 patients experiencing a range of cancers. The band was worn at the beginning of the chemotherapy session for 5 days. Both groups received an anti-emetics regimen that was consistent with the ASCO recommendation. The active ReliefBand group indicated significantly less overall vomiting ($p = 0.05$), overall retching ($p = 0.05$), and overall nausea severity ($p = 0.01$) over the five-day study period compared to the controls with sham ReliefBand. Furthermore, utilizing active ReliefBand significantly reduced delayed vomiting ($p = 0.032$) and acute nausea ($p = 0.028$) and delayed nausea ($p = 0.02$) periods. However, due to the small sample size, this result should be treated cautiously. The authors suggested larger and well-designed RCTs are required to build a strong evidence base.

The following three studies did not find any significant benefits of acustimulation for CINV at any time during the designated study periods.

The study by Roscoe et al. (2003) has already been addressed in the section on acupressure. The study failed to demonstrate that acustimulation had any positive effects in reducing CINV.

Another study by Roscoe et al. (2005) was reviewed by Chao et al. (2009). The study compared acustimulation wrist band (ReliefBand) with active stimulation, sham acustimulation, and no acustimulation in 96 women experiencing breast cancer. No significant difference was found in any outcomes including acute nausea, delayed nausea, vomiting, quality of life (QoL) and total amount of anti-emetic medication used.

A final study included in the Cochrane SR was conducted by McMillan et al. (1991). The study also compared TENS stimulation on PC6 and anti-emetics consisting of only 16 patients receiving chemotherapy for 5 consecutive days. The result failed to demonstrate that TENS had a significant benefit in reducing acute nausea (SMD −0.16; 95% CI −1.14 to 0.82).

6.3.6.1 Effects on Acute Nausea and Vomiting

The Cochrane SR pooled the data from five studies to determine the effect of non-invasive electrostimulation for reducing chemotherapy-induced acute nausea. The analysis showed no statistically significant effect (SMD −0.07; 95% CI −0.23 to 0.10; $p = 0.43$).

The data from two studies (Pearl et al. 1999; Roscoe et al. 2002) were pooled to determine the effect of non-invasive electrostimulation for reducing acute vomiting. The incident rate of acute vomiting in each group was 22% in the intervention group and 24% in the control group. No statistically significant effect was found (RR 0.90; 95% CI 0.67 to 1.19; $p = 0.45$) between the groups.

The later study by Roscoe et al. (2005) also reported that acustimulation for acute nausea and vomiting elicited a non-significant effect.

Based on these results, the following evidence statement can be made:

- There is no evidence to encourage the use of non-invasive electrostimulation for reducing chemotherapy-induced acute nausea and vomiting.

6.3.6.2 Effects on Delayed Nausea and Vomiting

The meta-analysis of all four studies demonstrated no significantly positive effects of non-invasive electrostimulation for delayed nausea (SMD 0.03; 95% CI −0.14 to 0.19; $p = 0.73$).

The data from two studies (Pearl et al. 1999; Roscoe et al. 2002) were pooled to determine the effect of non-invasive electrostimulation for delayed vomiting. The meta-analysis showed that non-invasive electrostimulation had no positive effects over the control group (SMD 0.06; 95% CI −0.11 to 0.22; $p = 0.49$) in regard to reducing delayed vomiting.

From these results, the following evidence statement can be made as follows:

- There is no evidence to encourage the use of non-invasive electrostimulation for reducing chemotherapy-induced delayed nausea and/or delayed vomiting.

6.3.7 All Acupoint-stimulation Methods

The Cochrane SR also pooled the data from all 11 studies to assess whether acupoint-stimulation regardless type of method, is effective in reducing CINV. The result showed that the incidence of acute vomiting had a statistically significant reduction (RR 0.82; 95% CI 0.69 to 0.99; $p = 0.04$). No significant reduction was reported in other outcomes including delayed vomiting, acute nausea and delayed nausea.

Based on this result, the following evidence statement can be established:

- Acupoint-stimulation regardless of type of stimulation method, may reduce chemotherapy-induced acute vomiting. However, it should be noted that any beneficial effects of each method have not yet been demonstrated yet except for electroacupuncture and acupressure.

6.3.8 Acupuncture for Pediatric Patients

One newly identified study examined whether acupuncture can reduce the necessity to use rescue anti-emetics for CINV in pediatric oncology patients.

Reindl et al. (2006) presented the preliminary results of their multicenter cross-over study at five tertiary hospitals in Germany. This was completed in 2008 and published in Gottschling et al. (2008). Therefore, the data from Reindl et al. (2006) was not reviewed. Nonetheless the report demonstrated promising findings that encourage the use of acupuncture in pediatric oncology.

In a cross-over trial reported by Gottschling et al. (2008), 23 children (13.6 ± 2.9 years of age) with solid malignant tumor were randomly allocated to acupuncture treatment during either the second or third identical chemotherapy course. All patients received standard anti-emetics. The acupuncture required significantly less rescue anti-emetics compared to the control ($p = 0.001$). Significantly fewer occurrences of vomiting were also reported ($p = 0.01$). Only four out of 23 patients reported pain from receiving a needle.

Based on this result, the following evidence statement can be developed:

- Acupuncture as a supportive anti-emetic approach may reduce the need for anti-emetic rescue medication during highly emetogenic chemotherapy in pediatric cancer patients. However, trials with a large sample size are required to develop a solid evidence base.

6.3.9 Safety of Acupoint-stimulation

One SR and one new trial reported on side effects caused by acupuncture. Overall, the studies found that acupuncture is safe to use for most patients.

Jindal et al.'s review (2008) of commonly reported adverse reactions caused by acupuncture was based on 22 clinical trials for patients of any age range and conditions. These included the following scenarios: sedation (32.05%), needle pain (26.33%), neuropathy/nervous system-related issues (15.96%), MSK/connective tissue-related issues (14.22%), puncture redness/irritation (6.94%), hematomas

Table 6.4 Primary studies from a systematic review: adverse events

Author(s) and year of publication	Total treatment number (acupoint-stimulation group plus sham group)	Type of acupoint-stimulation	Adverse events
Reindl et al. (2006)	11	Acupuncture	Needle pain ($n = 1$)
Butkovic et al. (2005)	120	Laser acupuncture	No AE reported
Wang and Kain (2002)	187	Acupuncture	No AE reported
Rusy et al. (2002)	80	Electroacupuncture	No AE reported
Somri et al. (2001)	30	Acupuncture	Unscheduled overnight hospital admission ($n = 1$)
Shenkman et al. (1999)	100	Acupressure and acupuncture	Puncture redness and irritation ($n = 10$ from experimental group) Puncture redness ($n = 8$ from sham group)
Schlager et al. (1998)	80	Laser acupuncture	No AE reported
Ng et al. (2004)	1,008	Acupuncture	Numbness at acupuncture site (Experimental group $n = 3$), headache ($n = 1$), light headedness ($n = 1$) Numbness at acupuncture site from sham acupuncture group ($n = 2$)
Radmayr et al. (2001)	249	Laser acupuncture	Light headedness ($n = 2$)

AE adverse event

(1.04%), feelings of faintness/sycope (1.04%), vascular disorder (0.69%), hysterectomy (0.35%), headache (0.35%) and unscheduled overnight hospital admission (0.35%).

From nine clinical trials involving 782 pediatric patients (2–18 years of age) (Schlager et al. 1998; Shenkman et al. 1999; Radmayr et al. 2001; Somri et al. 2001; Rusy et al. 2002; Wang and Kain 2002; Alimi et al. 2003; Butkovic et al. 2005; Reindl et al. 2006), a total of 29 acupuncture/sham adverse events were reported caused by acupuncture (incidence rate 1.55 per 100 acupuncture treatments). The most common adverse reaction in pediatric patients was puncture redness. The risk of serious adverse event was 5.36/10,000 treatments in pediatrics and 0.05/10,000 treatments in the overall population. The details of nine studies are presented in Table 6.4.

Table 6.5 An included systematic review: moxibustion

Author(s) and year of publication	Included study design(s)	Number of included studies	Type of cancer	Intervention(s)	Outcome measures
Lee et al. (2010b)	RCTs	In total five studies were reviewed and two studies reported on nausea and vomiting	Any type of cancer	Moxibustion as an adjunct therapy for conventional medicine	Chemotherapy induced nausea and vomiting, response rate, quality of life

RCT randomized controlled trial

A more recently published retrospective chart review (Ladas et al. 2010) concerned 32 patients (237 acupuncture sessions) undergoing treatment for cancer or stem cell transplantation. Japanese J-type Seirin needles were inserted at 0.5-cun depth, with mild manual stimulation. Of these patients, many had thrombocytopenia including severe (20%), moderate (8%) and mild (19%) thrombocytopenia. However, no bleeding side effects were reported.

From these results, the following evidence statement is developed:

- Acupuncture can be considered a safe treatment method for both adults and pediatric patients. However, clinicians should be aware of possible adverse events so that they can provide timely interventions.

6.4 Results for Moxibustion

Lee et al. (2010a) published a SR of clinical trials examining the effectiveness of moxibustion for managing cancer. In addition, Lee et al. (2010b) recently published an umbrella review of existing SRs on various clinical conditions. Because of overlapping and duplication of findings on nausea and vomiting in anticancer treatment, only the data from the first SR (Lee et al. 2010a) is reported here. The detailed information on the SR (Lee et al. 2010a) is summarised in Table 6.5.

Further information on the included primary studies in the SR by Lee et al. (2010b) is presented in Table 6.6.

6.4.1 A Systematic Review by Lee et al. (2010)

The major databases searched included MEDLINE, EMBASE, AMED, Cochrane Library, Scopus and CINAHL for studies published up to June 2007. The review identified the following two trials.

One RCT by Chen et al. (2000) compared salt-separated moxibustion on Shenque (CV8) with control. Fifty-six patients with stages III and IV of nasopharyngeal carcinoma were involved and all underwent radiotherapy and chemotherapy according to

Table 6.6 Primary studies from a systematic review: effectiveness of moxibustion

Author(s) and year of publication	Included SR	Study design	Number of participants	Patients type	Intervention(s)	Use of sham	Control	Outcome measures	Adverse event
Chen et al. (2000)	Lee et al. (2010b)	RCT	56	Gastric cancer patients receiving chemotherapy and radiotherapy	Moxibustion once a day for 30 days. Plus antiemetics	No	Antiemetics	Nausea and vomiting	Not reported
Cao et al. (1997)	Lee et al. (2010b)	RCT	36	Gastric cancer patients receiving chemotherapy	Moxibustion three times per week	No	Antiemetics	Nausea and vomiting	Not reported

RCT randomized controlled trial

the AD protocol. The experimental group received the moxibustion on 30 occasions from the beginning of the radiotherapy and chemotherapy sessions. The experimental group showed significantly less occurrence of side effects than the control group ($p < 0.05$).

The other study concerned a three-armed trial involving 36 patients with gastric cancer (Cao et al. 1997). The patients were randomly assigned to the following groups: moxibustion on CV8 three times per week, control, and drug therapies for side effects. The analysis showed that the moxibustion group received a significant benefit ($p < 0.05$) compared to the other groups.

6.4.1.1 Effects of Moxibustion

The data from the two trials were pooled to determine the effectiveness of moxibustion for reducing cancer treatment-induced nausea and vomiting. A moxibustion group ($n = 80$) experienced significantly less frequency of nausea and vomiting caused by chemotherapy (RR 0.38, 95% CI 0.22 to 0.65; $p = 0.0005$, heterogeneity: chi square 0.18, $p = 0.67$, $I^2 = 0\%$).

From these results, the following evidence statement is developed:

- The use of moxibustion may be effective for reducing nausea and vomiting induced by cancer therapies. However, the methodological quality of the included two studies is not high. More RCTs with large sample sizes are required to develop a strong evidence base to justify the use of moxibustion in cancer care.

6.4.2 *Safety of Moxibustion*

The existing trials did not report on adverse effects caused by moxibustion. High quality clinical trials are required to determine the safety of moxibustion for cancer patients who undergo chemotherapy.

6.5 Mechanism of Acupuncture and Moxibustion on Anti-nausea and Vomiting

The mechanisms behind the beneficial anti-emetic impacts of acupuncture are well explained by Takahashi (2011), largely based on its neuromodulation effect in the gut. This paper proposes that acupuncture stimulation of somatosensory neurons activates various nuclei at the CNS, including the nucleus tractus solitarius (NTS), the dorsal motor nucleus of vagi (DMV), the rostral ventrolateral medulla (RVLM), and periaqueductal gray (PAG). Activation of the NTS, DMV and RVLM modulates the imbalance between sympathetic and parasympathetic activity. Opioid released from the PAG is involved in mediating the anti-emetic and anti-nociceptive effects of acupuncture.

Acupuncture treatment involves the insertion of thin needles into the skin and underlying muscle and the subsequent manual or electrical stimulation of the needles. Thus, acupuncture stimulates the somatic afferent nerves of the skin and muscles. Somatic sensory information from the body is carried to the cortex area of the brain. Somatic sensory fibers also project to the various nuclei at the brain stem and hypothalamus. Through the process of somato-autonomic reflex, acupuncture modulates various biomechanical responses, such as prokinetic, anti-emetic, and anti-nociceptive effects (Takahashi 2011).

The role of polymodal receptors (PMRs) has also been emphasized based on the fact that PMRs are responsive to both acupuncture and moxibustion stimuli. Thermal sensitivity is essential in moxibustion therapy, and the characteristics of acupuncture points and trigger points are similar to those of sensitized PMRs. Axon reflexes mediated by PMRs may represent the mechanism whereby acupuncture and moxibustion trigger immediate action (Lin and Chen 2008).

Experiments in healthy human subjects have shown that electrical stimulation of acupuncture points may enhance the regularity of gastric myoelectrical activity. For example electroacupuncture at PC6 reduces gastric tachyarrhymia in vection-induced motion sickness in healthy volunteers (Hu et al. 1992). Combined acupuncture at ST36 and PC6 increases the percentage of regular slow waves, resulting in the normalization of arrhythmia in healthy humans (Lin et al. 1997). However, the mechanisms of acupuncture's anti-emetic effect were not explained in these studies.

Published data from experimental studies imply the evidence that acupuncture does have an anti-emetic effect. The level of plasma arginine vasopressin is rapidly elevated in response to diverse emetic stimuli such as motion stimuli (Kim et al. 1997) and anticancer drugs (Edwards et al. 1989; Cubeddu et al. 1990). Intravenous injection of vasopressin results in vomiting and retching in humans (Kim et al. 1997) and dogs (Carpenter et al. 1984; Chen et al. 2003). Acupuncture at ST36 and PC6 attenuates symptom scores of emesis induced by vasopressin infusion in dogs (Chen et al. 2003). Retrograde propulsive movement is closely linked to the frequency of retching and vomiting. Electroacupuncture at PC6 reduces the frequency of retrograde propulsive movement induced by vasopressin in dogs (Tatewaki et al. 2005).

Studies investigating the relationship between acupuncture and endogenous opiates (beta-endorphin, enkephalin, endomorphin and dynorphin) agreed with the contention that in normal animal models, lower frequency electroacupuncture stimulates the release of beta-endorphin, enkephalin and endomorphin, which in turn activates the mu- and delta-opioid receptors. Further higher frequency electroacupuncture stimulates dynorphin which activates the kappa-opioid receptor (Lin and Chen 2008). Opioids have dual effects—an anti-emetic effect as well as an emetic effect. It has been shown that central opioid plays a major role in mediating the anti-emetic effect (Costello and Borison 1977). The emetic effect is mediated *via* the chemoreceptor trigger zone (CTZ), whereas the anti-emetic effect is mediated *via* the vomiting center (Costello and Borison 1977; Blancquaert et al. 1986; Foss et al. 1998). The CTZ is contained in the area postrema on the caudal margin of the fourth ventricle. Since the area postrema has no blood brain barrier, naloxone methiodide (a peripheral opioid antagonist) can antagonize the emetic effect of opioid mediated *via* the CTZ. In contrast, the vomiting center is located deep beneath the solitary

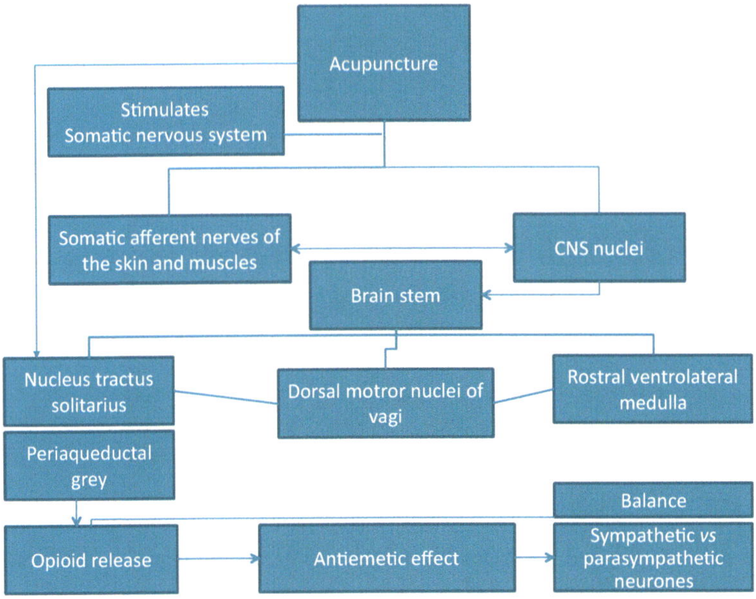

Fig. 6.1 Illustration of anti-emetic mechanism of acupuncture point stimulation

tract of the caudal brain stem. Both the emetic and anti-emetic effects of opioid can be blocked by naloxone, because naloxone can cross the blood brain barrier (Foss et al. 1998).

Naloxone hydrochloride, but not naloxone methiodide, abolishes the anti-emetic effect of electroacupuncture at PC6 in dogs (Tatewaki et al. 2005). This suggests that the anti-emetic effect of electroacupuncture at PC6 is mediated *via* the central opioid pathway.

Figure 6.1 is a visual presentation of the anti-emetic mechanism of acupuncture point stimulation.

To sum up, it has been stated with reference to traditional Chinese medicine, that "acupuncture is believed to restore the balance of yin and yang". This has been translated into Western medical terminology as meaning: "Acupuncture modulates the imbalance between parasympathetic and sympathetic activity" (Takahashi 2011). Acupuncture may be effective in patients with functional gastrointestinal (GI) disorders and in particular nausea and vomiting due to chemotherapy. This is because it has a neuromodulation effect on GI motility and the mechanism involving endogenous opiates (Takahashi 2011).

6.6 Practical Guidelines for Clinicians

The best-practical methods/procedures for various types of acupoint-stimulation have not been fully investigated using a rigorous scientific approach. More well-designed studies are required to determine factors related to the best outcomes such as best timing, length, duration and frequency for providing such interventions to reduce anticancer treatment-induced nausea and vomiting. The following guideline has been developed based on the reviewed trials and available guidelines provided by various professional bodies.

For any type of acupressure-point stimulation, patients should be fully informed about the benefits and possible harm. Clinicians should be aware of the risk of a serious adverse event such as pneumothorax and appropriate safeguards should be in place.

6.6.1 Practical Guideline for Manual or Electroacupuncture

Based on the available evidence, the following recommendations can be made for reducing CINV:

- **Patient type:** Patients with breast cancer, testicular cancer or possibly other types of cancer. Cancer patients with prior history of CINV. WHO (http://apps.who.int/medicinedocs/en/d/Js4926e/6.html) also recommends the use for radiotherapy-induced nausea and vomiting. Contraindication could be the site of a tumor or metastatic limbs with lymphedema, areas with considerable anatomic distortion due to surgery. Careful consideration is required in applying to patients with thrombocytopenia, coagulatopathy or nuetropenia.
- **Acupuncture point(s):** PC6 alone or with ST36.
- **Needle type:** Sterile single use needles.
- **Insertion technique:** From available studies, no strong scientific evidence was found regarding insertion technique. However, Deqi sensation should be elicited.
- **Length and timing of procedure:** Preferably before chemotherapy (5 min to 2 h before chemotherapy) for 20 min for 5 days or longer.
- **Electrostimulation:** 2 to 10 Hz.
- **Anti-emetics:** The anti-emetics should be provided following the ASCO guideline.

6.6.2 Practical Guideline for Acupressure

Based on the available evidence, the following recommendations can be drawn for reducing CINV:

- **Patient type:** Patients with breast cancer or patients with cancer who receive doxorubicin or cisplatin. Patients with prior history of chemotherapy induced nausea and vomiting.
- **Acupuncture point(s):** PC6 or possibly with ST36.

- **Length and timing of procedure:** Acupressure band or self acupressure device should be used before the commencement of chemotherapy for 3–6 min. Patients should be encouraged to use the acupressure as desired for 5 days or longer.
- **Others:** The anti-emetics should be provided following the ASCO guideline.

6.6.3 Practical Guideline for Non-invasive Electrostimulation

Due to the lack of scientific evidence on the efficacy of non-invasive electrostimulation for controlling anticancer treatment-induced nausea and vomiting, clinicians' judgement is required when introducing non-invasive electrostimulation for patients. Other types of acupuncture-point stimulation are recommended including electroacupuncture and acupressure based on available evidence:

- **Patient type:** Patients with breast cancer, lung cancer, gynaecologic cancer, or colorectal cancer patients who had previous history of CINV. Possibly patients with other types of cancer may be also considered.
- **Acupuncture point:** PC6.
- **Length and timing of procedure:** TENS device such as a ReliefBand should be worn before chemotherapy or soon after chemotherapy for 5–7 days or as long as patient feels that it is helping.
- **Intensity of stimulation:** Patients should be allowed to adjust the strength by turning the dial from 10–35 mA.
- **Others:** The anti-emetics should be provided in accordance with the ASCO guideline.

6.6.4 Practical Guideline for Pediatric Patients

Based on the available evidence, the following recommendations can be made for clinicians:

- **Patient type:** Patients aged from six to eighteen with solid malignant tumor or possibly other types of cancer.
- **Acupuncture point:** PC6.
- **Length and timing of procedure:** Acupuncture (or laser acupuncture if needle pain is felt) for 20 min on a first day preferably before chemotherapy starts, and every day throughout the chemotherapy course.
- The standard anti-emetics based on the ASCO guideline should be administered.

6.6.5 Practical Guideline for Moxibustion

Again, due to the extremely limited number of high quality studies reporting on the efficacy of moxibustion and the effective practical methods for applying moxibustion, strong recommendations are not possible. Again, well-designed large scale studies are required to develop the scientific evidence base to promote the use of moxibustion for oncological care:

- **Patients:** Patients who undergo anticancer treatments such as chemotherapy and/or radiotherapy for nasopharyngeal cancer, gastric cancer or possibly other types of cancer.
- **Moxibustion point:** CV8.
- **Type of moxibustion treatment:** Only "indirect method" was reported (indirect placement of moxibustion on some insulating material such as ginger, sale or others).
- **Timing and frequency:** At the beginning of the anticancer treatment, three times or more up to around 30 times throughout the treatment.
- **Types of grass:** No sufficient evidence was identified from available reports but salt-separated moxibustion was used.

6.7 Conclusion

This chapter has provided a review of currently available evidence on the efficacy and safety of acupuncture and moxibustion for reducing anticancer treatment-induced nausea and vomiting. All trials accessed acupuncture-point stimulation as an adjunct therapy for standardized anti-emetic drugs. Overall, evidence supports the use of acupoint-stimulation for reducing CINV in both adult and pediatric cancer patients with very low risk of serious adverse events. However, reasonably strong evidence is available only for electroacupuncture and acupressure on PC6. Electroacupuncture on PC6 can reduce acute nausea and vomiting while acupressure on PC6 is effective for reducing acute nausea. No indisputable scientific evidence was found to promote or discourage the use of manual acupuncture or non-invasive acupoint stimulation method. Some evidence supports the use of moxibustion but further studies are required to determine the levels of safety in clinical application. A lack of well-designed studies with a large sample size is a serious issue for developing a solid evidence base where acupuncture and moxibustion can be used widely.

References

Alimi, D., Rubino, C., Pichard-Léandri, E., Fermand-Brulé, S., Dubreuil-Lemaire, M. L., & Hill, C. (2003). Analgesic effect of auricular acupuncture for cancer pain: A randomized, blinded, controlled trial. *Journal of Clinical Oncology: Official Journal of the American Society of Clinical Oncology*, *21*, 4120–4126.

Allais, G., Rolando, S., Castagnoli, G. I., Burzio, C., Airola, G., Borgogno, P., et al. (2012). Acupressure in the control of migraine-associated nausea. *Neurology Science*, *33*, S207–S210.

Blancquaert, J., Lefebvre, R. A., & Willems, J. L. (1986). Emetic and antiemetic effects of opioids in the dog. *European Journal of Pharmacology*, *128*, 143–150.

Butkovic, D., Toljan, S., Matolic, M., Kralik, S., & Radesić, L. (2005). Comparison of laser acupuncture and metoclopramide in PONV prevention in children. *Paediatric Anaesthesia, 15*, 37–40.

Cao, J., Xiao, X. H., & Tang, X. Y. (1997). Elemene fluorouracil Moxibustion "Shenque" effect in the treatment of advanced gastric cancer observed. *Chinese Journal of Clinical Oncology, 24*, 549–550.

Carpenter, D., Briggs, D. B., & Strominger, N. (1984). Peptide-induced emesis in dogs. *Behavioural Brain Research, 11*, 277–281.

Cassileth, B., Deng, G. E., Gomez, J. E., Johnstone, P. A., Kumar, N., & Vickers, A. J. (2007). American College of Chest Physicians. Complementary therapies and integrative oncology in lung cancer: ACCP evidence-based clinical practice guidelines (2nd ed.). *Chest, 132*, 340S–354S.

Chao, L., Zhang, A. L., Liu, H. E., Cheng, M. H., Lam, H. B., & Lo, S. K. (2009). The efficacy of acupoint stimulation for the management of therapy-related adverse events in patients with breast cancer: A systematic review. *Breast Cancer Research and Treatment, 118*, 255–267.

Chen, K., Jiang, Y., Wen, H., Lu, X. Z., Lu, L., Wang, H. et al. (2000). Clinical study on treatment of nasopharyngeal carcinoma by radio and chemotherapy with supplementary moxibustion on Shenque point. *Chinese Journal of Integrative Medicine, 20*, 733–735.

Choo, S., Kong, K., Lim, W., Gao, F., Chua, K., & Leong, S. (2006). Electroacupuncture for Refractory Acute Emesis Caused by Chemotherapy. *The Journal of Alternative and Complementary Medicine, 12*, 963–969.

Chen, J., Qian, L., Ouyang, H., & Yin, J. (2003). Gastric electrical stimulation with short pulses reduces vomiting but not dysrhythmias in dogs. *Gastroenterology, 124*, 401–409.

Costello, D. J., & Borison, H. L. (1977). Naloxone antagonizes narcotic self blockade of emesis in the cat. *The Journal of Pharmacology and Experimental Therapeutics, 203*, 222–230.

Cubeddu, L., Lindley, C. M., Wetsel, W., Carl, P. L., & Negro-Vilar, A. (1990). Role of angiotensin II and vasopressin in cisplatin-induced emesis. *Life Sciences, 46*, 699–705.

Deng, G., Cassileth, B. R., Cohen, L., Gubili, J., Johnstone, P. A., & Kumar, N. (2007). Society for integrative oncology executive committee. Integrative oncology practice guidelines. *Journal of the Society for Integrative Oncology, 5*, 65–84.

Dibble, S. L., Chapman, J., Mack, K. A., & Shih, A. S. (2000). Acupressure for nausea: Results of a pilot study. *Oncology Nursing Forum, 27*, 41–47.

Dibble, S. L., Luce, J., Cooper, B. A., Israel, J., Cohen, M., Nussey, B., et al. (2007) Acupressure for chemotherapy induced nausea and vomiting: A randomized clinical trial. *Oncology Nursing Forum, 34*, 813–820.

Dundee, J., Ghaly, R. G., Fitzpatrick, K. T., Lynch, G. A., & Abram, W. P. (1987). Acupuncture to prevent cisplatin-associated vomiting. *Lancet, 1*, 1083.

Dundee, J., Sourial, F. B., Ghaly, R. G., & Bell, P. F. (1988). P6 acupressure reduces morning sickness. *Journal of the Royal Society of Medicine, 81*, 456–457.

Edwards, C., Carmichael, J., Baylis, P. H., & Harris, A. L. (1989). Arginine vasopressin—a mediator of chemotherapy induced emesis? *British Journal of Cancer, 59*, 467–470.

Ezzo, J., Richardso, M. A., Vickers, A., Allen, C., Dibble, S. L., Issell, B. F., et al. (2006). Acupuncture-point stimulation for chemotherapy-induced nausea or vomiting. *Cochrane Database of Systematic Reviews (Online), 19*, CD002285.

Foss, J., Yuan, C. S., Roizen, M. F., & Goldberg, L. P. (1998). Prevention of apomorphine- or cisplatin-induced emesis in the dog by a combination of methylnaltrexone and morphine. *Cancer Chemotherapy and Pharmacology, 42*, 287–291.

Gottschling, S., Reindl, T. K., Meyer, S., Berrang, J., Henze, G., Graeber, S., et al. (2008). Acupuncture to alleviate chemotherapy-induced nausea and vomiting in pediatric oncology—a randomized multicenter crossover pilot trial. *Klinische Pädiatrie, 220*, 365–370.

Gu, S., Yang, J., & Zhang, M. (2007). Contrast study for the effects of different administration route of dexamethasone on gastrointestinal reaction induced by chemotherapy. *Advanced Nursing, 22*, 399–400.

Ho, Y. F. (2006). Acupressure and psychological intervention for emesis due to chemotherapy on the patients with mammary cancer. *Guangxi Medical Journal, 28*, 738–739.

Hu, S., Stern, R. M., & Koch, K. L. (1992). Electrical acustimulation relieves vection-induced motion sickness. *Gastroenterology, 102*, 1854–1858.

Jadad, A., Moore, R. A., Carroll, D., Jenkinson, C., Reynolds, D. J., Gavaghan, D. J., et al. (1996). Assessing the quality of reports of randomized clinical trials: Is blinding necessary? *Controlled Clinical Trials, 17*, 1–12.

Jindal, V., Ge, A., & Mansky, P. J. (2008). Safety and efficacy of acupuncture in children: A review of the evidence. *Journal of Pediatric Hematology/Oncology, 30*, 431–442.

Kim, M., Chey, W. D., Owyang, C., & Hasler, W. L. (1997). Role of plasma vasopressin as a mediator of nausea and gastric slow wave dysrhythmias in motion sickness. *The American Journal of Physiology, 272*, G853–G862.

Ladas, E., Rooney, D., Taromina, K., Ndao, D. H., & Kelly, K. M. (2010). The safety of acupuncture in children and adolescents with cancer therapy-related thrombocytopenia. *Supportive Care in Cancer: Official Journal of the Multinational Association of Supportive Care in Cancer, 18*, 1487–1490.

Lee, M., Choi, T. Y., Park, J. E., Lee, S. S., & Ernst, E. (2010a) Moxibustion for cancer care: A systematic review and meta-analysis. *BMC Cancer, 10*, 130.

Lee, M., Kang, J. W., & Ernst, E. (2010b) Does moxibustion work? An overview of systematic reviews. *BMC Research Notes, 3*, 284.

Lin, J., & Chen, W. (2008). Acupuncture analgesia: A review of its mechanisms of actions. *The American Journal of Chinese Medicine, 36*, 635–645.

Lin, X., Liang, J., Ren, J., Mu, F., Zhang, M., & Chen, J. (1997). Electrical stimulation of acupuncture points enhances gastric myoelectrical activity in humans. *American Journal of Gastroenterology, 92*, 1527–1530.

Ma, L. (2009) Acupuncture as a complementary therapy in chemotherapy-induced nausea and vomiting. *Proceedings of the Baylor University Medical Center, 22*, 138–141.

Manheimer, E., Wieland, S., Kimbrough, E., Cheng, K., & Berman, B. M. (2009). Evidence from the cochrane collaboration for traditional chinese medicine therapies. *The Journal of Alternative and Complementary Medicine, 15*, 1001–1014.

McMillan, C., Dundee, J. W., & Abram, W. P. (1991). Enhancement of the antiemetic action of ondansetron by transcutaneous electrical stimulation of the P6 antiemetic point, in patients having highly emetic cytotoxic drugs. *British Journal of Cancer, 64*, 971–972.

Melchart, D., Ihbe-Heffinger, A., Leps, B., von Schilling, C., & Linde, K. (2006). Acupuncture and acupressure for the prevention of chemotherapy-induced nausea-a randomised cross-over pilot study. *Supportive Care in Cancer: Official Journal of the Multinational Association of Supportive Care in Cancer, 14*, 878–882.

Molassiotis, A., Helin, A. M., Dabbour, R., & Hummerston, S. (2007). The effects of P6 acupressure in the prophylaxis of chemotherapy-related nausea and vomiting in breast cancer patients. *Complementary Therapies in Medicine, 15*, 3–12.

Ng, D. K., Chow, P., & Ming, S. (2004). A double-blind, randomized, placebo-controlled trial of acupuncture for the treatment of childhood persistent allergic rhinitis. *Pediatrics, 114*, 1242–1247.

Ning, C. H. (2004). Contrast observation on injection metoclopramide in different acupuncture point for the treatment of emesis after chemical treatment to mammary cancer. *Guiding Journal of Traditional Chinese Medicine and Pharmacology, 10*, 39–41.

Noga, S., Tolman, A., & Roman, J. (2002). Acupressure as an adjunct to pharmacologic control of nausea, vomiting and retching (N/V) during blood and marrow transplantation (BMT): A randomized, placebo-controlled, algorithm based study. *Proceedings of the American Society of Clinical Oncology, 21*, 361a.

Nystrom, E., Ridderstrom, G., & Leffler, A. (2008). Manual acupuncture as an adjunctive treatment of nausea in patients with cancer in palliative care—a prospective, observational pilot study. *Acupuncture in Medicine, 26*, 27–32.

Pearl, M., Fischer, M., McCauley, D. L., Valea, F. A., & Chalas, E. (1999). Transcutaneous electrical nerve stimulation as an adjunct for controlling chemotherapy-induced nausea and vomiting in gynecologic oncology patients. *Cancer Nursing, 22*, 307–311.

Radmayr, C., Schlager, A., Studen, M., & Bartsch, G. (2001). Prospective randomized trial using laser acupuncture versus desmopressin in the treatment of nocturnal enuresis. *European Urology, 40*, 201–205.
Reindl, T., Geilen, W., Hartmann, R., Wiebelitz, K. R., Kan, G., Wilhelm, I., et al. (2006). Acupuncture against chemotherapy-induced nausea and vomiting in pediatric oncology. Interim results of a multicenter crossover study. *Support Care Cancer, 14*, 172–176.
Roscoe, J., Morrow, G., & Bushunow, P. (2002). Acustimulation wristbands for the relief of chemotherapy-induced nausea. *Alternative Therapies in Health and Medicine, 8*, 56–63.
Roscoe, J. A., Morrow, G. R., Hickok, J. T., Bushunow, P., Pierce, H. I., Flynn, P. J., et al. (2003). The efficacy of acupressure and acustimulation wrist bands for the relief of chemotherapy-induced nausea and vomiting. *Journal of Pain and Symptom Management, 26*, 731–742.
Roscoe, J., Matteson, S. E., Morrow, G. R., Hickok, J. T., Bushunow, P., Griggs, J., et al. (2005). Acustimulation wrist bands are not effective for the control of chemotherapy-induced nausea in women with breast cancer. *Journal of Pain and Symptom Management, 29*, 376–384.
Rusy, L. M., Hoffman, G. M., & Weisman, S. J. (2002). Electroacupuncture prophylaxis of postoperative nausea and vomiting following pediatric tonsillectomy with or without adenoidectomy. *Anesthesiology, 96*, 300–305.
Schlager, A., Offer, T., & Baldissera, I. (1998). Laser stimulation of acupuncture point P6 reduces postoperative vomiting in children undergoing strabismus surgery. *British Journal of Anaesthesia, 81*, 529–532.
Shen, J., Wenger, N., Glaspy, J., Hays, R. D., Albert, P. S., Choi, C., et al. (2000). Electroacupuncture for control of myeloablative chemotherapy-induced emesis: A randomized controlled trial. *JAMA: The Journal of the American Medical Association, 284*, 2755–2761.
Shenkman, Z., Holzman, R. S., Kim, C., Ferrari, L. R., DiCanzio, J., Highfield, E. S., et al. (1999). Acupressure-acupuncture antiemetic prophylaxis in children undergoing tonsillectomy. *Anesthesiology, 90*, 1311–1316.
Somri, M., Vaida, S. J., Sabo, E., Yassain, G., Gankin, I., & Gaitini, L. A. (2001). Acupuncture versus ondansetron in the prevention of postoperative vomiting. A study of children undergoing dental surgery. *Anaesthesia, 56*, 972–932.
Streitberger, K., Friedrich-Rust, M., Bardenheuer, H., Unnebrink, K., Windeler, J., Goldschmidt, H., et al. (2003). Effect of acupuncture compared with placebo-acupuncture at P6 as additional antiemetic prophylaxis in high-dose chemotherapy and autologous peripheral blood stem cell transplantation: A randomized controlled single-blind trial. *Clinical Cancer Research: An Official Journal of The American Association for Cancer Research, 9*, 2538–2544.
Takahashi, T. (2011). Mechanism of acupuncture on neuromodulation in the gut—a review. *Neuromodulation, 14*, 8–12 (discussion 12).
Tatewaki, M., Strickland, C. & Fukuda, H. (2005). Effects of acupuncture on vasopressin-induced emesis in conscious dogs. *American Journal of Physiology, Regulatory, Integrative and Comparative Physiology, 288*, R401–R408.
Treish, I., Shord, S., Valgus, J., Harvey, D., Nagy, J., Stegal, J., et al. (2003). Randomized double-blind study of the Reliefband as an adjunct to standard antiemetics in patients receiving moderately-high to highly emetogenic chemotherapy. *Support Care Cancer, 11*, 516–521.
Urroz, P., Colagiuri, B., Smith, C. A., & Cheema, B. S. (2012). Effect of acute acupuncture treatment on exercise performance and postexercise recovery: a systematic review. *Journal of Alternative and Complementary Medicine*, in press.
Wang, S. M., & Kain, Z. N. (2002). P6 acupoint injections are as effective as droperidol in controlling early postoperative nausea and vomiting in children. *Anesthesiology, 97*, 359–366.
World Health Organization. (2003). Acupuncture: Review and analysis of reports on controlled clinical trials: 87. Geneva: World Health Organization.
Xu, Y., Wang, J. L., & Du, H. Y. (2005). Contrast observation on injection metoclopramide in acupuncture point for the treatment of emesis after chemical treatment to 100 patients with cancer. *Central Plains Medical Journal, 32*, 58.
Zhang, J., Shang, H., Gao, X., & Ernst, E. (2010). Acupuncture-related adverse events: A systematic review of the Chinese literature. *Bull World Health Organ, 88*, 915C–921C.

Chapter 7
Acupuncture and Moxibustion for Side Effects of Chemotherapy in Cancer Patients

Jillian L. Capodice, Mitchell C. Benson and Dawn L. Hershman

Abstract This chapter introduces the major classes of chemotherapeutic drugs, including the alkylating agents, antimetabolites, vinca alkaloids, taxanes, antibiotics, hormone analogs and targeted drugs. The mechanisms of a number of chemotherapy-induced side effects such as nausea and emesis, cancer-related pain, peripheral neuropathy and vasomotor symptoms (e.g. hot flashes) are outlined. A detailed literature review expounds some of the major studies that have tested acupuncture and moxibustion as potential treatments for chemotherapy-induced side effects, including the use of acupuncture and moxibustion for chemotherapy-induced nausea and vomiting, peripheral neuropathy in patients receiving platinum and taxane-based regimens, vasomotor symptoms (hot flashes) in breast cancer patients receiving adjuvant hormonal therapy and prostate cancer patients receiving androgen deprivation therapy.

7.1 Introduction

Conventional treatment of cancer includes surgery, radiation, chemotherapy, immunotherapy and an array of other therapies such as bone marrow transplantation and gene therapy. Chemotherapy is the administration of drugs aimed at destroying cancer cells in order to have a beneficial effect on the history of the illness. Chemotherapy aims to arrest tumor progression and the ultimate goal of chemotherapy is a cure, defined as long-term, disease-free survival (Longo et al. 2012).

The landscape and practice of medical oncology has changed in the past 20 years as curative treatments have been discovered for several malignancies including testicular cancer and some leukemias and lymphomas (Brunton et al. 2011). Neo-adjuvant, adjuvant chemotherapy and hormonal treatments have been shown to increase disease-free survival and reduce recurrence in many cancers such as breast, colorectal and lung cancers. Molecular targeted drugs and immunotherapy are the newest medicines in the armamentarium of cancer chemotherapy treatments.

J. L. Capodice (✉) · M. C. Benson · D. L. Hershman
Department of Medicine, Columbia University, 10th Floor,
161 Fort Washington Avenue, New York, NY 10032, USA
e-mail: jc2346@columbia.edu

W. C. S. Cho (ed.), *Acupuncture and Moxibustion as an Evidence-based Therapy for Cancer,* Evidence-based Anticancer Complementary and Alternative Medicine 3,
DOI 10.1007/978-94-007-4833-0_7, © Springer Science+Business Media Dordrecht 2012

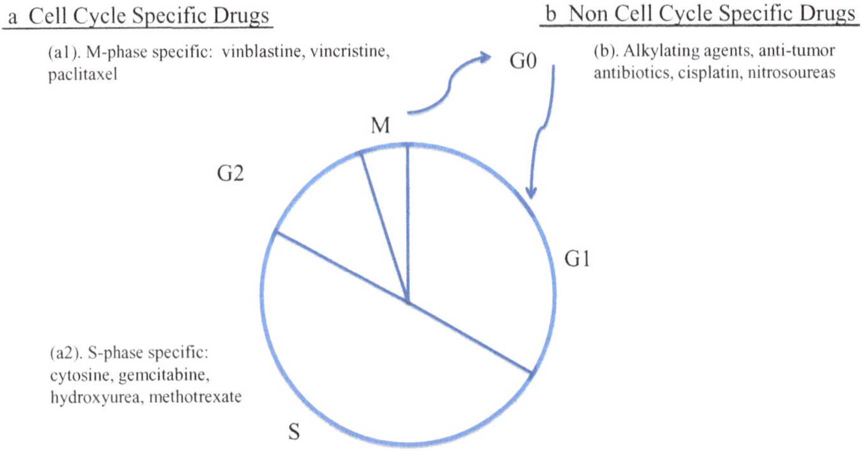

Fig. 7.1 The various phases of the cell cycle. The fundamental cell cycle events of DNA replication and cell division occur during interphase and mitosis, respectively. Interphase is the longer phase and includes the subphases G1, S and G2. G0 corresponds to cells that are withdrawn from the cycle into a resting state (G0). Cell cycle specific drugs include those that affect the cell during the M (a1) or S (a2) phase. Noncell cycle specific drugs (b) may act at any point in the cell cycle

A basic understanding of chemotherapy requires familiarity with the cell cycle as most chemotherapeutic drugs strive to cause cytotoxicity to the cancer cell either at specific or non-specific phases of the cycle. Drugs targets are often metabolic sites crucial to cell replication and the fraction of cancer cells in the replicative cycle is what makes them susceptible to chemotherapy. All dividing cells consist of three subpopulations: non-dividing cells that are terminally differentiated, proliferating cells, and resting cells that may be recruited into the cell cycle. In tumor cells, all three populations exist (Kufe 2010).

The cell cycle is composed of four phases during which the cell prepares for mitosis. Cells committed to divide enter the G1 phase, cellular processes prepare the cell for deoxyribonucelic acid (DNA) synthesis, the S phase, a second resting phase, G2, and subsequent mitosis, the M phase. The M phase is where the chromosomes condense and the cell separates into two daughter cells. Figure 7.1 depicts the cell cycle and the specificity of some cytotoxic agents. Cellular checkpoints also require a multiplicity of players and signaling events such as proteins, cyclin-dependent kinases and ion-signaling events and molecules that are crucial for cell replication. Many of the molecular-targeted drugs that have been designed are due to our increased knowledge of these players and targets.

Tumor kinetics and the effect of various chemotherapeutic drugs must also be understood. The growth rates of cancer cells are due to proportions between the number of actively dividing cells, the doubling time of the cell cycle and the rate of cell loss. Therefore, variations in these proportions are factors responsible for both the rate of tumor growth and the effect that a chemotherapeutic agent may have on a tumor. Cell cycle phase specific drugs have a plateau with respect to tumor cell killing ability whereas non cell cycle specific drugs have a linear dose-response curve. The concept of achieving cell kill in a logarithmic fashion is the fundamental of chemotherapeutic dosing concepts (Brunton et al. 2011).

The current major classes of anticancer drugs include the alkylating agents, antimetabolite analogs, vinca alkaloids, taxanes, antibiotics, hormones and hormone antagonists and other agents such as enzymes and molecular-targeted drugs. Table 7.1 lists the major chemotherapy drug classes' mode of action and frequent indications.

7.2 Anticancer Drugs

7.2.1 Alkylating Agents

The mechanism of action of alkylating agents is to impair cell function by binding to nucleophilic groups that interfere with the integrity and function of DNA inducing cell death (Brunton et al. 2011). The most important alkylation sites are DNA, RNA and proteins. Alkylating agents are non cell cycle specific but are dependent on cellular proliferation and are most toxic to rapidly dividing cells. Alkylating agents are used to treat a variety of solid and hematologic cancers. Acute toxicities of alkylating agents are largely due to their delayed effect on tissues with low mitotic indices including the liver, kidney and mature lymphocytes. The most common toxicities include bone marrow depression (dose limiting), neurotoxicity, other organ toxicity (e.g. pulmonary fibrosis, hepatotoxicity and gonadal dysfunction), nausea and vomiting, stomatitis and alopecia. The alkylating agents are further subdivided into classes according to their structure and mechanisms and include the nitrogen mustards, nitrosoureas and platinum coordination complexes (Kufe 2010).

Nitrogen mustards are non cell cycle specific alkylating agents. Their main mechanism of action is to break down and covalently modify DNA bases. Overall, the nitrogen mustards are strong local vesicants and require quick administration. They are most frequently used in treatment of hematologic malignancies. Cyclophosphamide is commonly used in combination to treat acute myelogenous leukemia (AML), acute lymphoblastic leukemia (ALL), chronic lymphocytic leukemia (CLL) and Hodgkin's and non-Hodgkin's lymphomas (Longo et al. 2012). The nitrogen mustard ifosfamide is used in combination treatment for testicular cancer (Siegert et al. 1994).

The nitrosoureas are known for their lipid solubility and instability. Their lipophilic nature enables them to rapidly penetrate the blood-brain barrier thus they are commonly used to treat a variety of brain tumors. Nitrosoureas may also cause delayed and bone marrow depression and kidney damage. Carmustine is used as an intravenous administration to treat brain tumors and as an implant (polifeprosan 20 with carmustine implant) in the adjuvant treatment of high-grade and recurrent malignant glioma and glioblastoma multiforme (Brem et al. 1995).

The platinum coordination complexes have broad anticancer activity and are used in the treatment of many solid tumors including head and neck, esophageal, lung,

Table 7.1 Classification of major chemotherapeutic drugs

Drug (class)	Mode of action and frequent indications
Nitrogen mustards (alkylating agent)	Kill cells by attacking DNA Used to treat acute chronic leukemias, Hodgkin's disease, lymphomas, and certain cancers of the lung, breast, prostate, ovary and testis Cyclophosphamide is a common nitrogen mustard that acts by cross-linking DNA
Nitrosoureas (alkylating agent)	Subgroup of alkylating agents that act to inhibit changes necessary for DNA repair Cross the blood-brain barrier and are commonly used to treat brain cancers Carmustine and lomustine are the major drugs in this group
Platinum coordination complexes (alkylating agent)	Normally used to treat many solid tumors including lung, ovarian, colon, testicular, bladder, esophageal, breast and head and neck cancers Cisplatin, carboplatin and oxaliplatin are the major platinum agents
Folic acid, pyrimidine and purine analogs (anti-metabolites)	Block cell growth by interfering with certain activities, usually DNA synthesis Broken down in to folic acid, purine and pyrimidine analogs Used to treat acute and chronic leukemias, choriocarcinoma, and some tumors of the gastrointestinal tract, breast, and ovary Methotrexate is the most common folic acid analog that acts to inhibit dihydrofolate reductase 6-mercaptopurine and 5-fluorouracil are the most commonly used purine and pyrimidine analogs respectively
Anticancer antibiotics (natural products)	Diverse group of compounds that generally act by binding with DNA and preventing RNA synthesis Widely used to treat a variety of solid and hematologic malignancies Doxorubicin, dactinomycin, mitomycin and bleomycin are the most frequently used drugs in this category
Vinca alkaloids (natural products)	Act by blocking cell division during mitosis Commonly used to treat acute lymphocytic leukemia, Hodgkin's and non-Hodgkin's lymphomas, neuroblastomas, Wilms' tumor, and cancers of the lung, breast and testis Vincristine, vinblastine and vinorelbine are the main agents in this group All bind tubulin and prevent microtubule assembly causing arrest in metaphase
Taxanes (natural products)	Act by blocking cell division during mitosis *via* prevention of microtubule depolymerization Commonly used to treat breast, ovarian, lung, head and neck, bladder and prostate cancers Paclitaxel and docetaxel are the two major taxanes
Hormonal agents	Includes corticosteroids, estrogens, anti-estrogens, and anti-androgens that modify the growth of certain hormone-dependent cancers such as breast and prostate Tamoxifen for breast cancer and leuprolide for prostate cancer are common examples
Molecular targeted drugs	Act by altering molecular pathways and/or cell signaling molecules Imatinib is a common tyrosine kinase inhibitor Rituximab is a common monoclonal antibody that binds CD20 antigen on B-lymphocytes Trastuzumab binds the HER2 receptor

bladder, colon and ovarian cancers. Their general mechanism of action is to covalently bind to nucleophilic sites on DNA causing DNA cross-links that inhibit synthesis of DNA, RNA and proteins. The most commonly used platinum complexes are carboplatin, cisplatin and oxaliplatin. Clinical toxicities include bone marrow depression, renal damage, ototoxicity, nausea and vomiting and peripheral neuropathy. Specifically, carboplatin is generally better tolerated and it has been noted that while it may not be as effective as cisplatin in the treatment of testicular, head and neck and esophageal cancers, it may be an effective alternative for patients that have cisplatin toxicities (Go and Adjei 1999; Brunton et al. 2011). Oxaliplatin, widely used in the treatment of colorectal and gastric cancers causes dose limiting toxicities of bone marrow depression and diarrhea as well as peripheral neuropathy often triggered by exposure to cold liquids in the mouth and throat and paresthesia in the upper and/or lower extremities (Goyle and Maraveyas 2005; Dolan and Fitch 2007; Sharma et al. 2007).

7.2.2 Anti-metabolites

Anti-metabolites are drugs that are analogs to naturally occurring metabolites of DNA and RNA synthesis. In the history of cancer treatment, the anti-metabolite folic acid analogs produced the earliest temporary remissions in leukemia and the first cure of a solid tumor (Farber and Diamond 1948; Berlin et al. 1963). Anti-metabolites interfere with the availability of normal purine or pyrimidine nucleotide precursors and act to inhibit or compete in DNA or RNA synthesis. They are cell cycle specific, exerting their maximal cytotoxic effects in the S phase of the cell cycle. The major classes of anti-metabolites include the folic acid, purine, pyrimidine and cytidine analogs.

Of the folic acid analogs, methotrexate is the most commonly used and its mechanism of action is as an inhibitor of dihydrofolate reductase that then inhibits folate-dependent enzymes of purine synthesis. Methotrexate is currently used in the management of ALL in children (Pui et al. 2004) and as a component in a number of combination chemotherapy regimens used to treat breast, bladder, ovarian, and head and neck cancers (Longo et al. 2012). Common methotrexate toxicities include bone marrow depression, dermatitis, nephrotoxicity, gonadal dysfunction and hepatic fibrosis and cirrhosis.

Purine and pyrimidine analogs are a diverse group of anti-metabolites that inhibit RNA and DNA function. The most common pyrimidine analogs are fluorouracil (5-FU), capecitabine, gemcitabine and floxuridine. 5-FU is commonly used as an adjuvant combination treatment with oxaliplatin or irinotecan and clinical toxicities include anorexia, nausea, stomatitis, diarrhea and bone marrow depression. The most common purine analogs are 6-mercaptopurine (6-MP) and 6-thioguanine (6-TG) and both are used in the treatment of ALL, AML and chronic myleogenous leukemia (CML) (Kufe 2010).

7.2.3 Natural Products

The category of natural products in chemotherapy refers to a variety of chemotherapeutic compounds that have been isolated from natural substances including plants, bacteria and fungi. These include the vinca alkaloids, anti-tumor antibiotics, taxanes, epipodophyllotoxins and camptothecin analogs.

7.2.3.1 Vinca Alkaloids

Vinca alkaloids are chemotherapeutic agents isolated from the periwinkle plant, *Catharanthus roseus*, a species of myrtle. The main vinca alkaloids used today, vincristine, vinblastine and vinorelbine, are used to treat various leukemias, lymphomas, lung, breast, and testicular cancers. The mechanism of action vinca alkaloids is cell cycle specific as they block cells in mitosis and impair the formation of mitotic spindles. The key side effects of vinca alkaloids include bone marrow depression, nausea and vomiting, diarrhea and peripheral neuropathy.

Specifically, vinblastine is normally used in combination with cisplatin and bleomycin for the curative treatment of testicular cancer (Einhorn 1997) and as a component in the regimen for Hodgkin's disease (Batty et al. 2012). Vincristine is regularly used in combination with glucocorticoids in the treatment of childhood leukemias and pediatric sarcomas as it is thought to be better tolerated by children than adults. Vinorelbine is used in combination with cisplatin in the treatment of non-small cell lung cancer (NSCLC) and is in Phase III studies in an oral dose form for NSCLC (Krzakowski et al. 2008).

7.2.3.2 Taxanes

Taxanes are semi-synthetic chemotherapeutic agents derived from the Western yew tree. The major compounds in this group include paclitaxel, nab-paclitaxel, and docetaxel. Taxanes also cause mitotic inhibition and conversely to vinca alkaloids, promote microtubulin-formation-induced mitotic arrest. Taxanes are widely used to treat ovarian, breast, lung, gastrointestinal, head and neck and genitourinary cancers. The most common toxicities of taxanes include bone marrow depression, allergic hypersensitivity reaction, fluid retention, myalgia and sensory peripheral neuropathy (Brunton et al. 2011).

7.2.3.3 Anti-tumor Antibiotics

Anticancer antibiotics are grouped according to their structure and chemistry and include dactinomycin and the anthracyclines such as idarubicin, epirubicin, and doxorubicin. The anthracyclines are derived from the fungus *Streptomyces peuceutius* and the structures of anticancer antibiotics vary slightly in comparison to their clinical activity. Idarubicin is primarily used in the treatment of acute leukemias and doxorubicin and epirubicin are more active in solid tumors. As a group, the primary mechanism of action is blocking DNA transcription or complexing with DNA topoisomerase II, an enzyme crucial for replication and repair. Clinical toxicities include bone marrow depression, stomatitis, alopecia, gastrointestinal (GI) disturbances and rashes (Brunton et al. 2011).

Specifically, bleomycin is used in combination to treat testicular, penile, cervical, head and neck cancers and Hodgkin's disease (Grimison et al. 2010; Meyer et al. 2012). Doxorubicin is used in combination treatment for ALL, AML, breast, ovarian and bladder cancers (Leone et al. 2011). Mitomycin is used for the treatment of gastric and bladder cancers (Shariat et al. 2010; Hamaguchi et al. 2011). Mitoxantrone is used to treat AML and prostate cancers (Ho et al. 1998; Sartor et al. 2011).

7.2.4 Hormones

A variety of cancers including breast, uterine and prostate, have been found to be hormone dependant and research into the understanding of the endocrine pathways implicated in the development of these cancers led to the identification and use of hormone analogs as chemotherapeutic treatments. The general mechanisms of hormonal agents in the treatment of cancer are to alter neuroendocrine signaling pathways, compete with receptors, or block genes that have been found to promote tumor growth and survival. The main categories of drugs in this class include glucocorticoids, anti-estrogens, aromatase inhibitors (AIs), anti-androgens, and gonadotropin-releasing hormone agonists and antagonists.

7.2.4.1 Glucocorticoids

The use of glucocorticoids in the treatment of neoplastic disease is based on their ability to induce anti-proliferative and/or apoptotic signals in sensitive cells as well as their ability to suppress mitosis in lymphocytes. They are normally used in the treatment of childhood and adult acute leukemias and lymphomas. For example, induction treatment of ALL in children includes administration of prednisone and vincristine (Eden et al. 2010).

7.2.4.2 Anti-estrogens and Aromatase Inhibitors

Anti-estrogens and AIs are primarily used as treatment for breast cancer following the discovery of the role of estrogen in the development of breast cancer and supporting evidence from epidemiologic studies and preclinical research that showed that estradiol promotes estrogen receptor (ER) positive breast cancer cell growth (Kufe 2010). The anti-estrogen treatments for hormone receptor positive breast cancer include the selective estrogen-receptor modulators (SERMs), the selective estrogen-receptor down regulators (SERDs) and the AIs. The mechanism of action of a SERM is to bind the ER and exert therapeutic effect by competitively inhibiting estradiol. Tamoxifen is the most frequently used SERM and its side effect profile includes hot flashes, vaginal atrophy, alopecia and nausea and vomiting. SERDs are pure anti-estrogens and do not have any estrogen agonist activity. Fulvestrant is only agent currently approved by the United States Food and Drug Administration (FDA) in this class although a number of agents are being tested in current clinical trials. Fulvestrant is generally well tolerated and the most common side effects are nausea, pain, vasomotor symptoms and headache (Brunton et al. 2011).

AIs block the function of the aromatase enzyme responsible for converting androgens to estrogens. AIs are now used as adjuvant treatment for post-menopausal women with HR-positive breast cancer. AIs are classified into first-, second- and third-generations according to potency, specificity and mechanism of action. The most commonly used AIs include anastrozole, letrozole and exemestane. The side effects of AIs vary slightly compared to the SERMs with regard to lower incidence of vaginal bleeding and hot flashes but higher incidence of musculoskeletal disorders and myalgias (Bonneterre et al. 2001). Other side effects include osteoporosis, fatigue and peripheral edema.

7.2.4.3 Anti-androgens and Gonadotropin-releasing Hormone Agonists and Antagonists

Anti-androgens and gonadotropin-releasing hormone (GnRH) agonists and antagonists are primarily used in the treatment of advanced prostate cancer; the collective term is androgen-deprivation therapy (ADT). ADT can alleviate cancer-related symptoms, normalize serum prostate-specific antigen, reduce bone pain and prolong survival in men with advanced prostate cancer (Sharifi et al. 2005). The most common GnRH agonists are leuprolide, goserelin and triptorelin and these agents act on the hypothalamic-pituitary-gonadal axis *via* a negative feedback mechanism which triggers the secretion of luteinizing hormone (LH) which causes a testosterone surge for about 1 to 2 weeks followed by suppression of LH with chronic GnRH administration (Conn and Crowley 1991). In 2009, a new GnRH antagonist, degarelix was approved by the FDA for the treatment of advanced prostate cancer. GnRH antagonists do not cause a hormone flare following administration (Klotz et al. 2008). Non-steroidal anti-androgens include flutamide, bicalutamide and nilutamide and these agents are most frequently used in combination ADT. Side effects of ADT in men with prostate cancer include hot flashes, fatigue, gynecomastia, anemia, weight gain, osteoporosis and decreased insulin sensitivity.

7.2.5 *Targeted Drugs*

The field of chemotherapy has evolved due to our increased knowledge about the molecular basis of cancer and spawned a new category of targeted molecular drugs such as tyrosine kinase inhibitors, monoclonal antibodies and cytokines. The fundamental mechanisms of these agents are based on targeting players in pertinent molecular cascades and/or mutation pathways that proliferate specific cancers and turn signals on or off to elicit tumor arrest.

Research on the use of targeted molecular agents and in particular, monoclonal antibodies, has largely increased over the past 30 years following seminal work by Kohler and Milstein (1975). The use of molecular-targeted drugs is now common for the management of certain cancers including some leukemias and lymphomas, breast, lung, colon and head and neck cancers (Harris 2004; Derby and Czuczman 2011). Some of the most common molecular-targeted drugs that have fundamentally impacted cancer treatment include rituximab, a chimeric monoclonal antibody against CD20 lymphocytes for non-Hodgkin's lymphoma; trastuzumab, a monoclonal antibody directed against the HER-2 membrane receptor for HER-2 receptor positive breast cancer; bevacizumab, a monoclonal antibody against vascular endothelial growth factor A for colon, non-small cell lung and breast cancers; and imatinib, a selective inhibitor of the BCR-ABL tyrosine kinase for the treatment CML and gastrointestinal stromal tumor (McLaughlin et al. 1998; Slamon et al. 2001; van Oosterom et al. 2001; Savage and Antman 2002; Talpaz et al. 2002).

7.3 Side Effects of Chemotherapy

One of the most important problems secondary to drug resistance, are the toxicities and side effects of chemotherapy. It is well known that any agent targeted to kill rapidly proliferating neoplastic cells will also affect normal cells. Cells undergoing rapid transformation such as buccal mucosal, hair, gastrointestinal mucosal cells and the hematopoietic system are most often affected and most toxicity is reversible. However toxicities affecting organs such as the lung, kidneys and heart must be monitored for toxicities to these organs can be irreversible if recognized too late.

The term supportive care refers to principles and care given to improve the quality of life of a patient. The National Cancer Institute defined supportive care as follows; "The goal of supportive care is to prevent or treat as early as possible the symptoms of a disease, side effects caused by treatment of a disease, and psychological, social, and spiritual problems related to a disease or its treatment" (http://cancer.gov/). Conventional treatments for chemotherapeutic toxicities include antibiotics, anti-emetics, growth factors and blood transfusions. In addition supportive care interventions include complementary and alternative medicine practices and procedures such as acupuncture. Practices with level 1 evidence are frequently termed "integrative" by the National Center for Complementary and Alternative Medicine (NCCAM) division of the National Institutes of Health (NIH) (http://nccam.nih.gov/).

Complementary therapies including acupuncture and moxibustion have been recently studied as potentially valuable supportive care interventions and research has been done testing acupuncture and moxibustion for a number of side effects commonly experienced during chemotherapy including nausea and vomiting, pain, neuropathy and vasomotor symptoms. Many of these symptoms are thought to be at least partially mediated by the central or peripheral nervous systems and though all of the mechanisms of action of acupuncture and moxibustion have not been elucidated, acupuncture has been proven to have a number of neuromodulatory effects as demonstrated by basic science and large multicenter clinical trials (NIH 1998).

The pathophysiology of each abovementioned chemotherapy-induced side effect will be detailed, followed by an in depth review of the supporting literature on acupuncture and moxibustion for the treatment of each named side effect.

7.4 Pathophysiology of Chemotherapy-induced Nausea and Emesis

Nausea and emesis (vomiting) refers to nausea, vomiting and retching. Nausea is defined as a "subjectively unpleasant sensation associated with flushing, tachycardia and an awareness of the urge to vomit" (American Society of Health-System Pharmacists (ASHP) 1999). Vomiting is defined as a contraction of the abdominal muscles, descent of the diaphragm and opening of the gastric cardia that result in an expulsion of the stomach contents from the mouth. Retching is defined as spasmodic contractions of the diaphragm, thoracic and abdominal wall muscles without expulsion of the gastric contents (ASHP 1999). All three may exist as a sequence or as individual events that are not predictive of one another. Nausea is the most difficult to define and characterize as it is largely subjective. While physiologic signs such as tachycardia and increased salivation may be concurrent during an episode of nausea, they are not universally present.

Vomiting and retching are easier to quantify as both produce physical signs such as contraction of the abdominal walls, shifting of the diaphragm, and expulsion of stomach contents. The purpose of vomiting is to expel noxious contents from the gastrointestinal tract and most often (but not always) vomiting is preceded by nausea. Three vomiting phases have been characterized, a prodromal, ejection and post-ejection phase (ASHP 1999). These phases are defined physiologically. The prodromal phase is the coordinated interplay between the vomiting center and the gastrointestinal tract in order to prepare it for emesis. During this phase, vagal afferents stimulate the proximal stomach and are also partly mediated by vasoactive intestinal polypeptide in the gut. Finally initiation of retrograde contraction moves the contents of the upper small intestine to the stomach and corrals any noxious contents to be ejected. It also directs any remaining contents of the lower small intestine into the stomach and commences the prodromal phase. The ejection phase refers to the actual expulsion of stomach contents *via* coordinated contraction of the muscular stomach, net compression of the stomach, and ejection of the stomach contents. Finally the post-ejection phase refers to the cessation of vomiting, cessation of nausea (if previously present) and generally, the person feeling better (Baker et al. 2005).

7.4.1 Neural Components and Neurotransmitters Involved in Vomiting

The aforementioned events are controlled by the vomiting center (VC), a collection of neurons in the medulla oblongata that was characterized by Borison and Wang (1953). Both the VC and the gut are associated with neurotransmitters such as serotonin, dopamine, histamine, acetylcholine and substance P that propagate signals to the VC and circulate in the brain. Serotonin and substance P are thought to be primary and dopamine, a secondary mediator of the nausea and vomiting response respectively (Faerber et al. 2007; Tipton et al. 2007). Enterochromaffin cells (EC) in the gut have also been demonstrated to respond to toxic substances and may release serotonin *via* the hepatic portal system to the chemoreceptor trigger zone (CTZ) that is located in the area postrema (AP) region in the bottom edge of the fourth ventricle. Finally, the nucleus tractus solitarius (NTS) and the dorsal motor nucleus of the vagus nerve also act as relay stations to coordinate an emetic response (Miller and Leslie 1994; Leslie and James 2000; Hornby 2001; Chin et al. 2006). While these mechanisms have been proposed, the exact organization and propagation of signals to the CTZ are not fully characterized. Moreover the AP is a unique area that is situated between the fourth ventricle that remains unprotected by the blood-brain barrier but in communication with the cerebrospinal fluid (CSF). It is this characteristic that is thought to significantly contribute to chemotherapy-induced nausea and vomiting (CINV) due to its exposure and ability to circulate potentially emetic toxins to the brain (Miller and Leslie 1994; Hornby 2001). Neural influences that convey the sensation of nausea such as emotion, olfaction and visual signals are also difficult to characterize and higher cerebral control is thought to be an important factor regulating nausea. Differences in the efficacy of standard anti-emetic drugs for nausea such as serotonin (5-HT) *vs* neurokinin (NK_1) receptor antagonists (the latter superior for nausea), implies that multiple neurotransmitters and cerebral responses coordinate nausea. Activation of the limbic system, vestibular system, and the hypothalamic-pituitary axis are also areas where sensations of nausea may be experienced in the cortex; however these have yet to be defined and may vary depending on the particular stimuli eliciting nausea (Sanger et al. 2006).

The main stimuli inducing CINV is the absorption of cytotoxic chemotherapy in the gut and resulting local (chemoreceptors, gut afferents) and central (CTZ, VC, AP, neurotransmitters, higher cortical functions) effects. It has been proposed that the pathomechanism of CINV is initiated by the presence and absorption of chemotherapeutic drugs in the gut and gut signaling to vagal afferents and the brainstem *via* the NTS and AP. Locally, cytotoxic drugs stimulate luminal cells that likely activate EC of the gastric mucosal layer and neurotransmitters including serotonin, substance P and cholecystokinin (Racke et al. 1996). Another proposed mechanism of CINV is thought to be the role of cytotoxic drugs on the CSF and its effect on the CTZ, NTS, AP and higher brain function (Racke et al. 1996). Figure 7.2 details systems thought to be involved in the pathogenesis of CINV.

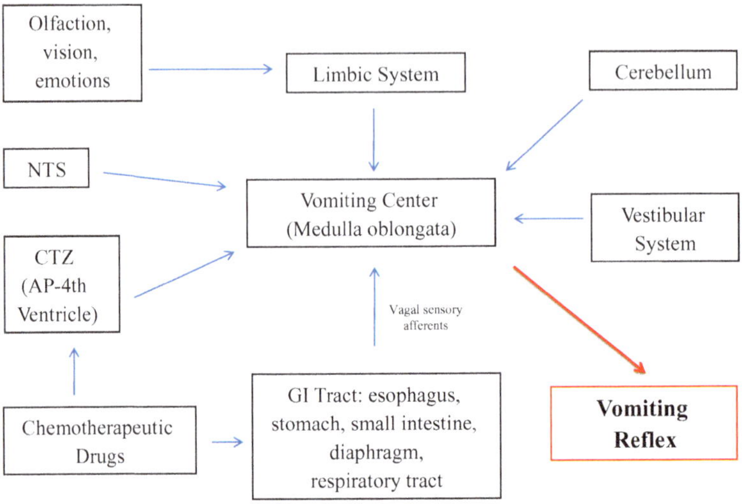

Fig. 7.2 The numerous systems thought to be involved in the pathogenesis of chemotherapy-induced nausea and vomiting. *AP* area postrema, *CTZ* chemoreceptor trigger zone, *GI* gastrointestinal, *NTS* nucleus tractus solitarius

7.4.2 Conventional Anti-emetics

The development of pharmaceutical anti-emetics has made a huge contribution to our knowledge and treatment of CINV. The use of modern anti-emetics can prevent vomiting in up to 70–80% of patients (Morrow et al. 2002). The four main anti-emetic drugs classes are: receptor antagonists, 5-hydroxytryptamine-3 (5-HT_3) receptor antagonists, NK_1 receptor antagonists, and corticosteroids. Other drugs less frequently used and not discussed here include neuroleptics, benzodiazepines, cannabinoids, substituted benzamides, anti-histamines and botanicals such as ginger and mint.

7.4.2.1 Dopamine Receptor Antagonists

The dopamine receptor antagonists were the first main class of agents used for CINV. Most are either non-selective for dopamine $(D)_1$ and D_2 receptors are or D_2 receptor specific. D_2 receptor antagonists are thought to act by antagonizing D_2 receptors in the AP. However it is not known whether an increased circulation of dopamine is provoked by cytotoxic chemotherapy or if dopamine is released into the blood or AP. Finally, it is also know that cisplatin induced nausea and vomiting is non-responsive to D_2 receptor antagonist drugs (Ettinger et al. 2005).

7.4.2.2 5-HT_3 Receptor Antagonists

5-HT_3 receptor antagonists work by blocking 5-HT_3 receptors which may be activated and contribute to CINV due to potentially increased amounts of serotonin from

EC in the gut mucosa and systemically circulating 5-HT (Morrow et al. 2002). It is also thought that they are important in de-sensitizing the vagus nerve that may be prone to activation by other excitatory substances released from EC cells such as substance P. 5-HT_3 receptor antagonists seem to provide superior relief in the acute phase of emesis (0–24 h) and less relief for delayed vomiting (24–120 h) and nausea (Kufe 2010). 5-HT_3 receptor antagonists are commonly used in combination with NK_1 antagonists or corticosteroids. The 5-HT_3 receptor antagonists in use include granisetron, ondansetron, tropisetron, dolasetron and palonosetron. Reported side effects of 5-HT_3 drugs include headache, constipation, diarrhea and asthenia.

7.4.2.3 NK_1 Receptor Antagonists

Preclinical studies demonstrated the potential of NK_1 receptor antagonist drug administration for the treatment of CINV. NK_1 receptors act by blocking NK_1 receptors in the CTZ, NTS and gastrointestinal tract binding of substance P. In clinical studies the use of NK_1 receptor antagonists have demonstrated their superiority in treating delayed vomiting and as abovementioned, they are often used as combination treatment with 5-HT_3 drugs for acute and delayed CINV. Side effects of NK_1 receptor antagonists include headache, abdominal pain, dizziness, anorexia, hiccups and mild transaminase elevation (Campos et al. 2001; Cocquyt et al. 2001; Van Belle et al. 2002).

7.4.2.4 Corticosteroids

Dexamethasone was the first reported corticosteroid to be used as an anti-emetic for cisplatin induced nausea and vomiting and post-operative nausea and vomiting (Ettinger et al. 2005). Despite their widespread use and ability to raise the emetic threshold, the anti-emetic mechanism of action of corticosteroids is unknown. Possible explanations include anti-inflammatory modulation such as modulation of cortisol levels and eicosanoid metabolism, modification of the blood-cerebrospinal fluid barrier or inhibition of cortical input to the VC (Ettinger et al. 2005). In general, steroids are considered to be safe anti-emetics and common side effects include insomnia, indigestion and weight gain.

7.4.3 Acupuncture for CINV

Acupuncture is the insertion of fine, single-use, sterile needles into points in the body as determined by a system of acupuncture points and meridians. As a modality, it is often oriented in a traditional medicine framework as it is one of the most frequent procedures employed in the practice of traditional Chinese medicine (TCM). Acupuncture has become an accepted therapy for a variety of conditions including

CINV in adult and pediatric cancer patients (Shen et al. 2000; Ezzo et al. 2006; Reindl et al. 2006). Research on the potential mechanisms of action of acupuncture date back to the 1970s and one of the earliest proven mechanisms of acupuncture is the liberation of β-endorphin by acupuncture needling (Peets and Pomeranz 1978; Malizia et al. 1979). Numerous studies have since examined the other potential mechanisms of action of acupuncture and it has been demonstrated that acupuncture has an effect on endogenous opioids, various neurotransmitters, and cortical areas including the hypothalamus and amygdala (Gao et al. 1994; Hsieh et al. 2001; Chen et al. 2006). Other research has showed that acupuncture needling affects multiple ion channels and stimulates fibroblast, and local connective tissue responses (Langevin et al. 2007). Researchers are also analyzing acupuncture point-specific treatment effects and the morphology of acupuncture points and meridians (Ahn et al. 2008). There are also many studies on the various practices of acupuncture and how these may be correlated in a treatment effect (Langevin et al. 2011).

Acupuncture has been proven to treat a number of conditions including low back pain and CINV (NIH 1998). Studies on acupuncture for general nausea and vomiting and CINV often utilize the acupuncture point, Neiguan (PC6). PC6 is located on the anterior surface of the wrist between the tendons flexor carpi radialis and palmaris longus. It is measured by the proportional *cun* measurement system as three finger breaths from the wrist crease which corresponds as 2 *cun* (Chen 1999). Other commonly studied acupuncture points for nausea and emesis include Zusanli (ST36), Zhongwan (CV12), Weishu (UB21) and Hegu (LI4) (Lee and Fan 2009).

All of the large randomized controlled trials that have demonstrated the effectiveness of acupuncture in controlling nausea and vomiting have used the acupuncture point PC6 (Vickers 1996; Lee and Fan 2009). The largest systematic review of acupuncture for CINV scrutinized randomized trials of acupuncture point stimulation by any method (e.g. needling, electrical stimulation, magnets and acupressure) for the treatment of CINV (Ezzo et al. 2006). The authors included eleven trials ($n = 1{,}247$) in their assessment and demonstrated that acupuncture point stimulation reduced the incidence of acute vomiting (RR 0.82; 95% CI 0.69 to 0.99; $p = 0.04$). Acupuncture needle stimulation also reduced the portion of acute vomiting but not acute nausea compared to electroacupuncture and electroacupuncture reduced the proportion of acute vomiting more than manual acupuncture (RR 0.76; 95% CI 0.60 to 0.97; $p = 0.02$) (Ezzo et al. 2006).

The exact physiologic mechanism of action of acupuncture for CINV is still under investigation. The most recent studies suggest various mechanisms for the anti-nausea and anti-emetic effects of acupuncture including the ability of acupuncture to release neurotransmitters, the influence of acupuncture on peripheral nervous system (PNS) nerve transmission, and the effect of acupuncture on higher central nervous system (CNS) functions such as emotion and expectancy (Wayne et al. 2005; Streitberger et al. 2006; Enblom et al. 2011). Recent studies in animal models have looked at the effect of electroacupuncture on emesis in conscious dogs (Tatewaki et al 2005). These investigators demonstrated reduced episodes of vomiting following electroacupuncture at PC6 in vasopressin-induced emesis in dogs. This effect was reversible by naloxone suggesting the potential mechanism of action of acupuncture needling is its effect on the endogenous opioid system. Other experiments proposed that the anti-emetic effect of acupuncture may be *via* decreasing transient lower esophageal sphincter relaxations (TLESRs). Zou et al. (2005) examined the effect of electroacupuncture on TLESRs in healthy human subjects. These investigators demonstrated that electroacupuncture at PC6 decreased the rate of TLESRs ($p < 0.02$) however this effect was not reversible by naloxone suggesting a non-opioid receptor mechanism. A third study looked electroacupuncture administration in cats and found that electroacupuncture at PC6 significantly reduced TLESRs *vs* sham stimulation ($p < 0.05$). This response was restored following infusion of a cholecystokinin-A receptor antagonist (CCK octapeptide) ($p < 0.05$) and naloxone ($p < 0.05$) but not phaclofen or tacrine (GABA antagonist and cholinesterase inhibitor respectively) (Wang et al. 2007).

Experimentation on the point specificity of PC6 utilizing functional magnetic resonance imaging (fMRI) has also been done. Yoo et al. (2004) demonstrated that acupuncture needling at PC6 resulted in activation of the left superior frontal gyrus, anterior cingulate gyrus and dorsomedial nucleus of the thalamus *vs* sham acupuncture. Bai et al. (2010) examined point specificity of acupuncture at PC6 *vs* an anti-emetic-irrelevant acupuncture point, Guangming (GB37) and found that there were distinct hemodynamic responses (as measured by fMRI) in subjects receiving stimulation at PC6 *vs* GB37. In particular, acupuncture stimulation at PC6 produced significant signal decreases in the amygdala, insula, perieacueductal gray (PAG) and the folcculonodular lobe of the cerebellum (nodulus and uvula) *vs* signal increases in the occipital cortex that occurred following GB37 needle stimulation. This study supports the distinct centrally mediated acupuncture point specificity of PC6.

7.4.4 Acupressure and CINV

Acupressure is based on meridian theory and is defined as the application of pressure to a specific meridian point by the use of the finger, hand, elbow, foot and/or acupressure band. A recent literature review of acupressure for CINV found a variety of studies, some that supported the use of acupressure for CINV and a few that showed no significant differences (Dibble et al. 2000; Melchart et al. 2006; Lee and Frazier 2011). Gardani et al. (2007) found that acupressure at PC6 controlled emetic symptomology in 68% of patients. There was no significant difference in efficacy related to tumor histotype but a trend showing decreased efficacy in patients receiving anthracyclines *vs* those receiving non-anthracycline containing combinations. Dibble et al. (2007) performed a multicenter, longitudinal randomized clinical trial of acupressure in women receiving chemotherapy for breast cancer. Their results demonstrated that there was a significant decline in the incidence of emesis for the PC6 acupressure group *vs* the placebo ($p = 0.002$) or usual care group ($p < 0.0001$) in delayed nausea (days 2–10). Overall, no prospective studies have analyzed differences between methodology and application of acupressure for CINV and more controlled studies are needed.

7.4.5 Moxibustion for CINV

Moxibustion is the use of heat to stimulate acupuncture points generated by preparations of the herb, *Artemisia vulgaris* (Chen 1999). Moxibustion has been widely used in many countries and is considered an important modality of traditional Chinese medicine (TCM) but there are fewer studies on moxibustion's mechanism of action and its role in treating CINV. Moxibustion (moxa) preparations include moxa-stick, -cone and -herbal cake applications. Moxa-stick moxibustion is performed by holding an ignited moxa stick a distance above the skin and warming the spot but not burning it. Herbal cake moxibustion is performed by placing an herbal cake on an acupuncture point(s), followed by the placement and ignition of moxa cones. Direct moxibustion is ignition of moxa cones or threads directly on the epidermis with or without the application of an emollient-type burn ointment. This type of moxibustion can cause scarring.

Research has suggested that moxibustion may have an anti-inflammatory mechanism of action and a recent study of moxibustion in mice demonstrated decreased levels of substance P, STAT6, NF-κB and iNOS in the nasal mucosa of mice that had received local moxibustion (Jung et al. 2012). Another study suggested that moxibustion may mediate mast cell morphology. These investigators administered moxibustion to a trinitro-benzene-sulfonic acid-induced rat model of colitis and demonstrated that the degranulation ratio of mast cells was higher in rats receiving moxibustion *vs* controls ($p<0.05$) indicating a correlation between the effect of moxibustion on mast cells (Shi et al. 2011).

There are no basic scientific studies on the anti-emetic specific mechanisms of moxibustion however there have been a number of clinical trials. Lee and colleagues recently performed a systematic review of five clinical trials of moxibustion and CINV (Lee et al. 2010). The review assessed the trials based on outcomes including response rates, side effects, and quality of life. Of the four randomized controlled trials of moxibustion that fit the inclusion criteria, all failed to show any beneficial effect of moxibustion on tumor response rate. Of the two trials that assessed the frequency of CINV in patients treated with moxibustion, both studies reported significantly fewer episodes of nausea and emesis in subjects receiving moxibustion and meta-analysis showed significantly less nausea and vomiting in patients receiving moxibustion ($n = 80$; RR 0.38; 95% CI 0.22 to 0.65; $p = 0.0005$; heterogeneity $\chi^2 = 0.18$, $p = 0.67$, $I^2 = 0\%$) (Lee et al. 2010). The first of these two trials by Chen et al. tested moxibustion on the acupuncture point, Shenque (CV8) in subjects with nasopharyngeal cancer following radiation (Chen et al. 2000). The second study examined the effect of moxibustion treatment in subjects with advanced gastric cancers (Cao et al. 1997). Note, the full text of both of these articles is in the Chinese language so only the abstract was assessed. While there are a number of other studies on moxibustion in the literature, there is a paucity of research on moxibustion and it is clear that more studies are desperately needed.

7.5 Acupuncture for Chemotherapy-induced Pain and Neuropathy

Cancer pain is a significant problem in oncology and it is a debilitating side effect. Effective conventional treatments for cancer-related pain include pharmacotherapy and physical therapy. Acupuncture is becoming more widely used to treat chemotherapy-induced cancer pain and a number of well-designed studies have been recently published.

7.5.1 Acupuncture for AI-induced Arthralgia

Increase in breast cancer survival is largely due to the benefit of the hormonal therapies such as tamoxifen and AIs. Large clinical trials have demonstrated that AIs are associated with increased frequency of musculoskeletal disorders including myalgias and arthralgias and pain commonly affects joints including hands and knees. It has also been reported that the severity of arthralgias can cause up to 5% of patients to discontinue AI therapy. While the mechanism of AI-induced joint pain is still unclear, a variety of treatments including acupuncture are currently being tested in order to determine if they provide substantial and durable pain relief so that women can remain on these life saving drugs. Recent clinical trials by Mao et al. (2009) and Crew et al. (2010) have examined the effectiveness of acupuncture for the treatment of AI-induced arthralgia.

In the study by Crew et al. (2010), manual full body and auricular acupuncture *vs* sham acupuncture was administered to women with moderate to severe, self-reported musculoskeletal pain related to AI use for at least 3 months in duration. Outcome measures were the Brief Pain Inventory-Short Form (BPI-SF), Western Ontario and McMaster Universities Osteoarthritis Index and the Modified Score for the Assessment of Chronic Rheumatoid Affections of the Hands. Data was obtained at baseline (week 0), weeks 3 and 6 (endpoint). The results demonstrated that of 38 evaluable subjects, the difference in mean BPI-SF worst pain scores at 6 weeks was significantly lower in the true *vs* sham acupuncture group ($p < 0.001$). Differences between true and sham acupuncture with regard to pain related interference and pain severity ($p = 0.002$ and $p = 0.003$, respectively) were also reported.

Mao et al. (2009) similarly tested the subjects with the same inclusion criteria as Crew et al. (2010) but Mao's team utilized electroacupuncture. Of the 12 subjects enrolled and analyzed, reduction in pain severity as measured by the BPI-SF was found in women receiving electroacupuncture ($p < 0.001$). An additional secondary outcome, the Patient Global Impression of Change (PGIC) also demonstrated that there was a significant reduction in scores after 6 weeks of treatment with electroacupuncture.

Table 7.2 Chemotherapeutic drugs that may induce neuropathy

Drug (class)	Primary mechanism	Type and features of neuropathy
Bortezomib (targeted drug)	Unknown	Predominately distal sensory
Cisplatin, oxaliplatin (platinum coordination complex)	Damage to dorsal root ganglia, possible inhibition of axonal transport and DNA cross-linking	Predominately sensory neuropathy with sensory ataxia, sensory neuropathy induced by cold (oxaliplatin only)
Paclitaxel, docetaxel (taxanes)	Promotes microtubule assembly, possible damage to dorsal root ganglia and interference with axonal transport	Predominately sensory
Vincristine, vinblastine, vinorelbine (vinca alkaloids)	Interference with axonal microtubule assembly, impairs axonal transport	Sensorimotor and distal sensory

7.5.2 Acupuncture for Chemotherapy-induced Peripheral Neuropathy

Peripheral neuropathy (PN) is a common side effect of chemotherapy and its pathogenesis is poorly understood. PN most frequently occurs with administration of taxanes, platinum-based agents and vinca alkaloids (Table 7.2). PN can affect either sensory or motor axons and neuropathies are generally classified by which area of the cell body they affect as well as the main cause of the neuropathy. It is also known that risk of developing a toxic neuropathy is greater in patients with pre-existing neuropathy or in those taking other neurotoxic drugs. Chemotherapy-induced peripheral neuropathy (CIPN) is categorized as a toxic neuropathy that is associated with malignancy and is the direct effect of a toxic treatment. Other neuropathies associated with malignancies can be due to the cancer itself, as a consequence of a compromised immune system or as a paraneoplastic effect (Longo et al. 2012).

The neurotoxicity in CIPN (regardless of the agent that causes it) is a predominantly distal sensory neuropathy, characterized by pain, numbness, tingling and reduced functional capacity in the extremities (Henderson et al. 2003). Other symptoms can include paresthesias, ataxia, impaired vibration and joint position sense and loss of tendon reflexes. The severity and frequency of the neuropathy are related to the dose level, cumulative dose, dose-intensity, and infusion times, with more rapid infusions associated with higher incidences (Sparano et al. 2008). Neurotoxicity also appears to be more frequent when the agent is used in combination with other potentially neurotoxic agents and in patients with pre-existing neuropathy, e.g. diabetic or alcohol induced neuropathy (Henderson et al. 2003). CIPN can be dose limiting and may lead to dose reduction or cessation of therapy.

The pathogenesis of taxane-induced peripheral neuropathy is thought to be due to abnormal aggregation of microtubules in neuronal cells that cause neurosensory symptoms. It has also been demonstrated that paclitaxel accumulates in the dorsal root ganglia leading to disturbances of cellular metabolism and axonal transport. The prevalence of peripheral neuropathy in patients treated with taxanes is about 30% (Theiss and Meller 2000; Quaasthoff and Hartung 2002) and symptoms have been reported to persist for up to 18 months after the cessation of taxane-based chemotherapy (Nakata and Yoriguji 1999).

The pathogenesis of cisplatin-induced neuropathy is due to its preferential uptake in the dorsal root ganglia that produces a dose-related sensory neuropathy (Cavaletti et al. 2004). Symptoms can include distal paresthesias and numbness, Lhermitte's sign and sensory ataxia. Cisplatin-induced sensory neuropathy most often occurs after a cumulative dose of at least 300 mg/m^2 but can occur with lower doses (Windebank et al. 1994; Albers et al. 2011).

Bortezomib-induced peripheral neuropathy (BIPN) is poorly understood and the incidence of peripheral neuropathy was reported in the Phase I studies of the drug (Aghajanian et al. 2002). The pathogenesis of BIPN is thought to be cumulative and dose related and prevalence has been reported to increase throughout the first five treatment cycles (Richardson et al. 2006). In a recent study by Richardson et al. (2006), 81% of patients reported BIPN and 71% experienced improvement after dose-modification or completion of therapy. Similar to the other chemotherapeutic agents, pre-existing neuropathy or concurrent use of other potentially neurotoxic drugs may increase the likelihood of onset of BIPN.

Recent reports suggest that nerve growth factor (NGF) may play a role in CIPN as mice treated with NGF, a putative neuroprotectant, demonstrated a reduction in the severity of oxaliplatin-induced neuropathy (Scuteri et al. 2010). Moreover, an inverse association between circulating levels of NGF and the severity of CIPN in cancer patients has been demonstrated (Lee and Swain 2006).

CIPN is difficult to prevent and treat. Symptomatic treatments include anti-depressants, anti-convulsants, non-narcotic and narcotic analgesics (Abuaisha et al. 1998). However, drug treatments are generally ineffective and limited by side effects. Acupuncture has been increasingly applied to the alleviation of pain, particularly among cancer patients and recently a few pilot studies have demonstrated that acupuncture may be beneficial in the treatment of this debilitating condition (Xu et al. 2010; Donald et al. 2011).

Donald et al. (2011) performed a retrospective evaluation of eighteen subjects that had be referred for acupuncture treatment with pre-existing PN after completing various chemotherapeutic regimens for hematologic and solid malignancies multiple myeloma (MM), ALL, CML, GI, breast and gynecological). The results demonstrated that 82% of patients (14 of 18) reported an improvement in symptoms following a course of 6-weeks of manual acupuncture. Patients were given individualized treatments however the most frequent acupuncture points used were Sanyinjiao (SP6), ST36, Taichong (LV3), LI4, Kunlun (UB60) and the Bafeng (EX-LE10) and Baxie (EX-UE9) points. Xu et al. (2010) performed a clinical trial of acupuncture treatment in 64 patients with paclitaxel or oxaliplatin induced peripheral neuropathy and found that acupuncture was superior to intramuscular injection of cobamamide ($p < 0.05$) though both were effective treatments. The acupuncture points utilized in this study included LI4, LV3, ST36, Qihai (CV6) and Quchi (LI11).

7.6 Acupuncture for Chemotherapy-induced Vasomotor Symptoms

7.6.1 Chemotherapy-induced Vasomotor Symptoms

The incidence of vasomotor symptoms due to hormonal treatment for breast or prostate cancer is common. In breast cancer patients, vasomotor symptoms are commonly reported in patients receiving adjuvant hormonal therapy with SERMs or AIs. The prevalence of vasomotor symptoms in women receiving SERMs has been reported to be as high as 80% (Jin et al. 2008) and up to 46% in women receiving AIs (Fallowfield et al. 2006). The pathomechanism of vasomotor symptoms (commonly called hot flashes or hot flushes) experienced by women receiving SERMs is due to the competitive inhibition of the drug (e.g. tamoxifen) to ER and blockage of the conversion of androgens to estrogens respectively. In women taking AIs, the suppression of peripheral aromatase leads to estrogen deprivation and both SERMs and AIs result in depletion of ERs and estradiol that are thought to be the main cause of the hot flashes. In men with prostate cancer, the pathomechanism of hot flashes is thought to be due to the decrease in circulating LH and follicle stimulating hormone (FSH) (Anderson 2003). The incidence of hot flashes in prostate cancer patients receiving ADT is close to 80% and it has been reported that hot flashes may persist up to 5 years after cessation of ADT (Higano 2003).

7.6.2 Acupuncture for the Treatment of Hormone Therapy-induced Hot Flashes

7.6.2.1 Breast Cancer

Only a few randomized controlled clinical trials of acupuncture for the treatment of hormone therapy induced hot flashes in breast cancer patients have been performed. Hervik and Mjåland (2009) initiated a prospective controlled clinical trial of 59 women receiving adjuvant therapy with tamoxifen and suffering from hot flashes and randomized them to true or sham acupuncture. A standardized acupuncture point protocol was administered and points included: LV3, Fengchi (GB20), Lieque (LU7), Taixi (KI3), SP6, Guanyuan (CV4), Daling (PC7) and Ququan (LV8). Over the 10-week period, the mean number of hot flashes was significantly reduced by almost 50% in the acupuncture group ($p<0.001$) *vs* the sham group. A further 30% reduction was seen in the 12-week follow up period ($p<0.017$). 22 of 30 patients experienced a reduction by at least 50% in the active treatment group, compared to 3 of 28 in the sham group ($p = 0.002$).

Nedstrand et al. (2005) randomized 38 patients with breast cancer and vasomotor symptoms to 12 weeks of electroacupuncture and 6 weeks of follow-up. The acupuncture points used in this study were Xinshu (UB15), Shenshu (UB23), Ciliao (UB32), Shenmen (HT7), SP6, LV3, PC6 and Baihui (GV20). In this study only five women were actively using adjuvant hormonal therapy with tamoxifen throughout the study period and there was no difference in the mean number of hot flashes at baseline between the women receiving or not receiving tamoxifen treatment. However in women that were not receiving tamoxifen, a reduction in mean number of hot flashes was seen after 4 weeks of treatment *vs* 12 weeks in the women who were undergoing adjuvant hormonal therapy ($p<0.05$).

Walker et al. (2010) recently performed a randomized controlled trial of acupuncture *vs* venlafaxine for the management of vasomotor symptoms in breast cancer patients receiving adjuvant hormonal therapy with either tamoxifen or AIs. 50 patients were randomly assigned to receive 12 weeks of acupuncture or venlafaxine and were followed up for 1 year post-treatment. All patients in the acupuncture arm were treated using a standardized protocol and a secondary protocol that allowed for selection of additional acupuncture points. The primary standardized acupuncture point protocol was UB23, KI3 and SP6. The secondary points that were used as needed according to the TCM diagnosis were Dazhui (GV14), GB20, Taiyuan (LU9), LV3, GV20, ST36, PC7 and HT7. The primary outcome, hot flash frequency, demonstrated a significant effect as both the acupuncture and venlafaxine groups experienced a decrease in hot flashes by about 50% and a return toward the baseline at follow up. This study also showed that there was a significant difference in adverse events (AE) in the venlafaxine group *vs* the acupuncture group ($p<0.002$) as there were 18 incidences of AEs in the venlafaxine group and zero in the acupuncture group.

7.6.2.2 Prostate Cancer

There have been a few clinical trials of acupuncture for the treatment of ADT induced hot flashes in prostate cancer patients. Capodice et al. (2011) performed a pilot study of acupuncture in 16 men with prostate cancer experiencing hot flashes. The results demonstrated that at 7 weeks, patients reported a significant decrease in hot flashes ($p = 0.04$) with an average of 6.00 ± 2.40 (mean $\pm$ standard deviation) hot flashes per day as compared to 9.57 ± 3.98 at baseline. Decreasing frequency of hot flashes continued at the 14 week follow-up with patients reporting an average of 2.63 ± 1.20 hot flashes per day ($p = 0.001$). Decreased hot flash frequency was maintained over a follow up period of 14 weeks without acupuncture treatments, and at the 28-week follow-up, the frequency of hot flashes was slightly increased but still significantly decreased as compared to baseline 3.2 ± 1.7 ($p=0.01$). The acupuncture points utilized in this study included full body standardized manual acupuncture and auricular acupuncture points including: SP6, UB15, UB23, Gaohuang (UB43), LV3, Zhaohai (KI6), LU7, HT7 (full body points) and auricular points including Shenmen, brain, kidney, liver and upper lung. Ashamalla et al. (2011) performed a pilot study in prostate cancer patients receiving ADT and found that acupuncture reduced the incidence of hot flashes from a mean of 28.3 hot flashes per day at baseline to 10.3 ($p = 0.0001$) at 2 weeks post-treatment, 7.5 ($p = 0.0001$) at 6 weeks and 7.0 ($p=0.001$) at 8 months. The acupuncture point protocol administered in this study included Yanglingquan (GB34), SP6, KI3, ST36, UB15, UB23, Taiyang (EX-HN5), HT7, PC6 and LI11.

7.7 Safety Profile of Acupuncture and Moxibustion in Oncology

Standard safety practices, practice guidelines and ongoing research continue to support the safety of acupuncture in the oncologic setting. Safety studies in the literature demonstrate that acupuncture is safe. Only six cases of potentially serious adverse events (SAE) were reported in a study of 97,733 patients receiving acupuncture in Germany. SAEs included exacerbation of depression, hypertensive crisis, vasovagal reaction, asthma attack and pneumothorax. Minor AEs included local bleeding and needling pain, both occurring in less than 0.05% of patients (Melchart et al. 2004). Another retrospective study estimated SAEs from acupuncture to be 0.05 per 10,000 treatments, and 0.55 per 10,000 individual patients respectively (White 2004).

Many clinical trials of acupuncture now follow both the Consolidated Standards of Reporting Trials (CONSORT) and Standards for Reporting Interventions in Clinical Trials of Acupuncture (STRICTA) guidelines. The CONSORT guidelines were comprised in the mid-1990s and act as a basic checklist for reporting in a randomized controlled trial (Altman et al. 2001). The STRICTA guidelines have improved both the design and reporting of clinical trials of acupuncture as they suggest that methodology specific to acupuncture including needling details, rationale and control to be interventions are to be reported (MacPherson et al. 2010).

In the clinic, cancer patients require specific care and it is important that clinicians are familiar with potential co-morbid conditions and toxicities. A guideline for the treatment of cancer patients with integrative therapies has been established by the Society for Integrative Oncology. The guidelines are based on grading recommendations according to the clinical encounter and intervention. Grade 1A evidence exists for acupuncture as a complementary therapy when pain is poorly controlled, for CINV and for post-operative nausea and vomiting (Deng et al. 2009). Updating the guidelines to include contraindications such as lower level of normal limits for platelet count, absolute neutrophil count and other reasons based on the judgment of the clinical team are warranted (Capodice 2010; Lu and Rosenthal 2010).

Practical issues related to administering acupuncture in the oncology clinic should also be mandated and Clean Needle Technique (CNT) is required by most state licensing boards in the United States. CNT mandates hand washing, universal precaution, immediate isolation of needles and use of sterile, disposable, guide-tube needles. The FDA regulates acupuncture needles as medical devices mandating device material biocompatibility and sterility (21CFR880.5580). However acupuncture as a term, is considered heterogeneous. The strict definition is the administration of thin, filiform needles intended to pierce the skin in the practice of acupuncture however acupuncture may be used as a term to encompass other procedures such as intradermal needles, injection of substances into acupuncture points, laser therapy, other perturbations of points and sometimes even moxibustion.

For moxibustion, there is no guideline for the administration of safe practices apart from textbooks of Chinese Medicine (Chen 1999). Moxibustion has important and unique practices and potential adverse events associated with it. Reported adverse events of moxibustion include burns, itching, infection, allergy, respiratory tract sensitivity and xerophthalmia (Park et al. 2010).

Moxibustion, a modality that involves burning an herb over selected acupuncture points is an area where more research is needed in order to make treatment recommendations and safety guidelines.

7.8 Conclusion

The administration of chemotherapy is life saving treatment for adults and children with solid and/or hematologic malignancies. The most common side effects and toxicities of chemotherapy include alopecia, bone marrow depression, nausea and vomiting, pain and vasomotor symptoms. While many of these side effects are reversible, in some cases, symptoms can persist for a number of years following chemotherapy treatment and can be dependent on both the pathomechanism of the side effect and/or the physiologic state of the host. Acupuncture, an integrative therapy, has been widely studied for its potential to ameliorate chemotherapy-induced side effects and has been proven to have neuromodulatory effects. Many of these side effects are likely mediated and/or propagated through the central and peripheral nervous systems and thus are effectively treated with acupuncture. Acupuncture is safe when performed by qualified practitioners and it is important to have safe and effective supportive care treatments for persons with cancer enabling the curative goal of cancer treatment, long-term, disease free survival.

References

Abuaisha, B. B., Constanzi, J. B., & Boulton, A. J. M. (1998). Acupuncture for the treatment of chronic painful peripheral diabetic neuropathy: A long term study. *Diabetes Research and Clinical Practice, 39,* 115–121.

Aghajanian, C., Soignet, S., Dizon, D. S., et al. (2002). A Phase I trial of the novel proteasome inhibitor PS341 in advanced solid tumor malignancies. *Clinical Cancer Research, 8,* 2505–2511.

Ahn, A. C., Colbert, A. P., Anderson, B. J., Martinsen, O. G., Hammerschlag, R., Cina, S., et al. (2008). Electrical properties of acupuncture points and meridians: A systematic review. *Bioelectromagnetics, 29,* 245–256.

Albers, J. W., Chaudhry, V., Cavaletti, G., & Donehower, R. C. (2011). Interventions for preventing neuropathy caused by cisplatin and related compounds. *Cochrane Database of Systematic Reviews, 16,* CD005228.

Altman, D. G., Schulz, K. F., Moher, D., Egger, M., Davidoff, F., Elbourne, D., et al. (2001). The revised CONSORT statement for reporting randomized trials: Explanation and elaboration. *Annals of Internal Medicine, 134,* 663–694.

American Society of Health-System Pharmacists (ASHP). (1999). ASHP therapeutic guidelines on the pharmacologic management of nausea and vomiting in adult and pediatric patients receiving chemotherapy or radiation therapy or undergoing surgery. *American Journal of Health-Systems Pharmacy, 56,* 729–764.

Anderson, J. (2003). The role of antiandrogen monotherapy in the treatment of prostate cancer. *BJU International, 91,* 455–461.

Ashamalla, H., Jiang, M. L., Guirguis, A., Peluso, F., & Ashamalla, M. (2011). Acupuncture for the alleviation of hot flashes in men treated with androgen ablation therapy. *International Journal of Radiation Oncology, Biology, Physics, 79,* 1358–1363.

Bai, L., Yan, H., Li, L., Qin, W., Chen, P., Liu, P., et al. (2010). Neural specificity of acupuncture stimulation at pericardium 6: Evidence from an FMRI study. *Journal of Magnetic Resonance Imaging: JMRI, 31*, 71–77.

Baker, P. D., Morzorati, S. L., & Ellett, M. L. (2005). The pathophysiology of chemotherapy-induced nausea and vomiting. *Gastroenterology Nursing, 28*, 469–480.

Batty, N., Hagemeister, F. B., Feng, L., Romaguera, J. E., Rodriguez, M. A., McLaughlin, P., et al. (2012). Doxorubicin, bleomycin, vinblastine and dacarbazine chemotherapy with interferon for advanced stage classic Hodgkin lymphoma: A 10-year follow-up study. *Leukemia and Lymphoma, 53* 801–806.

Berlin, N. I., Rall, D., Mead, J. A., Freireich, E. J., Vanscott, E., Hertz, R. et al. (1963). Folic acid antagonist. Effects on the cell and the patient. Combined clinical staff conference at the National Institutes of Health. *Annals of Internal Medicine, 59*, 931–956.

Bonneterre, J., Buzdar, A., Nabholtz, J. M., Robertson, J. F., Thürlimann, B., & von Euler, M. (2001). Anastrozole is superior to tamoxifen as first-line therapy in hormone receptor positive advanced breast carcinoma. *Cancer, 92*, 2247–2258.

Borison, H. L., & Wang, S. C. (1953). Physiology and pharmacology of vomiting. *Pharmacological Reviews, 5*, 193–230.

Brem, H., Piantadosi, S., Burger, P. C., Walker, M., Selker, R., Vick, N. A., et al. (1995). Placebo-controlled trial of safety and efficacy of intraoperative controlled delivery by biodegradable polymers of chemotherapy for recurrent gliomas. *Lancet, 345*, 1008–1012.

Brunton, L. L., Chabner, B. A., & Knollmann, B. C. (Eds.). (2011). Goodman & Gilman's the pharmacological basis of therapeutics (12th ed.). New York: McGraw-Hill Medical.

Campos, D., Pereira, J. R., Reinhardt, R. R., Carracedo, C., Poli, S., Vogel, C., et al. (2001). Prevention of cisplatin-induced emesis by the oral neurokinin-1 antagonist, MK-869, in combination with granisetron and dexamethasone or with dexamethasone alone. *Journal of Clinical Oncology, 19*, 1759–1767.

Cao, J. X., Xiao, X. H., & Tang, X. Y. (1997). Elemene fluorouracil Moxibustion "Shenque" effect in the treatment of advanced gastric cancer observed. *Chinese Journal of Clinical Oncology, 24*, 549–550.

Capodice, J. L. (2010). Acupuncture in the oncology setting: Clinical trial update. *Current Treatment Options in Oncology, 11*, 87–94.

Capodice, J. L., Cheetham, P., Benson, M. C., McKiernan, J. M., & Katz, A. E. (2011). Acupuncture for the treatment of hot flashes in men with advanced prostate cancer. *International Journal of Clinical Medicine, 2*, 51–55.

Cavaletti, G., Marmiroli, P., Cavaletti, G., & Marmiroli, P. (2004). Chemotherapy-induced peripheral neurotoxicity. *Expert Opinion on Drug Safety, 3*, 535–546.

Chen, X. (1999). *Chinese acupuncture and moxibustion*. Beijing: Foreign Languages Press.

Chen, K., Jiang, Y., Wen, H., Lu, X. Z., Lu, L., Wang, H., et al. (2000). Clinical study on treatment of nasopharyngeal carcinoma by radio and chemotherapy with supplementary moxibustion on Shenque point. *Chinese Journal of Integrative Medicine, 20*, 733–735.

Chen, J. X., Ibe, B. O., & Ma, S. X. (2006). Nitric oxide modulation of norepinephrine production in acupuncture points. *Life Sciences, 79*, 2157–2164.

Chin, C. L, Fox, G. B, Hradil, V. P., Osinski, M. A., McGaraughty, S. P., Skoubis, P. D. et al. (2006). Pharmacological MRI in awake rats reveals neural activity in area postrema and nucleus tractus solitarius: Relevance as a potential biomarker for detecting drug-induced emesis. *Neuroimage, 33*, 1152–1160.

Cocquyt, V., Van Belle, S., Reinhardt, R. R., Decramer, M. L., O'Brien, M., Schellens, J. H., et al. (2001). Comparison of L-758,298, a prodrug for the selective neurokinin-1 antagonist, L-754,030, with ondansetron for the prevention of cisplatin-induced emesis. *European Journal of Cancer, 37*, 835–842.

Conn, P. M., & Crowley, W. F. Jr. (1991). Gonadotropin-releasing hormone and its analogues. *The New England Journal of Medicine, 324*, 93–103.

Crew, K. D., Capodice, J. L., Greenlee, H., Brafman, L., Fuentes, D., Awad, D., et al. (2010). Randomized, blinded, sham-controlled trial of acupuncture for the management of aromatase inhibitor-associated joint symptoms in women with early-stage breast cancer. *Journal of Clinical Oncology, 28*, 1154–1160.

Deng, G. E., Frenkel, M., Cohen, L., Cassileth, B. R., Abrams, D. I., Capodice, J. L., et al. (2009). Society for integrative oncology. Evidence-based clinical practice guidelines for integrative oncology: Complementary therapies and botanicals. *Journal of the Society for Integrative Oncology, 7*, 85–120.

Derby, L., & Czuczman, M. S. (2011). Update on novel monoclonal antibodies and immunoconjugates for the treatment of lymphoproliferative disorders. *Future Oncology, 7*, 963–979.

Dibble, S. L., Chapman, J., Mack, K. A., & Shih, A. S. (2000). Acupressure for nausea: Results of a pilot study. *Oncology Nursing Forum, 27*, 41–47.

Dibble, S. L., Luce, J., Cooper, B. A., Israel, J., Cohen, M., Nussey, B., et al. (2007). Acupressure for chemotherapy-induced nausea and vomiting: A randomized clinical trial. *Oncology Nursing Forum, 34*, 813–820.

Dolan, S., & Fitch, M. (2007). The management of venous thromboembolism in cancer patients. *British Journal of Nursing, 16*, 1308–1312.

Donald, G. K., Tobin, I., & Stringer, J. (2011). Evaluation of acupuncture in the management of chemotherapy-induced peripheral neuropathy. *Acupuncture in Medicine, 29*, 230–233.

Eden, T. O., Pieters, R., & Richards, S. (2010). Childhood Acute Lymphoblastic Leukaemia Collaborative Group (CALLCG). Systematic review of the addition of vincristine plus steroid pulses in maintenance treatment for childhood acute lymphoblastic leukaemia—an individual patient data meta-analysis involving 5,659 children. *British Journal of Haematology, 149*, 722–733.

Einhorn, E. H. (1997). Testicular cancer: An oncological success story. *Clinical Cancer Research, 3*, 2630–2632.

Enblom, A., Lekander, M., Hammar, M., Johnsson, A., Onelöv, E., Ingvar, M., et al. (2011). Getting the grip on nonspecific treatment effects: Emesis in patients randomized to acupuncture or sham compared to patients receiving standard care. *PLoS ONE, 6*, e14766.

Ettinger, D. S., Dwight, D., & Kris, M. G. (Eds.). (2005). *National comprehensive cancer network: Antiemesis, clinical practice guidelines in oncology*. Jenkintown: NCCN.

Ezzo, J. M., Richardson, M. A., Vickers, A., Allen, C., Dibble, S. L., Issell, B. F., et al. (2006). Acupuncture-point stimulation for chemotherapy-induced nausea or vomiting. *Cochrane Database of Systematic Reviews, 19*, CD002285.

Faerber, L., Drechsler, S., Ladenburger, S., Gschaidmeier, H., & Fischer, W. (2007). The neuronal 5-HT3 receptor network after 20 years of research–evolving concepts in management of pain and inflammation. *European Journal of Pharmacology, 560*, 1–8.

Fallowfield, L. J., Bliss, J. M., Porter, L. S., Price, M. H., Snowdon, C. F., Jones, S. E., et al. (2006). Quality of life in the intergroup exemestane study: A randomized trial of exemestane versus continued tamoxifen after 2–3 years of tamoxifen in postmenopausal women with primary breast cancer. *Journal of Clinical Oncology, 24*, 910–917.

Farber, S., & Diamond, L. K. (1948). Temporary remissions in acute leukemia in children produced by folic antagonist 4-amethopteroylglutamic acid (aminopterin). *The New England Journal of Medicine, 238*, 787–793.

Gao, M., Xu, W., Chen, W., & He, L. (1994). Involvement of mu opioid receptors of periaqueductal gary (PAG) in acupuncture inhibition of noxious blood pressure response in rabbits. *Acupuncture & Electro-therapeutics Research, 19*, 81–88.

Gardani, G., Cerrone, R., Biella, C., Galbiati, G., Proserpio, E., Casiraghi, M., et al. (2007). A progress study of 100 cancer patients treated by acupressure for chemotherapy-induced vomiting after failure with the pharmacological approach. *Minerva Medica, 98*, 665–668.

Go, R. S., & Adjei, A. A. (1999). Review of the comparative pharmacology and clinical activity of cisplatin and carboplatin. *Journal of Clinical Oncology, 17*, 409–422.

Goyle, S., & Maraveyas, A. (2005). Chemotherapy for colorectal cancer. *Digestive Surgery, 22*, 401–414.

Grimison, P. S., Stockler, M. R., Thomson, D. B., Olver, I. N., Harvey, V. J., Gebski, V. J., et al. (2010). Comparison of two standard chemotherapy regimens for good-prognosis germ cell tumors: Updated analysis of a randomized trial. *Journal of the National Cancer Institute, 102*, 1253–1262.

Hamaguchi, T., Shirao, K., Ohtsu, A., Hyodo, I., Arai, Y., Takiuchi, H., et al. (2011). Gastrointestinal oncology study group of japan clinical oncology group. A Phase II study of biweekly mitomycin C and irinotecan combination therapy in patients with fluoropyrimidine-resistant advanced gastric cancer: A report from the gastrointestinal oncology group of the japan clinical oncology group (JCOG0109-DI Trial). *Gastric Cancer, 14*, 226–233.

Harris, M. (2004). Monoclonal antibodies as therapeutic agents for cancer. *Lancet, 5*, 292–302.

Henderson, I. C., Berry, D. A., Demetri, G. D., Cirrincione, C. T., Goldstein, L. J., Martino, S., et al. (2003). Improved outcomes from adding sequential paclitaxel but not from escalating doxorubicin dose in an adjuvant chemotherapy regimen for patients with node positive primary breast cancer. *Journal of Clinical Oncology, 21*, 976–983.

Hervik, J., & Mjåland, O. (2009). Acupuncture for the treatment of hot flashes in breast cancer patients, a randomized, controlled trial. *Breast Cancer Research and Treatment, 116*, 311–316.

Higano, C. S. (2003). Side effects of androgen deprivation therapy: Monitoring and minimizing toxicity. *Urology, 61*, 32–38.

Ho, A. D., Lipp, T., Ehninger, G., Illiger, H. J., Meyer, P., Freund, M. et al. (1998). Combination of mitoxantrone and etoposide in refractory acute myelogenous leukemia—an active and well-tolerated regimen. *Journal of Clinical Oncology, 6*, 213–217.

Hornby, P. J. (2001). Central neurocircuitry associated with emesis. *The American Journal of Medicine, 111*, 106S–112S.

Hsieh, J. C., Tu, C. H., Chen, F. P., Chen, M. C., Yeh, T. C., & Cheng, H. C., et al. (2001). Activation of the hypothalamus characterizes the acupuncture stimulation at the analgesic point in human: A positron emission tomography study. *Neuroscience Letters, 307*, 105–108.

Jin, Y., Hayes, D. F., Li, L., Robarge, J. D, Skaar, T. C., Philips, S., et al. (2008). Estrogen receptor genotypes influence hot flash prevalence and composite score before and after tamoxifen therapy. *Journal of Clinical Oncology, 26*, 5849–5854.

Jung, D., Lee, S., & Hong, S. (2012). Effects of acupuncture and moxibustion in a mouse model of allergic rhinitis. *Otolaryngology-Head and Neck Surgery, 146*, 19–25.

Klotz, L., Boccon-Gibod, L., Shore, N. D., Andreou, C., Persson, B. E., Cantor, P., et al. (2008). The efficacy and safety of degarelix: A 12-month, comparative, randomized, open-label, parallel-group Phase III study in patients with prostate cancer. *BJU International, 102*, 1531–1538.

Kohler, G, & Milstein, C. (1975). Continuous cultures of fused cells secreting antibody of predefined specificity. *Nature, 256*, 495–497

Krzakowski, M., Provencio, M., Utracka-Hutka, B., Villa, E., Codes, M., Kuten, A., et al. (2008). Oral vinorelbine and cisplatin as induction chemotherapy and concomitant chemoradiotherapy in stage III non-small cell lung cancer: Final results of an international Phase II trial. *Journal of Thoracic Oncology, 3*, 994–1002.

Kufe, D. W. (Ed.). (2010). *Holland-frei cancer medicine* (8th ed.). USA: People's Medical Publishing House.

Langevin, H. M., Bouffard, N. A., Churchill, D. L., & Badger, G. J. (2007). Connective tissue fibroblast response to acupuncture: Dose-dependent effect of bidirectional needle rotation. *Journal of Alternative and Complementary Medicine, 13*, 355–360.

Langevin, H. M., Wayne, P. M., Macpherson, H., Schnyer, R., Milley, R. M., Napadow, V., Lao, L., Park, J., Harris, R. E., Cohen, M., Sherman, K. J., Haramati, A., & Hammerschlag. R. (2010). Paradoxes in acupuncture research: Strategies for moving forward. *Evidence-Based Complementary and Alternative Medicine, 2011*, 180805.

Lee, A., & Fan, L. T. (2009). Stimulation of the wrist acupuncture point P6 for preventing postoperative nausea and vomiting. *Cochrane Database of Systematic Reviews, 2*, CD003281.

Lee, E. J., & Frazier, S. K. (2011). The efficacy of acupressure for symptom management: A systematic review. *Journal of Pain and Symptom Management, 42*, 589–603.

Lee, J., & Swain, S. (2006). Peripheral neuropathy induced by microtubule stabilizing agents. *Journal of Clinical Oncology, 24,* 19633–19642.

Lee, M. S., Choi, T. Y., Park, J. E., Lee, S. S., & Ernst, E. (2010). Moxibustion for cancer care: A systematic review and meta-analysis. *BMC Cancer, 10,* 130.

Leone, G., Fianchi, L., & Voso, M. T. (2011). Therapy-related myeloid neoplasms. *Current Opinion in Oncology, 23,* 672–680.

Leslie, R. A., & James, M. F. (2000). Pharmacological magnetic resonance imaging: A new application for functional MRI. *Trends in Pharmacological Sciences, 21,* 314–318.

Longo, D. L., Fauci, A. S., Kasper, D. L., Hauser, S. L., Jameson, J. L., & Loscalzo, J. (Eds.). (2012). *Harrison's principles of internal medicine* (18th ed.). New York: McGraw-Hill Medical

Lu, W., & Rosenthal, D. S. (2010). Recent advances in oncology acupuncture and safety considerations in practice. *Current Treatment Options in Oncology, 11,* 141–146.

MacPherson, H., Altman, D. G., Hammerschlag, R., Youping, L., Taixiang, W., White, A., et al. (2010). Revised standards for reporting interventions in clinical trials of acupuncture (STRICTA): Extending the CONSORT statement. *Journal of Evidence-based Medicine, 3,* 140–155.

Malizia, E., Andreucci, G., Paolucci, D., Crescenzi, F., Fabbri, A., & Fraioli, F. (1979). Electroacupuncture and peripheral beta-endorphin and ACTH levels. *Lancet, 2,* 535–536.

Mao, J. J., Bruner, D. W., Stricker, C., Farrar, J. T., Xie, S. X., Bowman, M. A., et al. (2009). Feasibility trial of electroacupuncture for aromatase inhibitor–related arthralgia in breast cancer survivors. *Integrative Cancer Therapies, 8,* 123–129.

McLaughlin, P., Grillo-López, A. J., Link, B. K., Levy, R., Czuczman, M. S., Williams, M. E., et al. (1998). Rituximab chimeric anti-CD20 monoclonal antibody therapy for relapsed indolent lymphoma: Half of patients respond to a four-dose treatment program. *Journal of Clinical Oncology, 16,* 2825–2833.

Melchart, D., Weidenhammer, W., Streng, A., Reitmayr, S., Hoppe, A., Ernst, E., et al. (2004). Prospective investigation of adverse effects of acupuncture in 97,733 patients. *Archives of Internal Medicine, 164,* 104–105.

Melchart, D., Ihbe-Heffinger, A., Leps, B., von Schilling, C., & Linde, K. (2006). Acupuncture and acupressure for the prevention of chemotherapy-induced nausea–a randomised cross-over pilot study. *Supportive Care in Cancer, 14,* 878–882.

Meyer, R. M., Gospodarowicz, M. K., Connors, J. M., Pearcey, R. G., Wells, W. A., et al. (2012). ABVD alone versus radiation-based therapy in limited-stage Hodgkin's lymphoma. *The New England Journal of Medicine, 366,* 399–408.

Miller, A. D., & Leslie, R. A. (1994). The area postrema and vomiting. *Frontiers in Neuro-endocrinology, 15,* 301–320.

Morrow, G. R., Roscoe, J. A., Hickok, J. T., Andrews, P. R., & Matteson, S. (2002). Nausea and emesis: Evidence for a biobehavioral perspective. *Supportive Care in Cancer, 10,* 96–105.

Nakata, T., & Yoriguji, H. (1999). Morphological evidence of the inhibitory effect of Taxol on the fast axonal transport. *Neuroscience Research, 35,* 113–122.

Nedstrand, E., Wijma, K., Wyon, Y., & Hammar, M. (2005). Vasomotor symptoms decrease in women with breast cancer randomized to treatment with applied relaxation or electro-acupuncture: A preliminary study. *Climacteric, 8,* 243–250.

NIH. (1998). NIH Consensus Conference. Acupuncture. *The Journal of the American Medical Association, 280,* 1518–1524.

Park, J. E., Lee, S. S., Lee, M. S., Choi, S. M., & Ernst, E. (2010). Adverse events of moxibustion: A systematic review. *Complementary Therapies in Medicine, 18,* 215–223.

Peets, J. M., & Pomeranz, B. (1978). CXBK mice deficient in opiate receptors show poor electroacupuncture analgesia. *Nature, 273,* 675–676.

Pui, C. H., Relling, M. V., & Downing, J. R. (2004). Mechanisms of disease: Acute lymphoblastic leukemia. *The New England Journal of Medicine, 350,* 1535–1548.

Quaasthoff, S., & Hartung, H. P. (2002). Chemotherapy induced peripheral neuropthay. *Journal of Neurology, 249,* 9–17.

Racke, K., Reimann, A., Schworer, H., & Kilbinger, H. (1996). Regulation of 5-HT release from enterochromaffin cells. *Behavioural Brain Research, 73*, 83–87.
Reindl, T. K., Geilen, W., Hartmann, R., Wiebelitz, K. R., Kan, G., Wilhelm, I., et al. (2006). Acupuncture against chemotherapy-induced nausea and vomiting in pediatric oncology Interim results of a multicenter crossover study. *Supportive Care in Cancer, 14*, 172–176.
Richardson, P. G., Briemberg, H., Jagannath, S., Wen, P. Y., Barlogie, B., Berenson, J., et al. (2006). Frequency, characteristics, and reversibility of peripheral neuropathy during treatment of advanced multiple myeloma with bortezomib. *Journal of Clinical Oncology, 24*, 3113–3120.
Sanger, G. J., & Andrews, P. L. (2006, October 30). Treatment of nausea and vomiting: Gaps in our knowledge. *Autonomic Neuroscience, 129*, 3–16.
Sartor, O., Michels, R. M., Massard, C., & de Bono, J. S. (2011). Novel therapeutic strategies for metastatic prostate cancer in the post-docetaxel setting. *Oncologist, 16*, 1487–1497.
Savage, D., & Antman, K. (2002). Imatinib mesylate. A new oral targeted therapy. *The New England Journal of Medicine, 346*, 683–693.
Scuteri, A., Galimberti, A., Ravasi, M., Pasini, S., Donzelli, E., Cavaletti, G., et al. (2010 Dec 17). NGF protects dorsal root ganglion neurons from oxaliplatin by modulating JNK/Sapk and ERK1/2. *Neuroscience Letters, 486*, 141–145.
Shariat, S. F., Chade, D. C., Karakiewicz, P. I., Scherr, D. S., & Dalbagni, G. (2010). Update on intravesical agents for non-muscle-invasive bladder cancer. *Immunotherapy, 2*, 381–392.
Sharifi, N., Gulley, J. L., & Dahut, W. L. (2005). Androgen deprivation therapy for prostate cancer. *The Journal of the American Medical Association, 294*, 238–244.
Sharma, S., Gong, P., Temple, B., Bhattacharyya, D., Dokholyan, N. V., Chaney, S. G. et al. (2007). Molecular dynamic simulations of cisplatin- and oxaliplatin-d(GG) intrastrand cross-links reveal differences in their conformational dynamics. *Journal of Molecular Biology, 373*, 1123–1140.
Shen, J., Wenger, N., Glaspy, J., Hays, R. D., Albert, P. S., Choi, C., et al. (2000). Electroacupuncture for control of myeloablative chemotherapy-induced emesis: A randomized controlled trial. *The Journal of the American Medical Association, 284*, 2755–2761.
Shi, Y., Qi, L., Wang, J., Xu, M. S., Zhang, D., Wu, L. Y. et al. (2011). Moxibustion activates mast cell degranulation at the ST25 in rats with colitis. *World Journal of Gastroenterology, 28*, 3733–3738.
Siegert, W., Beyer, J., Strohscheer, I., Baurmann, H., Oettle, H., Zingsem, J., et al. (1994). High-dose treatment with carboplatin, etoposide, and ifosfamide followed by autologous stem-cell transplantation in relapsed or refractory germ cell cancer: A Phase I/II study. The german testicular cancer cooperative study group. *Journal of Clinical Oncology, 12*, 1223–1231.
Slamon, D. J., Leyland-Jones, B., Shak, S., Fuchs, H., Paton, V., Bajamonde, A., et al. (2001). Use of chemotherapy plus a monoclonal antibody against HER2 for metastatic breast cancer that overexpresses HER2. *The New England Journal of Medicine, 344*, 783–792.
Sparano, J. A., Wang, M., Martino, S., Jones, V., Perez, E. A., Saphner, T., et al. (2008). Weekly paclitaxel in the adjuvant treatment of breast cancer. *The New England Journal of Medicine, 358*, 1663–1671.
Streitberger, K., Ezzo, J., & Schneider, A. (2006). Acupuncture for nausea and vomiting: An update of clinical and experimental studies. *Autonomic Neuroscience, 129*, 107–117.
Talpaz, M., Silver, R. T., Druker, B. J., Goldman, J. M., Gambacorti–Passerini, C., Guilhot, F., et al. (2002). Imatinib induces durable hematologic and cytogenic responses in patients with accelerated phase chronic myeloid leukemia: Results of a Phase 2 study. *Blood, 99*, 1928–1937.
Tatewaki, M., Strickland, C., Fukuda, H., Tsuchida, D., Hoshino, E., Pappas, T. N., et al. (2005). Effects of acupuncture on vasopressin-induced emesis in conscious dogs. *American Journal of Physiology. Regulatory, Integrative and Comparative Physiology, 288*, R401–R408.
Theiss, C., & Meller, K. (2000). Taxol impairs anterograde axonal transport of microinjected horseradish peroxidase in dorsal root ganglia neurons in vitro. *Cell and Tissue Research, 299*, 213–224.

Tipton, J. M., McDaniel, R. W., Barbourm, L., Johnston, M. P., Kayne, M., LeRoy, P., et al. (2007). Putting evidence into practice: Evidence-based interventions to prevent, manage, and treat chemotherapy-induced nausea and vomiting. *Clinical Journal of Oncology Nursing, 11*, 69–78.

Van Belle, S., Lichinitser, M. R., Navari, R. M., Garin, A. M., Decramer, M. L., Riviere, A., et al. (2002). Prevention of cisplatin-induced acute and delayed emesis by the selective neurokinin-1 antagonists, L-758,298 and MK-869. *Cancer, 94*, 3032–3041.

van Oosterom, A. T., Judson, I., Verweij, J., Stroobants, S., Donato di Paola, E., Dimitrijevic, S., et al. (2001). European organisation for research and treatment of cancer soft tissue and bone sarcoma group. Safety and efficacy of imatinib (STI571) in metastatic gastrointestinal stromal tumours: A Phase I study. *Lancet, 358*, 1421–1423.

Vickers, A. J. (1996). Can acupuncture have specific effects on health? A systematic review of acupuncture antiemesis trials. *Journal of the Royal Society of Medicine, 89*, 303–311.

Walker, E. M., Rodriguez, A. I., Kohn, B., Ball, R. M., Pegg, J., Pocock, J. R., et al. (2010). Acupuncture versus venlafaxine for the management of vasomotor symptoms in patients with hormone receptor-positive breast cancer: A randomized controlled trial. *Journal of Clinical Oncology, 28*, 634–640.

Wang, C., Zhou, D. F., Shuai, X. W., Liu, J. X., & Xie, P. Y. (2007). Effects and mechanisms of electroacupuncture at PC6 on frequency of transient lower esophageal sphincter relaxation in cats. *World Journal of Gastroenterology, 13*, 4873–4880.

Wayne, P. M., Krebs, D. E, Macklin, E. A., Schnyer, R., Kaptchuk, T. J., Parker, S. W., et al. (2005). Acupuncture for upper-extremity rehabilitation in chronic stroke: A randomized sham-controlled study. *Archives of Physical Medicine and Rehabilitation, 86*, 2248–2255.

White, A. (2004). A cumulative review of the range and incidence of significant adverse events associated with acupuncture. *Acupuncture in Medicine, 22*, 122–133.

Windebank, A. J., Smith, A. G., & Russell, J. W. (1994). The effect of nerve growth factor, ciliary neurotrophic factor, and ACTH analogs on cisplatin neurotoxicity in vitro. *Neurology, 44*, 488–494.

Xu, W. R., Hua, B. J., Hou, W., & Bao, Y. J. (2010). Clinical randomized controlled study on acupuncture for treatment of peripheral neuropathy induced by chemotherapeutic drugs. *Zhongguo Zhen Jiu, 30*, 457–460.

Yoo, S. S., Teh, E. K., Blinder, R. A., & Jolesz, F. A. (2004). Modulation of cerebellar activities by acupuncture stimulation: Evidence from fMRI study. *Neuroimage, 22*, 932–940.

Zou, D., Chen, W. H., Iwakiri, K., Rigda, R., Tippett, M., & Holloway, R. H. (2005). Inhibition of transient lower esophageal sphincter relaxations by electrical acupoint stimulation. *American Journal of Physiology. Gastrointestinal and Liver Physiology, 289*, G197–G201.

Chapter 8
Acupuncture for the Treatment of Symptoms Associated with Radiation Therapy

Jennifer A. Stone, Sarah C. Greene and Peter Johnstone

Abstract Radiation therapy (RT) is the standard therapy for many cancers. This chapter summarizes the various effects of RT on different tissues of the body and presents considerations for the use of acupuncture as an integrated treatment for symptoms referable to RT in terms of traditional Chinese medicine (TCM) and Western medicine. Many common side effects of RT are presented, including xerostomia, skin irritation and burns, nausea, vomiting, neutropenia and fatigue. The mechanisms of acupuncture's effects are discussed, including increase of fibroblast, decrease of inflammatory cytokines, as well as increase of T lymphocytes, adenosine, neuropeptides, opioid peptides and peptide hormones. A brief explanation is given on how TCM theory is applied to enhance a patient's overall wellness from both the TCM and Western medical perspectives. The concept of "symptom clusters" is addressed, showing how TCM is well-suited for this phenomenon. Acupuncture may be used as a safe adjunct to help preventing and minimizing the side effects of RT, enabling cancer patients to continue and complete their RT on schedule.

8.1 Radiation Effects

The effect of radiation on living tissue is broadly recognized as the discipline of Radiation Biology and clearly exceeds full description here. Readers are suggested to refer to Hall and Giaccia (2012) for more in-depth elucidation of concepts discussed in this section.

J. A. Stone (✉)
Department of Radiation Oncology, School of Medicine, Indiana University,
357 S. Landmark Ave. Suite B, Bloomington, IN 47403, USA
e-mail: jemeador@iupui.edu

S. C. Greene
Indiana University, 357 S. Landmark Ave.
Suite B, Bloomington, IN 47403, USA

P. Johnstone
Chair of the Department of Radiation Oncology,
535 Barnhill Drive RT041, Indianapolis, IN 46202, USA

W. C. S. Cho (ed.), *Acupuncture and Moxibustion as an Evidence-based Therapy for Cancer*, Evidence-based Anticancer Complementary and Alternative Medicine 3,
DOI 10.1007/978-94-007-4833-0_8,

Radiation is delivered clinically using either particles or photons. Regardless of which method used, once radiation enters the skin and subcutaneous tissue, it interacts with atoms and molecules resulting in a shower of electrons within the tissue: these then interact with DNA within the cells.

Much of this DNA damage is repaired by inherent mechanisms in the cell, although some is not. Some of the lingering DNA damage causes the cell to die, however some does not. A portion of the non-lethal effects are of no consequence, but some are quite important. The likelihood of radiation effect in any organ is thus related to the type of radiation, the dose of radiation, the inherent repair capacity of the organ, the percentage of the organ treated, and the specific effect of interest. As an example of the last point: the total radiation dose at which skin becomes erythematous is far lower than the dose required to produce a severe radiation burn or non-healing wound.

Tumors, as a rule, have less inherent repair capacity than normal tissue. Tumor cellular mechanisms are generally shifted to emphasize reproduction (i.e. making new tumor cells). For the purpose of this chapter, however, the effect of radiation on tumors is of less importance than its normal tissue effect.

The effect of radiation at the DNA/cellular level manifests variable morbidity at the organ level since different organs serve vastly different functions. The skin and the digestive system have large stem cell populations, as there is a constant sloughing of more superficial cells requiring replacement with new cells. In these organs, radiation effects are seen relatively quickly: erythema, in the oropharynx, usually begins within the first 3 weeks of a course of radiation therapy. Other organs (e.g. brain, spinal cord) seldom or never require new cells once they are mature. In these organs, radiation effects are generally seen months after therapy is completed. Note that the time at which radiation toxicity manifests is a unique function of each organ.

Similarly, each organ has a unique minimum radiation dose at which toxicity is noted. Some organs are far more sensitive than others. This is the case for tumors as well; radiation doses used to treat seminomas are different than those for lymphomas or carcinomas.

Thus, while the goal of RT appears deceptively simple: "Give enough doses to kill the entire tumor," each patient has a unique lesion surrounded by unique organs in a unique body. Radiation oncologists are limited by that normal tissue when they treat tumors. If the patient dies because of radiation's effect on normal tissue we clearly have not provided them a benefit. The benefit to patients comes from maximizing dose to tumor (thus potential for cure) while minimizing normal tissue effects (thus potential for toxicity).

A particular circumstance of radiation exposure contributing to a unique set of syndromes exists when the entire body is irradiated. Understandably, this has significant consequences even under the best of circumstances because the body's stem cell supply for white blood cells, among others, is quite limited. Whole-body radiation dose may produce fatalities after nuclear accidents and is the predominant medical concern in patients surviving the blast effect after nuclear explosions, yet this is routinely performed in the cancer clinic as pre-treatment prior to stem cell transplant for leukemias and similar diseases. In this context, patients are closely monitored and provided supportive medicines, etc. to minimize risk of fatality from the procedure. This is an extraordinarily complex procedure requiring significant integration of services within the hospital. Radiation doses are closely scrutinized to ensure they contribute solely to hematopoietic toxicity and remain below the threshold level for the gastrointestinal syndrome. Once that threshold is exceeded, and digestive system mucosa sloughs without stem cell regeneration, patients inevitably die of fluid loss and overwhelming sepsis. At higher doses seen only in radiation accidents or incidents, a CNS syndrome leads to much more rapid death, likely due to vascular disruption.

8.2 Complementary and Alternative Medicine (CAM) and Acupuncture

Natural tribal medicines and healing techniques practiced by different cultures for millennia that have survived today fall into the category of CAM. Some types of CAM include Ayurvedic medicine from India, Tibetan medicine, Native American medicine, and traditional Chinese medicine (TCM). These medicines and healing techniques exist today as a result of thousands of years of empirical evidence.

Integrative medicine (IM) refers to the types of CAM therapies that have been proven to be effective in modern rigorous clinical trials. Acupuncture is one of those therapies. The National Cancer Institute (NCI) provides an overview of the use of acupuncture as a treatment for individuals with cancer or cancer-related disorders. The summary includes a brief history of acupuncture practice, a review of laboratory and animal studies, the results of clinical observations and trials, and possible side effects of acupuncture therapy (http://www.cancer.gov/cancertopics/pdq/cam/acupuncture/healthprofessional).

Acupuncture has been practiced for over 3,500 years. It is a healing technique of puncturing the body with small needles for the intended relief or cure of symptoms and illness. According to TCM theory, acupuncture acts to restore a balance of Qi, the vital energy of the body. Qi is subcategorized into yin Qi and yang Qi. Yin Qi is feminine in nature and refers to the cool solid nurturing energy in the body nourished by the food and water the body receives. Yang Qi is masculine in nature and refers to the active warm energy that creates movement in the body and is nourished by the air we breathe. Each organ and system is considered either yin or yang. Solid organs such as spleen, liver, and kidney are yin organs. Hollow, more active organs are categorized as yang organs, such as stomach, intestines, and urinary bladder (Kaptchuk 2000).

Meridians are pathways of Qi that house the acupuncture points. There are 12 primary bilateral meridians that are associated with each organ and system. The acupuncture points located on these meridians are chosen to restore the balance of Qi in both the meridians and in the whole body system. Acupuncture used in TCM treatment strategy usually involves selecting points that will harmonize both the "root" of the problem (for example, increasing fluids and nutrients) and the "branch" (helping to deliver the fluids and nutrients to where they are needed) (Kaptchuk 2000).

8.2.1 Diagnosis in Acupuncture

TCM and its theories are a vast field (http://nccam.nih.gov/health/whatiscam/chinesemed.htm). A TCM diagnosis is made by collecting information, including medical history, symptoms, habits, and lifestyle. Examination involves looking at the patient to assess the sheen and color of the skin and the tongue and the shape of the body, listening to the sound and quality of the voice and the breathing, and by palpating the muscles, acupuncture points, abdomen and 12 radial pulses that correspond to each organ and system. Once the diagnosis of disharmony is made, acupuncture points are selected on the meridians affected.

8.2.2 Biological Mechanisms of Acupuncture and Acceptance in the West

Little is known about the biological mechanisms of action for the positive effects of acupuncture, though many studies have been conducted to provide a better explanation of the effectiveness of acupuncture from a Western medical perspective in recent years. Some of these mechanisms are noted here. A needle pricking the skin causes the body to react in defense of the invasion and stimulates a biochemical and bioelectric cascade of events, each of which could explain the effects. The body responds to the needle with the release of numerous chemical signals. Mast cells release histamine triggering dilation and increased permeability of the capillaries. Macrophages discharge prostaglandins, which promote blood flow to the site. The vascular changes and dilation of the capillaries allow larger antimicrobial proteins access to the site. Blood vessel endothelial cells secrete chemokines, which direct the migration of phagocytes and signal them to increase production (Campbell and Reece 2005). A recent review examines the effect of acupuncture on fibroblast cells, a decrease of inflammatory cytokines, an increase of T lymphocytes, and the increase of adenosine, neuropeptides, opioid peptides, peptide hormones, and stem cells (Stone and Johnstone 2010).

The exact mechanism of action for the positive effects of acupuncture in treating any symptom is unknown and likely a collection of events. One possible mechanism could be related to fibroblast cytoskeletal remodeling. Fibroblasts, the most common of connective tissue cells, secrete an extracellular matrix—a web rich in collagen and other macromolecules. These fibroblasts play an important role in wound healing.

An investigation of acupuncture's effect on connective tissue revealed that acupuncture induces extensive fibroblast spreading and lamellipodia formation (Langevin et al. 2006). Another possible mechanism could be an increased production and mobilization of stem cells. Though a very recent and limited area of research, it was reported that acupuncture induced mobilization of $CD133^{+}$ $CD34^{-}$ cells in healthy individuals following whole-body acupuncture for spinal cord injuries while using a spinal injury treatment regimen compared to sham treatment (Moldenhauer et al. 2010). $CD133^{+}$ and $CD34^{-}$ cells are young, non-differentiated progenitor or stem cells, which have the ability to proliferate and differentiate into several cell types depending on the growth factors present in an environment. The concentration of these cells in peripheral blood normally is very low. The results of this study indicate that acupuncture mobilized $CD133^{+}$ and $CD34^{-}$ cells. To confirm the possibility of acupuncture mobilizing stem cells, further studies should be done.

Acupuncture was validated in cancer-related symptoms in the US at a 1997 National Institutes of Health Consensus Conference (NIH Consensus Conference 1998). The conference consisted of a 12-member panel representing the areas of acupuncture, pain, psychology, psychiatry, physical medicine and rehabilitation, drug abuse, family practice, internal medicine, health policy, epidemiology, statistics, physiology, biophysics as well as representatives from the general public. During the conference, experts from these fields presented data to the panel and a conference audience.

A summary in the Journal of the American Medical Association in 1998 (NIH Consensus Conference 1998) reported that acupuncture was safe and effective in treating adult postoperative and chemotherapy nausea and vomiting and in postoperative dental pain. The report also discussed adjunct treatment or an acceptable alternative in a comprehensive medical program for addiction, stroke rehabilitation, headache, menstrual cramps, tennis elbow, fibromyalgia, myofascial pain, osteoarthritis, low back pain, carpal tunnel syndrome, and asthma. A list of credible websites for the evaluation of acupuncture for cancer patients are listed in Table 8.1.

As a result of this conference, the NIH funded more CAM and acupuncture research in medical schools and other institutions. The NCI, the Office of Cancer CAM (OCCAM), and the National Center for CAM (NCCAM) now provide grants specifically in this area. Today acupuncture is provided as an adjunct therapy for the relief of symptoms associated with cancer treatments in many well respected cancer treatment centers and academic health centers. A recent investigation by the author reveals that acupuncture to support cancer patients is provided at 26 of the 39 NCI's Designated Comprehensive Cancer Research Centers.

8.3 Radiation Therapy Side Effects

Although Western medicine regularly controls tumor growth, RT is not without potential side effects and risk. In most cases, radiation regimens are chosen for different types of cancers based on years of research and clinical trials. While it is critical for

Table 8.1 Websites about the evaluation of acupuncture for cancer patients

Credible websites for evaluation of acupuncture for cancer patients	Links
Society of Integrative Oncology	http://www.integrativeonc.org/
National Institutes of Health	http://nccam.nih.gov/health/acupuncture/
National Cancer Institute	http://www.cancer.gov/cancertopics/pdq/cam/acupuncture/healthprofessional/page1/AllPages
Consortium of Academic Health Centers for Integrative Medicine	http://www.imconsortium.org/members/home.html
NIH Consensus Conference Acupuncture	http://www.ncbi.nlm.nih.gov/pubmed/9809733

patients to follow the radiation schedule recommended by their radiation oncologist, sometimes RT side effects such as xerostomia, skin changes, nausea and vomiting, neutropenia and fatigue may be severe enough to necessitate a break in the radiation schedule to allow patients to heal before continuing. If this is the case, acupuncture may be considered to both prevent and heal these toxicities.

8.3.1 Xerostomia

Xerostomia is a frequent and potentially debilitating toxicity of RT for cancers of the head and neck. In normal use, adequate saliva is necessary to help process and swallow food. Saliva also prevents many infections of the mouth and throat and is crucial for proper dental hygiene. Patients who suffer from xerostomia, in addition to being uncomfortable due to this lack of saliva, are at risk for complications such as gingivitis and periodontal disease. There are many articles in the scientific literature supporting the use of acupuncture for xerostomia (Johnstone et al. 2001; Garcia et al. 2009; Braga Fdo et al. 2011; Meng et al. 2012).

One of the earliest topics of research in CAM for cancer symptom control was the use of acupuncture for xerostomia. In accordance with TCM theory, xerostomia is dryness of the stomach yin, causing dryness to rise into the throat and mouth. Since yin is nourished by nutrients and fluids, acupuncture treatment involves selection of points to nourish the yin, moisten the fluids, and extinguish and release heat and dryness. Many modern acupuncturists may provide additional needling locally around the salivary glands.

In a single institution study in pilocarpine resistant patients, it was found that acupuncture palliates xerostomia for many head and neck cancer patients following RT (Johnstone et al. 2001). A regimen of 3–4 weekly treatments followed by monthly sessions is now recommended, although some patients achieve lasting response without further therapy (Kahn and Johnstone 2005).

More recently, two prospective trials have been reported, concluding that doing acupuncture procedures while patients are on RT may reduce subsequent development of xerostomia (Braga Fdo et al. 2011). In the first, 24 consecutive patients scheduled to receive an RT dose > 50 Gy to the major salivary glands bilaterally were assigned to either the preventive acupuncture (PA) group ($n = 12$), treated with acupuncture before and during RT, or a control group ($n = 12$), treated with RT and not receiving acupuncture. Although all patients exhibited some degree of impairment in salivary gland functioning after RT, significant differences were found between the groups. Patients in the PA group showed improved salivary flow rates ($p < 0.001$) and decreased xerostomia-related symptoms ($p < 0.05$) compared with patients in the control group (Braga Fdo et al. 2011).

In addition, Dr Meng's group from Fudan University Shanghai Cancer Center collaborating with Dr Cohen's group from the University of Texas MD Anderson Cancer Center conducted a sham-controlled, randomized, feasibility trial of acupuncture for prevention of radiation-induced xerostomia (RIX) among patients with nasopharyngeal carcinoma. To determine feasibility of a sham procedure, 23 patients were randomized to real acupuncture ($n = 11$) or to sham acupuncture ($n = 12$). Patients were treated 3 times per week during their course of RT. It was concluded that true acupuncture given concurrently with RT significantly reduced xerostomia symptoms and improved QOL when compared with the sham acupuncture (Meng et al. 2012).

Previous studies on acupuncture for pilocarpine resistant xerostomia (Johnstone et al. 2001; Wong et al. 2003) and neuromuscular electrical stimulation to improve swallow function in patients with chronic dysphagia as a result of head and neck RT (Linkov et al. 2011) led to the development of a recently completed study protocol that produced positive results. The protocol was designed and developed by the Radiation Therapy Oncology Group (RTOG) of the American College of Radiology. Dr Wong and Dr Sagar conducted a feasibility study entitled "A Phase II/III study comparing acupuncture-like transcutaneous electrical nerve stimulation (ALTENS) *vs* pilocarpine in treating early RIX" (Wong et al. 2012). In a study from Stockholm, researchers designed a protocol to determine the long-term effects of acupuncture in patients with xerostomia of different etiologies. The data suggests that additional acupuncture therapy can maintain this improvement in salivary function rates for up to 3 years (Blom and Lundeberg 2000).

The exact mechanism of action for the positive effects of acupuncture on xerostomia is unknown and is likely a collection of events. The relation to a subtle stimulation of the autonomic nervous system is one possible mechanism. Concurrently, many patients who receive acupuncture for xerostomia due to Sjögren's syndrome also report improvement in dryness of eyes as well (Niemtzow et al. 2002). The mechanism for this effect is unclear, since the initial publication from San Diego included only patients resistant to the potent autonomic stimulant pilocarpine (Johnstone et al. 2001).

8.3.2 Radiation Erythema and Desquamation

Both sunlight and RT are forms of electromagnetic energy, thus the effect of both on skin will be indistinguishable. Radiation erythema and desquamation will be localized to the area that is being treated by the radiation. As a rule, radiation desquamation heals quickly but may be extremely uncomfortable for the patient. Erythema usually begins during the 3rd to 4th week of radiation, with progression to dry desquamation (flaking) and subsequently to moist desquamation. Desquamation is self-limited and will heal in 5–7 days if radiation is discontinued.

Traditional Chinese medicine theory describes a burn as toxic heat and fire at the skin level. The acupuncture points selected would attempt to nourish and cool yin and fluids in the whole body system, release and extinguish the yang heat and fire in the system, and harmonize and cool the lung, which, in TCM theory, has a direct impact on the skin and cools it as well.

There is limited evidence examining the effect of acupuncture on radiation burns in cancer patients. However, a Korean study examining the effect of acupuncture on mice shows promising results and may explain the mechanism of action for the positive effects (Lee et al. 2011). The effect of acupuncture on healing of deep second degree burns was compared to a conventional hydrocolloid dressing in mice. The expression level of inflammatory proteins were significantly reduced in the injured skin, and the number of eosinophils in blood decreased significantly following the acupuncture treatment compared to the dressing at 7 days after the burn. In addition, the acupuncture treatment was more effective in decreasing the wound size and inducing epidermal regeneration. Histological findings also revealed that there was less leukocyte infiltration and a greater reduction in the immunohistochemical reaction to macrophage inflammatory protein in the wounds treated with acupuncture *vs* dressing. This study thus demonstrates that acupuncture accelerates the skin regeneration process following deep second degree burns (Lee et al. 2011).

8.3.3 Radiation Fatigue

Radiation fatigue and the "brain fog" that accompanies it normally occur in the 3rd or 4th week of radiation (Nelson 2009). For patients who receive chemotherapy and radiation the fatigue is more pronounced. Cancer patients themselves report that the fatigue is extreme and overwhelming. Sources of fatigue are varied and may include anemia, psychological distress, concomitant symptoms and side effects, and concurrent medications. New preliminary data suggest that activation of the proinflammatory cytokine network may be responsible to some extent for fatigue that is experienced during radiotherapy (Nelson 2009).

According to a report in *Clinical Cancer Research*, there is an association between fatigue and biomarkers of cytokine activity. In particular, increased levels of the interleukin (IL)-6 cumulative exposure biomarker C-reactive protein and the IL-1β cumulative exposure biomarker IL-1 receptor antagonist were associated with a higher frequency and severity of fatigue (Nelson 2009).

The use of acupuncture to support fatigue in radiation patients is a relatively new area of research. According to TCM theory, fatigue is due to a deficiency in Qi and a disharmony of yin and yang. Diagnosis would involve determining the root of the Qi weakness and treating both the yin and yang organs and systems associated with the weakness. The root of the problem could be related to dehydration which would correspond to the kidney Qi or the lack of nutrition relating to the organs and systems that process and assimilate the food we ingest. Once the root of the problem is identified, treatment is designed to harmonize the organ or system involved to improve the yin Qi.

The branch of the TCM diagnosis would involve determining the deficiency of yang energy involved in the patient. Weakness in the lung which receives air and oxygen could be contributing to the fatigue, or a weakness or blockage in the circulatory system could be preventing the oxygen from arriving to the tissues. Acupuncture points would then be selected to harmonize both the root of the deficiency of the yin Qi and the branch of the disharmony which would circulate the oxygen and nutrients to the brain, bones, and tissues.

Evidence suggests that clinicians and cancer survivors may find benefit in considering acupuncture as an option for managing fatigue (Johnstone et al. 2003). The particular treatment described in the article "A prospective, randomized pilot trial of acupuncture of the kidney-bladder distinct meridian for the lower urinary tract symptoms" was bladder support *via* the Mingmen technique, and a positive effect was noted on coexistent hot flashes and fatigue. The exact mechanism explaining this effect is unknown, and it is likely that different mechanisms will be necessary to relieve different causes of the fatigue. If fatigue is due to psychological distress, the neuromodulatory effect of acupuncture could be a possible explanation (Wang et al. 2008); electroacupuncture stimulation protects dopaminergenic neurons (Liu et al. 2004). Another study (Shen and Lai 2007) examined the effect of six different acupoints on dopamine in the brains of rats. One of the points, Daling (PC7), stimulated dopamine in the brain. Further studies revealed that various frequencies of PC7 electrostimulation released varying levels of dopamine.

If inflammatory cytokines contribute to fatigue, acupuncture might act to modulate the inflammatory response. In recent studies acupuncture was found to have decreased the expression of three cytokines: IL-6, β-nerve growth factor and tissue inhibitors of metalloproteinase-1 (Chae et al. 2007).

Following a feasibility study to determine rationale for studying fatigue, clinical trials were conducted to determine effect size (Balk et al. 2009; Mao et al. 2009). In a pilot feasibility study involving 16 trial participants, the average fatigue and energy domains of the Lee fatigue scale (LFS) remained stable during and after RT without any expected statistical decline owing to RT (Mao et al. 2009). A modified, double-blind, randomized, placebo-controlled trial was conducted comparing a sham acupuncture treatment with a true acupuncture treatment. The sham treatment involved needling in non-specific acupuncture points unrelated to fatigue. The study was underpowered to find a statistically significant difference between the sham and the true acupuncture groups, possibly due to the biochemical and bioelectric effect of any needle invasion. Despite being underpowered, it appeared that subjects receiving the true acupuncture may benefit more than subjects receiving sham acupuncture (Balk et al. 2009). This finding may be due to the point selection of the true acupuncture which was designed to restore homeostasis in the system. Larger clinical trials are needed to further examine the impact of acupuncture on radiation fatigue.

Acupuncture is not routinely considered in mainstream discussions of options for fatigue management. While future research will more clearly determine its relative effectiveness, given the present options available, clinicians and cancer survivors may find benefit in considering and discussing acupuncture as an approach for managing persistent fatigue (Johnston et al. 2007).

Additional research is needed to evaluate the effectiveness of these therapies as well as other intervention strategies such as the use of antidepressant and psychostimulant medications (Jacobson and Thors 2003).

8.3.4 Neutropenia and Thrombocytopenia

Neutropenia and thrombocytopenia are constant concerns in cancer treatment and are a potential cause of treatment interruptions. Neutropenia is characterized as an abnormally low number of neutrophils—the most important type of white blood cell defense against infections. Thrombocytopenia refers to an abnormally low amount of platelets which are necessary for blood clotting. In cancer treatment, the most important risk factors for radiation therapy treatment interruptions with both thrombocytopenia and neutropenia are concurrent chemotherapy and percentage of marrow irradiated. Other significant factors in these groups are bone marrow metastases and previous chemotherapy (Mac Manus et al. 1997). Chemotherapy and radiation dosages have been adjusted through clinical trials and published experiences to reduce the risk of neutropenia and thrombocytopenia. However, due to the nature of chemotherapy and RT, these problems will always be a concern.

TCM theorizes that neutropenia and thrombocytopenia are due to deficient blood and yin. A physical examination is necessary to determine which organs and systems are responsible for that deficiency: it could be due to improper nutrition or an insufficiency of the digestive system to absorb and assimilate nutrients and fluids. It may also be due to a deficiency in the kidney Qi which supports the bones that make the marrow or it could be related to a stagnation of Qi that circulates the blood and the fluids. Acupoints are selected to support the identified root cause, and others are selected for supporting and making new blood. Once the root cause is established, appropriate treatment may be considered.

Until recently, acupuncture was considered to be contraindicated in patients with neutropenia and thrombocytopenia. It was previously not recommended for cancer patients undergoing chemotherapy and radiation. Studies have now shown that not only is acupuncture safe for pediatric, adolescent, and adult populations of cancer patients undergoing chemotherapy and radiation (Lu et al. 2009; Ladas et al. 2010), but it had been shown effective in improving neutropenia (Lu et al. 2009) and increasing immune cells (Okumura et al. 1999; Mori et al. 2002; Jong et al. 2006).

The mechanism of the effect of acupuncture on immune cells is still under investigation; however, flow cytometry reveals that acupuncture reduces levels of $CD4^+$ and $CD8^+$ cells, which are known to suppress overactive immune response and to increase cytotoxic NK cell activity (Okumura et al. 1999; Mori et al. 2010). An additional study revealed that immune related acupuncture points compared to non-immune related points modulated T cells. It also increased soluble IL-2 receptors and decreased IL-4 and IL-6. This indicates that acupuncture may modulate both peripheral blood lymphocyte populations and serum cytokine levels of the immune system (Jong et al. 2006).

8.3.5 Nausea and Vomiting

Gastrointestinal complaints, primarily nausea and vomiting, are a common problem for the cancer patient receiving chemotherapy or RT to the upper abdomen. The most thoroughly investigated acupuncture treatment for a cancer related symptom is the effect of acupuncture on hyper-emesis. This investigation is due in part to the 1998 report of the NIH consensus conference (NIH Consensus Conference 1998). Following this report many investigators have reported positive impact of acupuncture on both chemotherapy and radiation-induced nausea and vomiting (Melchart et al. 2006; Reindl et al. 2006; Enblom et al. 2011). For example, in a Swedish trial, patients undergoing abdominopelvic RT were randomized into two groups, receiving either true or sham acupuncture. All patients believed they had the true acupuncture and all experienced antiemetic effects. Most patients experienced relaxation as well as half pain-reduction and sleep improvement. Nausea was experienced by 20% of the acupuncture treated patients and 80% of the sham acupuncture treated patients (duration median 24% of the radiotherapy-days) (Enblom et al. 2011).

In 2002, researchers at the University of Rochester Cancer Center conducted a study examining the effect of acupressure bands at the location of acupuncture point Neiguan (PC6) on 739 patients undergoing chemotherapy. Data revealed that the acupressure bands decreased nausea and vomiting on the day of treatment but did not have a lasting effect (Roscoe et al. 2003). This study met the inclusion criteria to support a recommendation in clinical practice guidelines from the American Society of Clinical Oncology (Basch et al. 2011).

TCM theory refers to hyper-emesis as "reverse stomach Qi". In a healthy individual the Qi of the stomach directs downward. If there is an imbalance, the Qi will go backwards or up, and food, fluids and saliva will thus come back up. Reverse stomach Qi is a symptom and therefore a "branch" of the diagnosis. The root of the reverse stomach Qi might be yin and blood deficiency, stomach yin deficiency, liver fire blazing upward (e.g. in rupture of esophageal varices due to cirrhosis), or a combination of two or more root causes. TCM acupuncture point selection would be based on the appropriate root diagnosis and would describe acupoints to direct the stomach Qi downward again.

When considering factors that can influence nausea and vomiting, and the neural pathways that lead to the vomiting reflex, we can see how one study on anesthetized rats might help explain the effect of acupuncture on hyper-emesis (Fig. 8.1).

Strain gauge transducers were implanted on the serosal surface of the stomach to record circular muscle contractions during acupuncture in rats. Acupuncture caused

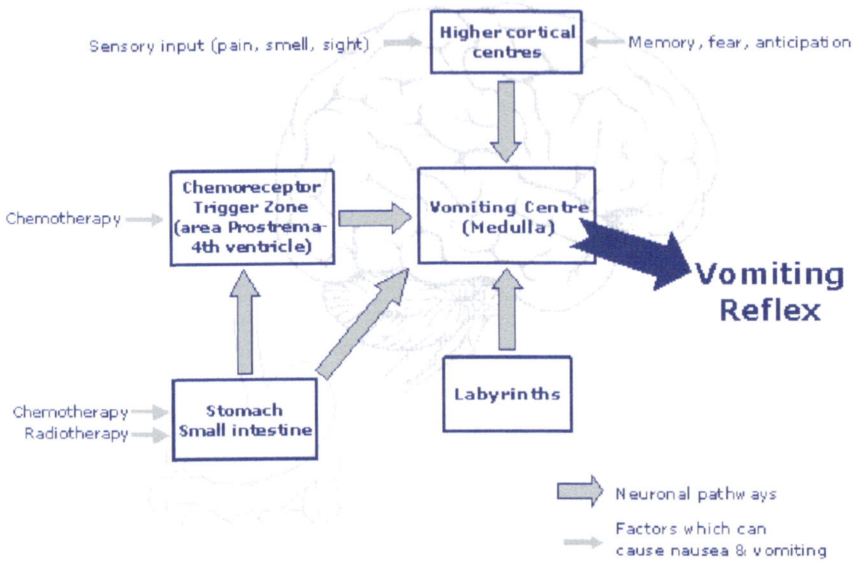

Fig. 8.1 Factors causing nausea and vomiting and neuronal pathways

transient relaxation of the stomach and increased the number of c-Fos immuno-positive cells, a marker of neuronal activity, at the ventrolateral medulla (VLM). Due to the control of blood pressure, the heart, blood vessels, swallowing and breathing all being dependent on the integrity of the VLM, researchers therefore concluded that acupuncture-induced gastric relaxations are mediated *via* the somatosympathetic reflex (Tada et al. 2003).

8.4 Symptom Clusters

A relatively new term in oncology is "symptom clusters" (Dodd et al. 2001). Most cancer patients undergo several types of treatments, and experience symptoms related both to their disease and to the treatments being received. Symptom clusters refer to patients suffering three or more related and concurrent symptoms. Defined in cancer, the symptoms may be due to any disease, to its treatment, or to some unique aspect of survivorship. Simple coexistence of symptoms at the same time is necessary but not sufficient, evidence of linkage or relationship is required (Johnstone 2011).

In 2003, the NIH sponsored a grant opportunity to examine symptom clusters and further characterize the concept. An interesting example of the NIH sponsored research was published by Chow et al. (2007) in 2007. Five hundred and eighteen patients with bone metastases completed baseline data using the Edmonton symptom assessment scale (ESAS) as a metric to investigate clustering of symptoms. The four most prevalent symptoms were poor sense of well-being (93.5%), fatigue (92.3%), pain (84.1%) and drowsiness (81.8%). Three clusters were identified and accounted for 66% of the total variance at baseline. In this study a cluster was defined as two or more symptoms that occur together, are stable, and are relatively independent of other clusters (Chow et al. 2010).

When treating symptom clusters, classic practice has been to treat each symptom separately although this contributes to polypharmacy and an increasing likelihood of drug interactions. Acupuncture presents a unique mechanism for a single therapy of symptom clusters due to the unique aspect of TCM diagnosis and treatment strategy and the reciprocal impact on the patient, the disease, and its symptoms.

8.5 Conclusion

TCM diagnosis considers the patient, the disease, the symptoms, the treatments and the psychosocial surroundings as a whole entity—a system within a universe. Underlying the practice of TCM is a unique view of the world and the human body that is markedly different from Western medicine concepts. This view is based on the ancient Chinese perception of humans as microcosms of the larger, surrounding universe—interconnected with nature and subject to its forces. The human body is regarded as an organic entity in which the various organs, tissues, and other parts have distinct functions but are all interdependent. In this view, health and disease relate to balance of the functions.

Acupuncture clearly is effective as a single modality within the whole medicine system of TCM. It is most effective in conjunction with the many therapies of the TCM system.

References

Balk, J., Day, R., Rosenzweig, M., Beriwal, S. (2009). Pilot, randomized, modified, double-blind, placebo-controlled trial of acupuncture for cancer-related fatigue. *Journal of the Society for Integrative Oncology, 7*, 4–11.

Basch, E., Prestrud, A. A., Hesketh, P. J. (2011). Antiemetics: American Society of Clinical Oncology Clinical Practice Guideline Update. http://www.asco.org/ASCOv2/Department%20Content/Cancer%20Policy%20and%20Clinical%20Affairs/Downloads/Guideline%20Tools%20and%20Resources/Antiemetics/2011/Antiemetics%20Full%20Guideline%2010.14.11.pdf.

Blom, M., Lundeberg, T. (2000). Long-term follow-up of patients treated with acupuncture for xerostomia and the influence of additional treatment. *Oral Diseases, 6*, 15–24.

Braga Fdo, P., Lemos, C. A. Jr., Alves, F.A., Migliari, D. A. (2011). Acupuncture for the prevention of radiation-induced xerostomia in patients with head and neck cancer. *Brazilian Oral Research, 25*, 180–185.

Campbell, N., Reece, J. (2005). Biology, 7th ed. San Francisco: Pearson Educational Inc., pp. 901–902.

Chae, Y., Hong, M. S., Kim, G. H. (2007). Protein array analysis of cytokine levels on the action of acupuncture in carrageenan-induced inflammation. *Neurological research, 29*(Suppl 1), S55–S58.

Chow, E., Fan, G., Hadi, S., Filipczak, L. (2007). Symptom clusters in cancer patients with bone metastases. *Supportive Care in Cancer, 15,* 1035e–1043e.
Dodd, M. J., Miaskowski, C., Paul, S. M. (2001). Symptom clusters and their effect on the functional status of patients with cancer. *Oncology Nursing Forum, 28,* 465–470.
Enblom, A., Tomasson, A., Hammar, M., Steineck, G., Borjeson, S. (2011). Pilot testing of methods for evaluation of acupuncture for emesis during radiotherapy: A randomised single subject experimental design. *Acupuncture in Medicine: Journal of the British Medical Acupuncture Society, 29,* 94–102.
Garcia, M. K., Chiang, J. S., Cohen, L., Liu, M., Palmer, J. L., Rosenthal, D. I., et al. (2009). Acupuncture for radiation-induced xerostomia in patients with cancer: A pilot study. *Head Neck-Journal for the Sciences and Specialities of the Head and Neck, 31,* 1360–1368.
Hall, E., Giaccia, A. (2012). Radiobiology for the radiologist 15th ed. Philadelphia: Lippincott Williams and Wilkins.
Jacobsen, P. B. & Thors, C. L. (2003). Fatigue in the radiation therapy patient: Current management and investigations. *Seminars in Radiation Oncology, 13,* 372–380.
Johnstone, P. A., Peng, P., May, B., Inouye, W. S., & Niemtzow, R. C. (2001). Acupuncture for pilocarpine-resistant Xerostomia following radiotherapy for head and neck malignancies. *International Journal of Radiation Oncology, Biology, Physics, 50,* 353–357.
Johnston, M. F., Xiao, B., Hui, K. K. (2007). Acupuncture and fatigue: Current basis for shared communication between breast cancer survivors and providers. *Journal of Cancer Survivorship, 1,* 306–312.
Johnstone, P. A., Polston, G. R., Niemtzow, R. C. (2002). Integration of acupuncture into the oncology clinic. *Palliative Medicine, 16,* 235–239.
Johnstone, P. A. S., Bloom, T. L., Niemtzow, R. C., Crain, D., Riffenburgh, R. H. (2003). A prospective, randomized pilot trial of acupuncture of the kidney-bladder distinct meridian for the lower urinary tract symptoms. *Journal of Urology, 169,* 1037–1039.
Johnstone, P. A. S. (2011). Acupuncture as cancer symptom therapy. What a difference a decade makes. *The Journal of Acupuncture and Meridian Studies, 4,* 209–213.
Jong, M. S., Hwang, S. J., Chen, F. P. (2006). Effects of electro-acupuncture on serum cytokine level and peripheral blood lymphocyte subpopulation at immune-related and non-immune-related points. *Acupuncture & Electro-therapeutics Research, 31,* 45–59.
Kahn, S. T., Johnstone, P. A. S. (2005). Management of xerostomia related to radiotherapy for head and neck cancer. *Oncology, 19,*1827–1832.
Kaptchuk, T. (2000). The web that has no weaver, Chicago: Contemporary books.
Ladas, E. J., Rooney, D., Taromina, K., Ndao, D. H., Kelly, K. M. (2010). The safety of acupuncture in children and adolescents with cancer therapy-related thrombocytopenia. *Supportive Care in Cancer, 18,* 1487–90.
Langevin, H. M., Bouffard, N. A., Badger, G. J., Churchill, D. L., Howe, A. K. (2006). Subcutaneoustissue fibroblast cytoskeletal remodeling induced by acupuncture: Evidence for a mechanotransductionbased mechanism. *Journal of Cellular Physiology, 207,* 767–774.
Lee, J. A., Jeong, H. J., Park, H. J., Jeon, S., Hong, S. U. (2011). Acupuncture accelerates wound healing in burn-injured mice. *Burns, 37,* 117–125.
Linkov, G., Branski, R. C., Amin, M., Chernichenko, N., Chen, C., Alon, G. et al. (2011). Murine model of neuromuscular electrical stimulation on squamous cell carcinoma: Potential implications for dysphagia therapy. *Head Neck-Journal for the Sciences and Specialities of the Head and Neck.* doi: 10.1002/hed.21935.
Liu, X. Y., Zhou, H. F., Pan, Y. L. (2004). Electro-acupuncture stimulation protects dopaminergic neurons from inflammation-mediated damage in medial forebrain bundle-transected rats. *Experimental Neurology, 189,* 189–196.
Lu, W., Matulonis, U. A., Doherty-Gilman, A., Lee, H., Dean-Clower, E., Rosulek, A., et al. (2009). Acupuncture for chemotherapy-induced neutropenia in patients with gynecologic malignancies: A pilot randomized, sham-controlled clinical trial. *Journal of Alternative and Complementary Medicine, 15,* 745–53.

Mac Manus, M., Lamborn, K., Khan, W., Varghese, A., Graef, L., Knox, S. (1997). Radiotherapy-associated neutropenia and thrombocytopenia: Analysis of risk factors and development of a predictive model. *Blood, 89*, 2303–2310.

Mao, J. J., Styles, T., Cheville, A., Wolf, J., Fernandes, S., Farrar, J. T. (2009). Acupuncture for nonpalliative radiation therapy-related fatigue: Feasibility study. *Journal of the Society for Integrative Oncology, 7*, 52–58.

Melchart, D., Ihbe-Heffinger, A., Leps, B., von Schilling, C., Linde, K. (2006). Acupuncture and acupressure for the prevention of chemotherapy-induced nausea–a randomised cross-over pilot study. *Supportive Care in Cancer, 14*, 878–882.

Meng, Z., Garcia, M. K., Hu, C. (2012). Randomized controlled trial of acupuncture for prevention of radiation-induced xerostomia among patients with nasopharyngeal carcinoma. *Cancer. 118*, 3337–3344.

Moldenhauer, S., Burgauner, M., Hellweg, R., Lun, A., Hohenböken, M., Dietz, E., et al. (2010). Mobilization of $CD133^{(+)}$CD34(2) cells in healthy individuals following whole-body acupuncture for spinal cord injuries. *Journal of Neuroscience Research, 88*, 1645–1650.

Mori, H., Nishijo, K., Kawamura, H., Abo, T. (2002). Unique immunomodulation by electro-acupuncture in humans possibly via stimulation of the autonomic nervous system. *Neuroscience Letters, 320*, 21–24.

Nelson, R. (2009). Radiation therapy-induced fatigue linked to inflammation. *Medscape Medical News*. http://www.medscape.com/viewarticle/707572.

Niemtzow, R. C., Kempf, K. J., & Johnstone, P. A. S. (2002). Acupuncture for Xerophthalmia. *Medical Acupuncture, 13*, 21–22.

NIH Consensus Conference (1998). Acupuncture. *JAMA, 280*, 1518–1524.

Okumura, M., Toriizuka, K., Iijima, K., Haruyama, K., Ishino, S., Cyong, J. C. (1999). Effects of acupuncture on peripheral T lymphocyte subpopulation and amounts of cerebral catecholamines in mice. *Acupuncture & Electro-therapeutics Research, 24*, 127–139.

Reindl, T. K., Geilen, W., Hartmann, R., Wiebelitz, K. R., Kan, G., Wilhelm, I., et al. (2006). Acupuncture against chemotherapy-induced nausea and vomiting in pediatric oncology. Interim results of a multicenter crossover study. *Supportive Care in Cancer, 14*, 172–176.

Roscoe, J. A., Morrow, G. R., Hickok, J. T. (2003). The efficacy of acupressure and acustimulation wrist bands for the relief of chemotherapy-induced nausea and vomiting. A University of Rochester Cancer Center Community Clinical Oncology Program multicenter study. *Journal of Pain and Symptom Management, 26*, 731–742.

Shen, E. Y., Lai, Y. J. (2007). The efficacy of frequency-specific acupuncture stimulation on extracellular dopamine concentration in striatum – a rat model study. *Neuroscience Letters, 415*, 179–184.

Stone, J. A., Johnstone, P. A. (2010). Mechanisms of action for acupuncture in the oncology setting. *Current treatment Options in Oncology, 11*, 118–127.

Tada, H., Fujita, M., Harris, M., Tatewaki, M., Nakagawa, K., Yamamura, T, et al. (2003). Neural mechanism of acupuncture-induced gastric relaxations in rats. *Digestive Diseases and Sciences, 48*, 59–68.

Wang, S. M., Kain, Z. N., White, P. (2008). Acupuncture analgesia. The scientific basis. *Anesthesia and Analgesia, 106*, 602–610.

Wong, R. K., Jones, G. W., Sagar, S. M., Babjak, A. F., Whelan, T. (2003). A Phase I–II study in the use of acupuncture-like transcutaneous nerve stimulation in the treatment of radiation-induced xerostomia in head-and-neck cancer patients treated with radical radiotherapy. *International Journal of Radiation, Oncology, Biology, Physics, 57*, 472–480.

Wong, R. K., James, J., Sagar, S., Wyatt, G., Nguyen-Tân, P. F., Singh, A. K., et al. (2012). A Phase 2/3 study comparing acupuncture-like transcutaneous electrical nerve stimulation versus pilocarpine in treating early radiation-induced xerostomia. *Cancer*. doi: 10.1002/cncr.27382.

Chapter 9
Quality of Life of Cancer Patients after Acupuncture and Moxibustion Treatment

Namie O. Sawada, Liyoko Okino and Adriana C. Nicolussi

Abstract The use of acupuncture and moxibustion can date back to primitive Chinese societies. Today, they are sometimes used in Western medicine, mainly in cancer patients, as a complementary treatment. Scientific evidence has shown their effects on various diseases and cancer treatment. This chapter discusses different acupuncture and moxibustion techniques and their applications in oncology. Acupuncture points can be stimulated through needles, pressure, electric stimulus, laser and local heat applications using herbs. Moxibustion techniques involve stimulating the points by burning herbs directly or indirectly. Scientific evidence demonstrates the action mechanisms of acupuncture and moxibustion that benefit cancer patients, relieving various collateral treatment effects and disease symptoms. Quality of life (QoL) assessments are meant to improve care for cancer patients and expand the parameters of the benefits provided by conventional and unconventional treatments, apart from assessing the disease-free survival and overall survival. There are several measures to evaluate QoL. The European Organization for Research and Treatment of Cancer—Quality of Life Questionnaire-Core30 (EORTC—QLQ-C30) and Functional Assessment Cancer Therapy-General (FACT-G) are the most commonly used tools. As QoL measure provides important information about treatment impact on patients, specific tools for measuring health-related QoL (HRQoL) is used to assess the impact of acupuncture and moxibustion. Acupuncture and moxibustion may be used as complementary treatments for cancer patients because they can help with symptom control and enhance patients' physical and emotional aspects.

9.1 Acupuncture and Moxibustion

Acupuncture is the insertion of needles with different shapes, sizes and materials on specific body points, extremities and the head. The origin of the word acupuncture derives from the Latin words *acus* (pointed or cutting) and *punctura* (puncture). Needles can be removed immediately, left in place for some time or turned a number of times, depending on the nature of the disease. Moxibustion is the application on the

N. O. Sawada (✉) · L. Okino · A. C. Nicolussi
College of Nursing at Ribeirão Preto, University of Sao Paulo,
Ribeirão Preto, SP, Brazil
e-mail: sawada@eerp.usp.br

W. C. S. Cho (ed.), *Acupuncture and Moxibustion as an Evidence-based Therapy for Cancer*, Evidence-based Anticancer Complementary and Alternative Medicine 3,
DOI 10.1007/978-94-007-4833-0_9,

skin of cones of dried or powdered *Artemisia vulgaris* leaves. These cones are lighted and burned for some time until a small blister develops. The word moxibustion is a contraction of moxa and combustion. Moxa derives from the Japanese expression mongusa, which means "burning herb". Moxibustion was enthusiastically received in Japan, where it is still practiced today in its original form, as an alternative or complement to acupuncture, independently of possible resulting burn scars. In China, on the other hand, moxibustion is used in a mitigated form, as the moxa is gradually removed from the skin, avoiding the burn. Today, it is used almost exclusively to warm the needles or warm the acupuncture points at a distance (Veith 1973).

9.1.1 Acupuncture and Moxibustion Modalities

Acupuncture and moxibustion are two different treatment methods. The first involves placing needles on energetic points, while the second comprises heat application on these points.

Although technically different, both methods exert the same therapeutic action. They act through the stimulation of acupunctural points on the meridians and organs, aimed at harmonizing the energy-blood circulation to regularize vital organic functions, reinforce defense mechanisms and neutralize aggressors.

These mechanisms put the organism in favorable conditions to fight diseases.

Acupunctural points are skin locations where the energy (Qi) of organs and intestines is manifested. When stimulated, they entail reactions of varying intensity levels, leading to the regularization of the organism's energy balance and, consequently, to the recovery of health. To stimulate these points, various traditional Chinese medicine (TCM) techniques are used, the most characteristic and frequent ones being acupuncture and moxibustion.

When metal needles are introduced in acupuncture, these can even provoke a typical pain reaction, a feeling of engorgement, weight and paresthesia.

Moxibustion is a traditional Chinese medicine method that uses burning herbal preparations with *Artemisia vulgaris* to stimulate the acupuncture points. According to World Health Organization (2007), two types of moxibustion exist: direct moxibustion—is applied directly on the skin surface on the acupuncture point; indirect moxibustion—some materials like ginger, salts and others are placed between the moxa cone and the skin.

Acupuncture instruments go through improvements depending on the cultural and economic development of society, ranging from the use of jade, metals like gold and silver to the stainless steel used today.

The needles placed on the points indicated to treat the disease and removed after 15–20 min can be stimulated manually or through polarized electrical stimuli, with frequencies and intensities chosen according to the desired result.

Press tack or wheat-shaped needles are used to remain inserted in the skin down to the subcutaneous level to treat chronic illnesses that need continuous stimulation, such as headache, insomnia, dysmenorrhea and asthma. Research has shown that auriculotherapy was as effective as systemic acupuncture to control preoperative anxiety (Wu et al. 2011) with a view to minimizing postoperative adverse effects.

The simplest means to stimulate acupuncture points is by pressing the points with the fingers, hand, elbow and foot—acupressure, aimed at stimulating the Qi energy flow. Acupressure can be an effective intervention for a range of symptoms people experience during the lifetime. It is a non-invasive and cheap intervention without adverse effects and useful for treating children (Jones et al. 2008). A review reports on different studies that have used this simple procedure to control post-surgery nausea and vomiting, motion sickness during pregnancy and pain during dysmenorrhea, labor, back pain and dyspnea. In fatigue cases, evidence of positive control was found, despite safeguards regarding better study design and randomization for future studies (Lee and Franzier 2011).

9.1.2 Auricular Point Stimulation

The application of electrical stimuli for pain relief goes back to 2500 BC, when the Egyptians used electric fish for pain treatment. In 1825, Salandière used galvanic stimulation in acupuncture to treat gout, but soon discovered that the galvanic current produces unwanted effects and even tissue necrosis, which made Duchenne (1849) use alternating faradic current for therapeutic ends (Macdonald and Coates 1995).

The use of transcutaneous electrical nerve stimulation (TENS) in acupuncture needles derived from the need to replace vigorous manual stimulation for at least 20 min to achieve surgically evoked pain suppression.

A study showed, depending on the stimulation frequency, the release of different endogenous opioid peptides (EOP). Thus, 2 Hz releases metenkephalin, 100 Hz dynorphins and 15 Hz a mixture of enkephalin and dynorphins (Han et al. 1984).

The application of low-frequency and high-intensity TENS produces its analgesic effect through the release of EOP at three sites:

- Dorsal horn: stimulating the sensory muscle afferents II and III releases enkephalin and dynorphins in the dorsal horn, leading to the blocking of any information the nociceptive system produces, transmitted through group IVU and C-polymodal muscle afferents of the skin.
- Midbrain: leads to the release of enkephalin that activates the pain inhibition system, mediated by the serotonergic system that descends from the periaqueductal gray through the lateral funiculus into the dorsal horns.
- Hypothalamus/hypophysis complex: releases the adrenocortical tropic hormone from the anterior hypophysis into the circulation and presumably releases cortisol, leading to anti-inflammatory and bronchodilator action, and the release of β-endorphin by the hypothalamus through its projection to the midbrain activates the pain inhibition system that descends from this site.

TENS stimulates A-BETA sensory afferents through high-frequency and low-intensity stimuli (40–150 Hz), which releases γ-aminobutyric acid and blocks intradorsal transmission of the information coming from group IV muscle fibers and C-nociceptors of the skin. Transcutaneous stimulation similar to acupuncture (L-TENS) uses low frequencies (1–5 Hz) and high intensity to simulate α-delta fibers and suppresses EOP mediated pain. A review on the use of TENS for cancer pain control demonstrates that pain can be neuropathic or nociceptive (Robb et al. 2009). Nociceptive pain results from the activation and sensitization of C-polymodal nociceptors on the skin and group IV muscle nociceptors, differently from neuropathic pain, which develops through the bad functioning of the central or peripheral nervous system. One reason for this is that neuropathic pain is much less responsive to acupuncture than nociceptive pain, in line with the findings of another study, which shows neuropathic pain's extreme resistance to opioid effects (Portenoy et al. 1990).

Cancer pain can be nociceptive or neuropathic, and this needs to be taken into account when deciding on the best way to relieve it (Banning et al. 1991). In cancer cases, it is important to remind that both types can coexist, as nociceptive pain can be due to trigger points (TP) in the muscle, so that it is shortened, compressing the underlying nervous roots or, on the opposite, when the cervical or lumbar nervous roots provoke the development of the trigger points.

The difference between both types can be described as follows:

The origin of nociceptive pain is myofascial. It is characterized by numb, diffuse pain with painful tissue sensitivity in the affected area and the presence of well-demarcated and very sensitive TP located at a certain distance from the site.

Neuropathic pain, which is due to peripheral nerve injury or dysfunction, is commonly described as burning or takes the form of very anguishing electric shocks.

Besides pain, various other frequent symptoms in cancer patients, whether undergoing chemotherapy or not, can be minimized or eliminated through acupuncture applications.

9.2 Health-related Quality of Life in Cancer

A study surveyed quality of life (QoL) research in the last 20 years and found that the development of more effective treatments and early cancer detection have increased cancer patients' survival (Meneses and Benz 2010). According to recent survival data by the National Cancer Institute, more than 11.4 million of cancer survivors exist in the USA. This number represents 3.8% of the population. About 14% of the 14 million cancer survivors had been diagnosed more than 20 years earlier and more than 60% of survivors had reached the age of 65 years. Cancer survival figures in the USA are increasing due to various factors, including gains in cancer prevention and early detection, target treatments and therapies, understanding about the biological bases of cancer, improved symptom control and cancer surveillance. Research about cancer survivors in the last 20 years has changed its focus from physical, psychosocial and economic sequelae during treatment to QoL changes after and at the end of treatment.

Today, it is no longer conceivable to increase cancer patients' years of life without granting them quality of life. Besides, according to Ferrans and Varrichio (2010), QoL assessment was used exclusively for cancer research 20 years ago, while QoL measures have been used to broaden the focus beyond clinical trials on tumor response and survival time today. QoL assessment in the current context has expanded into the clinical area, providing orientations for treatment decisions, intervention choices and efficacy assessment, and as a tool for medical care delivery in response to patient concerns.

One of the first instruments that broadened the assessment of patients beyond physiological and clinical examination was the Karnofsky performance status (KPS). This instrument was proposed for use in clinical settings in 1947, is a simple scale ranging from 0 for "dead" to 100 indicating "normal", no complaints, no evidence of disease. Over the years, several instruments have been constructed to evaluate functional abilities, physical functioning and activities of daily living (ADL), such as the Barthel Index. Although these questionnaires are sometimes described as QoL instruments, they capture only one aspect of it and provide an inadequate representation of patients' overall well-being and QoL (Fayers and Machin 2000).

The QoL measure in health has been called health-related QoL (HRQoL), and often in literature it appears as a synonym of perceived health status, whose main goal is to verify the extent to which the disease or chronic condition starts to interfere in an individual's daily life beyond its symptoms (Fayers and Machin 2007).

The most used instruments for HRQoL assessment in cancer survivors found in literature are European Organization for Research and Treatment of Cancer—Quality of Life Questionnaire-Core30 (EORTC—QLQ-C30), Functional Assessment Cancer Therapy-General (FACT-G), Functional Living Index-Cancer (FLI-C) and Cancer Rehabilitation Evaluation System (CARES) (Pearce et al. 2008). The authors highlight the need to test the reliability and validity of all instruments before their application to cancer survivors. As the QoL measure provides important information about treatment impact on patients' QoL, specific tools for measuring HRQoL should be used to assess the impact of acupuncture and moxibustion.

Various studies have demonstrated the effects of interventions that improve cancer patients' HRQoL, including a randomized and controlled clinical trial that tests the efficacy of an information intervention about the doubts of elderly long-term breast cancer survivors. The sample included 509 Caucasian and African women with non-metastatic disease between five and nine years after treatment. The subjects were allocated to the usual care or intervention group. Women in the intervention group were followed by telephone during 4 weeks. The nurses supported the survivors with the help of a cassette-tape that contained cognitive-behavioral strategies to manage doubts about relapse and a self-help manual to help the women understand the long-term collateral effects of treatment. The main hypothesis is that cancer survivors who received the intervention could experience significant knowledge improvements, cognitive resignification, problem solving and social support in comparison with the control group. The results demonstrated differences between the intervention and control groups ($p < 0.01$), supporting the research hypothesis (Mishel et al. 2005).

A clinical research was developed on the effects of a psycho-educational support intervention, including a breast cancer education intervention (BCEI) about the QoL of 256 female breast cancer survivors, in which participants were randomized into the intervention and control groups (Meneses et al. 2009). The BCEI consisted of three face-to-face meetings with 5 months of monitoring. The control group received 4 months of telephone care. Baseline QoL data were collected using the QoL-cancer survivors (QOL-CS) and profile of mood states (POMS) before the randomization, and three to 6 months after the start of the study. Initially, the important aspects were QoL and psychological, social and spiritual wellbeing. No baseline difference existed between both groups. The intervention group reported a better QoL after 3 months, while the control group reported a decline in QoL and treatment effects continued to exist between both groups 6 months later (Meneses et al. 2009).

A study was developed to investigate the use of acupuncture and moxibustion to improve the QoL of cancer survivors with lymphedema, involving breast and head and neck cancer patients with moderate lymphedema complications after less than 3 months of treatment. The patients received seven individualized acupuncture/moxibustion treatments (S1) and six optional treatments (S2). The instruments measure yourself medical outcome profile (MYMOP), medical study short form (SF-36) and positive and negative affect schedule (PANAS) were applied at baseline, during each series and at 4 and 12 months after the end of treatment. Out of 35 recruited patients, only 30 completed the research. The mean MYMOP score changed for breast cancer patients, with scores improving by 1.28 on a seven-point scale ($SD = 0.93$, $p < 0.0001$, $n = 25$) for S1 and 1.41 for S2 ($SD = 0.94$, $p < 0.0001$, $n = 24$). For head and neck cancer patients in S1, the score increased by 2.29 ($SD = 0.62$, $p < 0.0001$, $n = 7$), against 0.94 for S2 ($SD = 0.95$, $p < 0.06$, $n = 6$). Changes in SF-36 scores for breast cancer patients were significant after 4 weeks of treatment. No adverse effect was found. They concluded that, although the study was small, acupuncture/moxibustion showed to be an accepted adjuvant usual care treatment method for cancer survivors with lymphedema (Valois et al. 2012).

9.3 The Application of Acupuncture and Moxibustion in Cancer Treatment: Evidence from Systematic Reviews

Today, cancer patients increasingly turn to complementary treatments as adjuvant treatment, due to the different collateral effects conventional treatments cause (Lee et al. 2010; Reagan and Filshie 2010).

In this context, acupuncture and moxibustion treatments stand out, as scientific evidence already exists about these complementary therapies' effect on several symptoms cancer and its treatment cause. Next, systematic review results on the effects of acupuncture and moxibustion in cancer patients will be presented.

A study presents the action mechanisms of acupuncture in the oncology area (Stone et al. 2010) and highlights that evidence supports acupuncture use for chemotherapy-induced peripheral neuropathy (CIPN) in a case series of five patients with advanced gynecological cancer. The acupuncture protocol used was empirically developed and the points utilized were Qihai (CV6), Zusanli (ST36) and Quchi (LI11). The Hesea points of the stomach and Large Intestine meridians, respectively, were used to further tonify the Qi and blood. All five patients reported improvement of pain, numbness and tingling. The average pain score was reduced to 3 out of 10 (range 1–5). Symptom improvements were observed after the first treatment in one patient who had experienced 6 months of CIPN. The results suggest that the effect of an empirical protocol on CIPN is promising, although results need to be interpreted with caution because the sample included only five patients. A definitive conclusion that acupuncture is generally effective for CIPN needs to be proven in large trials. No mentions of adverse side effects were found (Wong and Sagar 2006).

A randomized controlled trial (Shen et al. 2000) demonstrated that in patients with breast cancer receiving high-dose chemotherapy, adjunct electroacupuncture was more effective in controlling emesis than minimal needling or anti-emetic pharmacotherapy alone in chemotherapy-associated nausea and vomiting. In that study, the objective was to compare the effectiveness of electroacupuncture *vs* minimal needling and mock electrical stimulation or anti-emetic medications alone in controlling emesis among patients undergoing a highly emetogenic chemotherapy regimen. The patients were randomly assigned to receive low-frequency electroacupuncture on classic anti-emetic acupuncture points once per day for 5 days ($n = 37$); minimal needling on control points with mock electrostimulation on the same schedule ($n = 33$) or no adjunct needling ($n = 34$). All patients received concurrent triple anti-emetic pharmacotherapy and high-dose chemotherapy (cyclophosphamide, cisplatin and carmustine). The results demonstrated that the number of emesis episodes occurring during the 5 days was lower for patients receiving electroacupuncture when compared with those receiving minimal needling or pharmacotherapy alone (median number of episodes of emesis 5, 10 and 15 respectively; $p < 0.001$). The electroacupuncture group experienced fewer episodes of emesis than the minimal needling group ($p < 0.001$), whereas the minimal needling group had fewer episodes of emesis than the group undergoing anti-emetic pharmacotherapy alone ($p = 0.01$). The differences among groups were not significant during the 9-day follow-up period ($p = 0.18$). The authors speculate that some observed effects may be manifested through the serotonin-and substance P-mediated components of the emetic reflex, as well as through the opiate μ receptor *via* its anti-emetic actions. They suggest future neurophysiological and neurochemical investigations, which may help us to further understand the complexity of emesis and broaden the current approach to the anti-emetic care spectrum. About adverse effects, two patients experienced these as a result of the electroacupuncture or minimal needling procedure, while one patient complained of an electrical shock sensation from the needle-and-stimulation apparatus at the end of the first treatment session and the equipment was immediately removed. The patient reported no complaints on subsequent treatment days. One patient who had residual peripheral neuropathy from prior chemotherapy, manifested as tingling and numbness, complained of an aggravated tingling sensation following each needling procedure.

A randomized and controlled clinical trial (Johnstone et al. 2002) involved 50 patients with xerostomy after radiation therapy, who were offered acupuncture as potential palliative therapy for their symptoms. The intervention involved a two-stage process. They needled three points in the bilateral ears and a single point in the distal radial aspect of the index finger. Concurrently, they provided the patient with a piece of sugar-free candy or a lozenge, which is used to "milk" the salivary glands. Although this is a known form of salivary stimulation, most patients with severe xerostomy are refractory to this intervention in the absence of acupuncture. As a result, great variability was observed in the number and dates of patients' acupuncture treatments. The median number of visits per patient over the history of the program to date was 5, with a range from 2 to 15. The median number of days between the first and second visits was 5 (range 0–168), and between the second and third visits 15 (range 1–169). In sum, 50 patients underwent 318 treatments, with a median follow-up since the first treatment of 224 days (range 9–455). Patient response to acupuncture occurred in 35 patients (70%), while 24 patients (48%) received a benefit of 10 points or more on the xerostomia inventory (XI). Duration of the effect is variable, but most patients require acupuncture monthly to bimonthly for continuing effects. For 13 patients (26%), the duration of the effect exceeded 3 months. Authors who explain the action mechanism of acupuncture according to Eastern philosophy would claim that a blockage of Qi was removed to relieve the xerostomy. No adverse events referable to acupuncture were noted.

A randomized and controlled clinical trial (Molassiotis et al. 2007) about chemotherapy-induced fatigue recruited 47 cancer patients with moderate to severe fatigue, randomized either to an acupuncture group ($n = 15$), an acupressure group ($n = 16$) or sham acupressure group ($n = 16$). The acupuncture group received six 20-min session over 2 weeks, while patients in the two acupressure groups were taught to massage/press the points and did so daily thereafter for 2 weeks on their own. The patients completed the multidimensional fatigue inventory before randomization and the end of the 2-week intervention and again about 2 weeks after the end of the intervention. The results demonstrated significant improvements in general fatigue ($p < 0.001$), physical fatigue ($p = 0.016$), activity ($p = 0.004$) and motivation ($p = 0.024$). At the end of the intervention, there was a 36% improvement in fatigue levels in the acupuncture group, while the acupressure group improved by 19% and sham acupressure by 0.6%. Improvements were observed even 2 weeks after treatments, although results were lower (22, 15 and 7%, respectively). Acupuncture was a more effective method than acupressure or sham acupressure. Side effects from the acupuncture included spot bleeding in 2 cases, bruise in one point in one patient, one patient feeling discomfort in one point Sanyinjiao (SP6), and one patient feeling nauseous after the end of the session. One patient felt nervous about needles, but still continued with all treatments. In the acupressure groups, only one patient complained about bruising from pressure, and one patient complained of pain in the points after pressure.

A randomized pilot clinical trial (Lu et al. 2009a) investigated the effect of acupuncture administered during myelosupressive chemotherapy on white blood cell (WBC) count and absolute neutrophil count (ANC) in patients with ovarian cancer. Patients received active acupuncture *vs* sham acupuncture while undergoing chemotherapy. A standardized acupuncture protocol was employed with manual and electrostimulation. The frequency of treatment was 2–3 times per week for a total of 10 sessions, starting 1 week before the second chemotherapy cycle. The results showed that the median leukocyte value in the acupuncture arm on the first day of the third chemotherapy cycle was significantly higher than in the control arm after adjusting for baseline values (8,600 cells/μL range 4,800–12,000 *vs* 4,400 cells/μL range 2,300–10,000) ($p = 0.046$). The incidence of grade 2–4 leukopenia was lower in the acupuncture arm than sham arm (30 *vs* 90%; $p = 0.02$). There were no statistically significant differences in plasma G-CSF between the two groups. The mechanism of neutrophil cell response to acupuncture suggested that growth factor priming could increase the number of myeloid precursors in the bone marrow and decrease the number of stem cells killed by chemotherapy to produce a myeloprotective effect. The adverse events during the study period were minimal. Two adverse events occurred, as well as one event in which a sham needle mistakenly was not removed from a subject at the completion of acupuncture. This caused some patient distress, but no physical harm. Another patient developed a local port infection and was removed from the study, but this was unrelated to acupuncture treatment.

Moxibustion and acupuncture are powerful interventions used to support conventional cancer treatment like surgery, chemotherapy and radiotherapy (Stabler 2009). That author provides an experience report on daily moxibustion use to relieve chemotherapy effects, especially in cases of leukopenia. The same author developed a protocol in which patients and caregivers were taught to use moxibustion at home every day during the entire chemotherapy treatment. The moxa is used on acupuncture points Geshu (BL17), Ganshu (BL18) and Pishu (BL20) to prevent leukopenia, for five minutes on each point until the skin turns bright read. The whole procedure takes about 30 min. The studies postulated that the toxic effect of chemotherapy causes injury to Qi and yin and results in Qi blood deficiency. They found that moxibustion on Dazui (GV14) and BL17 raises the WBC count, moxibustion on BL20 and Weishu (BL21) tonifies the source of Qi and blood and improves appetite, and moxibustion on Shensu (BL23) warms yang and tonifies the bone marrow. The author believes that moxibustion is beneficial rather than contraindicated during chemotherapy. The issue of whether the inhalation of moxa smoke is harmful to the patient (and the person applying it) has been raised in the past. It was suggested to solve the problem by applying a few ground rules and some common sense, i.e. the room should always be adequately ventilated. It was concluded that there are no contraindications for the use of daily moxibustion during chemotherapy.

A systematic review with meta-analysis about moxibustion in cancer care evidenced randomized and controlled clinical trials that compare moxibustion effects with conventional therapy. Four of these failed to demonstrate the favorable effect of moxibustion on the response rates in comparison with chemotherapy ($n = 229$, RR 1.04, 95% confidence interval (CI) 0.94 to 1.15, $p = 0.43$). Two clinical trials assessed collateral effects of chemotherapy and demonstrated the favorable effect of moxibustion. The meta-analysis demonstrated a significant decrease in the frequency of chemotherapy-caused nausea and vomiting in the moxibustion group ($n = 80$, RR 0.38, 95% CI 0.22 to 0.65, $p = 0.0005$; heterogeneity $\chi^2 = 0.18$, $p = 0.67$, $I^2 = 0\%$). The authors assumed that moxibustion is beneficial for cancer patients and might be safer than drug treatment. None of the included trials assessed adverse events. It was discussed that moxibustion may not only absorb moxa extract on acupuncture points, but also exert direct effects due to acupuncture point stimulation from heat. Some aspects of its mechanism may be similar to that of acupuncture. This includes that moxibustion may influence the multiple cortical, subcortical/limbic and brainstem areas. Another possible mechanism includes an influence on the heat shock proteins and the function of immune cells. The third hypothesis discussed is that the moxibustion improves the function of immune cells. The authors highlight that evidence is limited, that the studies entail high risks of bias, but suggest moxibustion as effective support treatment for nausea and vomiting and highlight the need for further research to better investigate the benefits of moxibustion in cancer care (Lee et al. 2010).

Another review (Ernst 2009), which used the Cochrane Library database, assessed all forms of acupuncture and found 32 systematic reviews about acupuncture in certain conditions, such as pain, and a review of all treatment types. It was concluded that, in 25 systematic reviews, the results were negative, against 5 positive and 2 inconclusive. The author discussed that, currently, there is sound evidence to support the existence of numerous Cochrane reviews: nausea/vomiting (Lee and Fan 2004; Ezzo et al. 2009). The same author appointed that the problem of adequately blinding patients and therapists in randomized controlled trials (RCT) about acupuncture is not fully resolved. It is therefore notoriously difficult to control for non-specific effects, and we can rarely be sure whether the therapeutic benefit derives from acupuncture *per se* or from a placebo effect that might be sizable.

The positive results of acupuncture were proven with regard to chemotherapy-induced nausea and vomiting symptoms (Ezzo et al. 2009); postoperative nausea and vomiting (Lee and Fan 2004). A systematic review (Ezzo et al. 2009) assessed the effectiveness of acupuncture-point stimulation on acute and delayed chemotherapy-induced nausea and vomiting in cancer patients. The results demonstrated that eleven studies ($n = 1{,}247$) were pooled. Overall, acupuncture point stimulation of all methods combined reduced the incidence of acute vomiting (RR 0.82, 95% CI 0.69 to 0.99; $p = 0.04$), but not acute or delayed nausea severity when compared to control. By modality, stimulation with needles reduced the proportion of acute vomiting (RR 0.74, 95% CI 0.58 to 0.94, $p = 0.01$), but not the severity of acute nausea. Electroacupuncture reduced the proportion of acute vomiting (RR 0.76, 95% CI 0.60 to 0.97, $p = 0.02$), but manual acupuncture did not; delayed symptoms were not reported for acupuncture. Acupressure reduced mean acute nausea severity (SMD -0.19; 95% CI -0.37 to -0.01, $p = 0.04$), but not acute vomiting or delayed symptoms. Non-invasive electrostimulation showed no benefit for any outcome. All trials used concomitant pharmacological anti-emetics, and all except electroacupuncture trials used state-of-the-art anti-emetics. The authors concluded that the review complements data on post-operative nausea and vomiting, suggesting a biologic effect of acupuncture-point stimulation. Electroacupuncture has demonstrated benefit for chemotherapy-induced acute vomiting, but studies with state-of-the-art anti-emetics, as well as studies for refractory symptoms, are needed to determine clinical relevance. Acupressure appears to reduce chemotherapy-induced acute nausea severity, though studies did not involve a placebo control. It seems unlikely that non-invasive electrostimulation has a clinically relevant impact when patients are given state-of-the-art pharmacologic anti-emetic therapy. Neither electrostimulation nor acupressure offered significant relief. Delayed data were not available. Acupuncture-point stimulation according to any method is safe, with minimal and rare side effects.

A systematic review was performed about acupuncture and moxibustion in chronic fatigue treatment. The main findings appoint that acupuncture and moxibustion more effectively reduced chronic fatigue than cortisone treatment. Combined acupuncture, i.e. acupuncture treatment associated with other therapies like Tuina, herbs, psychotherapy and music, is better than acupuncture alone. The experimental group with selected points is better than the group with non-selected points (control group). They pointed out the following limitation: quality of the studies included in the review were with poor methodologies that contained flawed study designs, non-randomized and non-controlled trials, without standardization of treatment protocols, non-standardized result measures and non-effective assessment methods. They suggested the need for randomized and controlled clinical trials to confirm the efficacy of acupuncture in chronic fatigue treatments (Wang et al. 2008) (Table 9.1).

The effectiveness of moxibustion was reported in a systematic review with all randomized controlled trials between January 1998 and July 2008. The results yielded 46 trials in which six moxibustion types were applied to 36 diseases ranging from breech presentation to digestive disorders. The six types were: direct moxibustion, indirect moxibustion, moxa stick, moxa rolls with herbs, natural moxibustion, and one study employed multiple moxibustion techniques. Moxibustion was compared to three types of control group: general care, Oriental medical therapies or wasting list. Moxibustion was superior to the control in 14 out of 54 control groups in 46 studies. There were no significant differences among groups in seven studies, and the outcome direction was not determined in 35 studies. Seven studies were included in a meta-analysis. Moxibustion was more effective than medication in two ulcerative colitis studies. Overall, the results did not support the effectiveness of moxibustion in specific diseases due to the limited number and low quality of the studies and inadequate use of controls.

9.4 The Application of Acupuncture and Moxibustion in Cancer Treatment: Evidence from Experimental Studies

We conducted a search in three databases: PubMed, Lilacs and SciELO. PubMed is an international literature database on the medical and biomedical area produced by National Library of Medicine (NLM), USA and contains bibliographic references and abstracts to over 5,000 journal titles published in the United States and in other

Table 9.1 A summary of the systematic reviews discussed in Sect. 9.3

Study	Study Design	Sample	Treatment interventions	Treatment Responses and efficacies	Adverse effects
Lee et al. 2010	Systematic review and meta-analysis of moxibustion	4 RCTs	The studies compared the effects of moxibustion with conventional therapy	4 RCTs failed to show favourable effects of moxibustion on response rate compared with chemotherapy 2 RCTs assessed the occurrence of side effects of chemotherapy and showed favourable effects of moxibustion A meta-analysis showed significantly lower frequency of nausea and vomiting from chemotherapy for moxibustion group	Mild or no adverse effect, one study concerned possible hazardous effects of smoke from mouldering moxibustion
Ernst 2009	Overview of Cochrane reviews of acupuncture	32 systematic reviews of 2 different types	Reviews of acupuncture for a certain condition Reviews of all treatment options, including acupuncture, for a certain condition	Only 5 reviews arrived at positive or tentatively positive conclusions for chemotherapy-induced nausea/vomiting, PONV and idiopathic headache	No adverse event was discussed
Ezzo et al. 2009	Systematic review	11 studies	Use of acupuncture-point stimulation on acute and delayed chemotherapy-induced nausea and vomiting in cancer patients	Acupuncture point stimulation of all methods combined reduced the incidence of acute vomiting, but not acute or delayed nausea severity compared to control	Minimal and rare side effects

Table 9.1 (continued)

Study	Study Design	Sample	Treatment interventions	Treatment Responses and efficacies	Adverse effects
Lee and Fan 2004	Systematic review	40 RCTs	Use of techniques intended to stimulate the Neiguan (PC6) acupoint: acupuncture, electroacupuncture, laser acupuncture, transcutaneous electrical stimulation, an acu-stimulation device, acupressure and capsicum plaster; *vs* sham treatment or drug therapy for the prevention of PONV	PC6 acupoint stimulation prevented PONV	The side effects associated with PC6 acupoint stimulation were minor and self-limiting (haematomas, mild cutaneous irritation, pain in the acupuncture site) No side effect was observed for patients receiving acupuncture; acupressure, in several trials; or transcutaneous electro-acupoint stimulation by a peripheral nerve stimulator
Wang et al. 2008	Systematic review of acupuncture and moxibustion	40 studies on the treatment of CFS with acupuncture and moxibustion	17 studies researched acupuncture and/or moxibustion 7 studied acupuncture and/or moxibustion plus cupping 2 studied acupuncture and/or moxibustion plus Tuina (massage) 3 studied acupuncture and/or moxibustion plus herbs 1 studied acupuncture plus Tuina and herbs 4 studied acupuncture and/or moxibustion plus other therapy 6 studied other acupuncture therapy	Acupuncture and/or moxibustion are effective treatments for CFS The effectiveness of acupuncture and/or moxibustion is better than the treatments with cortisone, ATP and herbs Combined treatment of acupuncture with augmentation treatment, such as Tuina, herbs, cupping, psychotherapy and music, is better than a single therapy, such as acupuncture alone or herbal medicine alone	Few studies described safety monitoring, and only one study reported that one patient fainted during an acupuncture treatment. In that study, the fainting episode was attended to and the patient continued to receive acupuncture treatment

Table 9.1 (continued)

Study	Study Design	Sample	Treatment interventions	Treatment Responses and efficacies	Adverse effects
Kim et al. 2011	Systematic review and meta-analysis of moxibustion	46 studies (seven studies were included in meta-analysis and 39 studies in second analysis)	Direct moxibustion was used in seven studies, indirect moxibustion was used in 19 studies, moxa stick was used in 19 studies, moxa rolls with herbs was used in one, natural moxibustion was used in one, and one study employed multiple moxibustion techniques. Moxibustion was compared to three types of control group: general care, Oriental medical therapies or wasting list.	Moxibustion was superior on the control in 14 out of 54 control groups in 46 studies. There were no significant differences among groups in seven studies, and the outcome direction was not determined in 35 studies. Seven studies were included in a meta-analysis. Moxibustion was more effective than medication in two ulcerative colitis studies. Overall, the results did not support the effectiveness of moxibustion in specific diseases due to the limited number and low quality of the studies and inadequate use of controls.	Only 12 studies commented on adverse events. Seven studies reported no adverse event. In a rheumatoid arthritis study, the patients had no appetite, abnormal taste, nausea, increased aminotransferase levels and trombocytopenia. One study reported slight burning and blistering. Two studies about nasopharyngeal carcinoma, the side effects were induced by radiotherapy or chemotherapy rather than moxibustion. And one study reported no adverse event associated with moxibustion, but with cases of premature rupture of the membranes and preterm delivery that were less in the moxibustion group compared to the waiting list control

CFS chronic fatigue syndrome, *PONV* post-operative nausea and vomiting, *RCT* randomized controlled trial

70 countries. It contains references to articles in several areas published from 1966 to date. This database is monthly updated. Latin American and Caribbean Health Sciences (LILACS) is a bibliographic index of literature on health sciences, published in the countries of Latin America and the Caribbean since 1982. It is a cooperative product of the VHL Network. In 2009, LILACS included 500,000 thousand bibliographic records of articles published in about 1,500 journals in health science, approximately 800 of which are currently indexed. LILACS also indexes other types of scientific and technical literature, such as theses, monographs, books and chapters of books, congress and conference proceedings, reports, governmental publications and regional international organizations' publications. Scientific Electronic Library Online (SciELO) is a consolidated electronic publication project of scientific journals following the Open Access model, which makes the full-text articles of more than 290 scientific journals from Brazil and other Latin America countries available on the internet, totally free of charge.

This search in PubMed, Lilacs and SciELO, using the descriptors quality of life, neoplasms, acupuncture therapy, moxibustion and complementary therapies, over a 10-year period (January 2000 to July 2011), revealed the following clinical trials:

One clinical trial (Sawada et al. 2010) with a quasi-experimental and longitudinal design aimed to describe the results of relaxation with visualization and acupuncture for the quality of life of adult cancer patients submitted to chemotherapy treatment. As a theoretical base, the authors used the body-mind model proposed by Candace Pert, who discovered the opiate receptor and many other peptide receptors in the brain and body and provided an understanding of the dislocation process of chemical substances between mind and body. Neuropeptides and their receptors constitute an information network inside the body, which enables the body to pay attention and react to what one is thinking and feeling. The acupuncture technique fits well within Pert's model of mind-body communication. It involves the insertion of fine needles in the skin and underlying tissues, on specific points (acupuncture points); its action mechanism is based on the stimulation and response of the neuro-endocrine and peripheral system, releasing endogenous substances like endorphins, met-enkephalin and dynorphins, serotonin, oxytocin and endogenous steroids that act in analgesia.

Two groups were recruited: intervention group (IG) with 38 patients and control group (CG) with 37 patients. Patients from the IG received relaxation with visualization sessions once per week and during the entire chemotherapy treatment, which took approximately 6 months. The acupuncture points were: PC6, ST36, Zhongwan (VC12), Danzhong (VC17), SP6, extra point Yintang (EX-HN3) and Xingjian (LR2). To assess the patients' QoL, the EORTC QLQ-C30 was used, properly validated for the Brazilian culture (Brabo et al. 2006). Results at the end of treatment demonstrated a significant increase in the intervention group for global health, emotional and social functions and decreased fatigue, nausea and vomiting, appetite loss, insomnia, pain, constipation and diarrhea, with statistical significance for fatigue and appetite loss ($p < 0.05$). The control group displayed increased global health scores, decreased cognitive function and increased symptoms like fatigue, nausea and vomiting, pain, insomnia and diarrhea, but without a statistically significant difference ($p < 0.05$), except for global health/QoL. When comparing the QoL scores between the CG and

IG, they found a statistically significant difference between the groups, demonstrating the IG's positive results for relaxation with visualization and acupuncture. They concluded that these two interventions influenced the improvement of chemotherapy patients' QoL (Sawada et al. 2010).

Another study, with an experimental and longitudinal design, aimed to assess the reliability and preliminary effects of acupuncture in patients with advanced-stage ovary and breast cancer patients. A sample of 40 patients was selected, who complied with the inclusion criteria: patients with advanced ovary or other types of cancer, using conventional palliative therapies, over 21 years of age, who had not received acupuncture treatment for 6 months, platelet levels higher than 25,000 cells/μL, absolute neutrophils higher than 500 cells/μL, without a history of blood disorders, without acute psychosis, KPS > 60. The following exclusion criteria were adopted: patients involved in other complementary therapies or QoL studies. Out of 40 patients involved in the study, 28 completed 4 weeks of treatment, 26 completed 8 weeks, 8 dropped out before they received acupuncture and 6 gave up treatment early due to the disease's progression. Acupuncture was applied for 8 weeks, with 2 sessions per week during the first 4 weeks and once per week during the other 4 weeks (totaling 12 sessions), with a baseline protocol of 10 acupuncture points on 17 sites. The results demonstrated, among the 32 patients assessed, self-reported improvement after anxiety, fatigue, pain and depression treatment and significant improvement over time for anxiety and depression patients. The QoL measures showed better pain, physical and psychological stress, satisfaction with life and mood status scores, with benefits continuing for 12 weeks. For QoL assessment, the brief pain inventory (BPI), Rotterdam symptom checklist (RSCL), satisfaction with life domains scale-cancer (SLDS-C), profile of mood states (PMOMS) and cancer coping methods were used. The patients completed the questionnaires at 5 times: baseline (before treatment), 4, 8, 9 and 12 weeks. The authors concluded that acupuncture for 8 weeks showed to be a reliable treatment form for symptom reduction in advanced cancer patients. As a study limitation, they highlight the lack of a control group and the Hawthorne effect (patients performing better because they are participating on a trial), as the significant findings cannot be directly attributed to acupuncture treatments. In other words, it is possible that patients improved because of the attentive presence of the acupuncturists, the relaxing environment, patients' desire to please the practitioners, concurrent cancer treatment, placebo effect, or a combination of these factors, which refers to the patient's improvement because they are participating in a clinical trial (Dean-Clower et al. 2010).

A randomized and controlled clinical trial assessed the effect of acupuncture on the reduction/elimination of vasomotor symptoms in breast cancer patients, comparing patients who received anti-estrogen hormone therapy with the drug venlafaxine, with a view to determining whether acupuncture causes less collateral effects than venlafaxine (Walker et al. 2010).

Fifty patients were randomized and 25 were included in the group that received acupuncture for 12 weeks, while the other 25 constituted the venlafaxine treatment group. The inclusion criteria were: patients with stage 0-III breast cancer in the pre or post-menopause, undergoing hormone therapy with tamoxifen or anastrozol, with episodes of $\geq$ 14 hot flashes per week, age $\geq$ 18 years, past treatment with surgery and/or radiotherapy and finished chemotherapy, could be undergoing radiotherapy but, if not, post-treatment should be 5 years or more, stable dose of hormone therapy during 4 weeks or more, without plans to quit treatment during the study, KPS >70, life expectancy >6 months. The acupuncture group received treatment twice per week during the first 4 weeks, once per week during the other 8 weeks, in 40-min sessions. The acupuncture point protocol included: Taichi (KI3), BL23, SP6, Fengshi (GB20), Dazhui (VG14), Baihui (VG20), ST36, Taichong (LR3), Shenmen (HT7), Dailing (PC7), Qihai (VC6) and Taiyuan (LU9). The results demonstrated a significant decrease in hot flashes, depressive symptoms and other QoL symptoms in both groups, including mental health improvements from pre to post-treatment. Two weeks after treatment, the venlafaxine group showed a significant increase in hot flashes while, in the acupuncture group, levels of hot flashes remained low. The venlafaxine group presented 18 adverse effect events, including nausea, dry mouth, dizziness and anxiety, while patients in the acupuncture group experienced no adverse negative effects. Besides, some women presented additional effects like increased sexual desire, improved energy levels, clear thinking and feeling of wellbeing. The authors concluded that acupuncture was as effective as venlafaxine medication therapy in breast cancer patients with vasomotor symptoms and that it can exert additional and long-term effects without adverse effects, demonstrating that the treatment is safe, effective and lasting for secondary vasomotor symptoms, including the long-term use of anti-estrogen hormones in breast cancer patients (Walker et al. 2010) (Table 9.2).

An exploratory single-arm observational clinical study, investigated using acupuncture and moxibustion (acu/moxa) in the management of cancer treatment-related upper body lymphoedema in two steps. The study included breast and head and neck cancer survivors with mild-and-moderate uncomplicated lymphoedema for $\geq$3 months, $\geq$3 months pos active-cancer treatment, no active cancer disease, undergoing routine lymphoedema maintenance. The participants received seven individualized treatments (S1) and six optional additional treatments (S2), Medical Outcome Profile (MYMOP), Medical Outcome Study Form (SF36), and Positive and Negative Affect Schedule (PANAS) were administered at baseline, during each series, and follow-up three and twelve weeks after end-of-treatment. The results demonstrated that 35 participants recruited: 30 completed S1 and S2, three completed S1, and two were lost to the study. Mean MYMOP profile change scores for breast cancer participants were 1.28 improvement on a seven-point scale (SD = 0.93, $p < 0.0001$, $n = 25$); 1.41 for S1 (SD = 0.94, $p < 0.0001$, $n = 7$) and 0.94 for S2 (SD = 0.95, $p < 0.06$, $n = 6$). Changes in some SF-36 scores for breast cancer participants were significant to four weeks after treatment. No serious adverse effects were reported (Valois et al. 2012).

9.5 Safety and Adverse Effects of Acupuncture and Moxibustion

When applying acupuncture and moxibustion in cancer patients, both safety and the monitoring of adverse effects should be guaranteed. The United States Food and Drug Administration has regulated acupuncture needles as a medical device. In

Table 9.2 A summary of the experimental studies discussed in Sect. 9.4

Study	Study Design	Sample	Treatment interventions	Treatment responses and efficacies	Adverse effects
Sawada et al. 2010	A quasi-experimental study	Patients with different types of cancer undergoing chemotherapy	The IG completed weekly relaxation with visualization and acupuncture sessions	Results evidenced an increase in global health and emotional and social functions and a decrease in fatigue and loss of appetite for the IG, and an increase in global health for the CG A highly significant difference was found when comparing the post-chemotherapy scores of the Quality of Life Questionnaire-Core30 in the global health domain between the CG and the IG indicating positive outcomes of the CAM intervention	No adverse event was observed
Dean-Clower et al. 2010	This is a pilot, single-armed prospective clinical trial for patients with advanced cancer	40 patients with advanced cancer	12 acupuncture sessions over 8 weeks with follow-up at weeks 9 and 12	There was self-reported improvement immediately post-treatment in anxiety, fatigue, pain, and depression and significant improvement over time for patients with anxiety ($p = 0.001$) and depression ($p = 0.02$)	No adverse event was discussed
Walker et al. 2010	RCT	50 patients in stage 0-III pre- or post-menopausal breast cancer on hormone therapy with tamoxifen or arimidex	12 weeks of acupuncture or venlafaxine treatment. Health outcomes were measured for up to 1 year post-treatment The study tested whether acupuncture reduces vasomotor symptoms and produces fewer adverse effects than venlafaxine	Both groups exhibited significant decreases in hot flashes, depressive symptoms, and other quality of life symptoms, including significant improvements in mental health from pre- to post-treatment. These changes were similar in both groups, indicating that acupuncture was as effective as venlafaxine	The venlafaxine group experienced 18 incidences of adverse effects (e.g. nausea, dry mouth, dizziness, anxiety), while the acupuncture group experienced no negative adverse effects

Table 9.2 (continued)

Study	Study Design	Sample	Treatment interventions	Treatment responses and efficacies	Adverse effects
Valois et al. 2012	Single-arm observational study with before and after measurements	27 patients with breast cancer and eight patients with head and neck cancer	Step 1 – seven sessions of acupuncture once weekly. Step 2 – participants could choose a further six sessions of acupuncture. Moxibustion was used as appropriate to the individual's presenting symptoms and priorities.	Results demonstrated changes in Medical Outcome Profile (MYMOP) scores, which were statistically to primary outcomes at all measurements points, except for changes in patients with head and neck cancer in the wellbeing scores for both series. They concluded that acupuncture and moxibustion may have a potential role in reducing the symptoms burden in cancer survivors with lymphoedema.	Two incidents of cellulitis were reported during the study but the nurse specialist confirmed that these were unrelated to acupuncture and moxa treatment.

CAM complementary and alternative medicine, *CG* control group, *IG* intervention group, *RCT* randomized controlled trial oncology, attention should be paid to the needle sites, professional preparation, and the patient needs continuous assessment; it can be counter-indicated in patients with active infections at the acupuncture sites, radiotherapy burns, in surgery dehiscences and metastatic tumor sites. Special attention is due with bleeding and coagulation disorder patients. According to Capodice (2010), only six cases of adverse events were reported in the study (Melchart et al. 2004), involving 97,733 patients who received acupuncture in Germany, mentioning effects like exacerbated depression, hypertensive crises, vasovagal reactions, asthma attack and pneumothorax; they also found that the most common and smallest adverse effects were bleeding and pain in the needling site.

The most common complications in acupuncture are infections, tissue and internal organ lesions (Lu et al. 2009b). It is highlighted that these adverse effect events can be minimized through safe practices, such as disposable needle use, hand washing and needle disposing in appropriate boxes immediately after usage, use of thin needles. Safety measures should be established for other acupuncture types, like moxibustion, and for needles containing medication. In addition, acupuncturists need solid knowledge and skills, experience in treating various cancer types and skills to interact with the multidisciplinary team. These authors do not recommend acupuncture in the following conditions: neutropenia, neutrophils below 500 cells/μL; platelet counts below 25,000 cells/μL, altered mental status, heart arrhythmia and other instability conditions, which should be considered base by case.

A study developed to test the toxicity of moxa burning, in which results revealed that only two volatile components were produced at levels equivalent to or higher than safe exposure levels, including the carbon monoxide level. One chemical group of aromatic amines, with known carcinogenous properties, did not reach approved security levels. The test results in the study were in line with levels found in urban environments. The authors concluded that there is no immediate concern attached to the continuous use of moxa as a treatment modality in Traditional Chinese Medicine. Further tests are needed to establish whether current recommendations for ventilation treatment and cleaning of room surfaces need to be revised. Stronger recommendations may also be necessary with regard to the inconvenience of using moxa on irritated skin (Wheeler et al. 2009).

In a systematic review realized to identify the adverse effects of moxibustion, it was found that these effects were reported in four randomized clinical trials, one controlled clinical trial, two non-controlled observational studies, 13 case studies and one prospective study. In these studies, the most common adverse effects were allergic reactions, burns, infections like cellulites and hepatitis C. Allergic reactions were found in six case studies, four of which also reported on infection and two on burns. The other case studies reported on xerophthalmia, xeroderma, hyperpigmentation spots, ptosis and eyelid eversion. In the clinical trials, various adverse events were identified, such as redness, blisters, itching, discomfort due to smoke, general fatigue, stomach problems, headaches and burns. They conclude that moxibustion is not totally risk-free, as it entails various potential risks, with adverse events like burns, allergy and infection. Today, the incidence of these events is unknown. To enhance patient safety, large prospective studies are needed, with strict designs to clarify this issue (Park et al. 2010).

9.6 Final Considerations

The use of acupuncture and moxibustion in cancer patient care is strongly developing, encouraged by scientific evidence that has demonstrated the benefits of this millenary practice in symptom management and control of chemotherapy and radiotherapy side effects, enhancing the physical and emotional aspects of cancer patients and, consequently, improving their QoL.

The evidence found in systematic reviews demonstrated that acupuncture effectively reduces chemotherapy-induced nausea, vomiting and fatigue and radiotherapy-induced xerostomy. Acupuncture and moxibustion showed their effectiveness to treat fatigue in chronic conditions and moxibustion was effective to treat pain, nausea and vomiting and intestinal constipation.

Experimental studies demonstrated that acupuncture decreased nausea and vomiting, fatigue, appetite loss, insomnia, pain, depression and anxiety, constipation, diarrhea and hot flashes, improving emotional and social functions and, consequently, chemotherapy and hormone therapy patients' QoL and satisfaction with life.

Acupuncture and moxibustion exert various effects in cancer symptom management and treatment, but evidence is limited, demanding randomized and controlled clinical trials with strict designs that produce stronger evidence. The authors unanimously consider that acupuncture and moxibustion should be used as complementary treatments in cancer patients, due to their effectiveness to decrease symptoms, improve physical and emotional aspects and reduce adverse effects.

Evidence also demonstrates the limited adverse effects of acupuncture and moxibustion, and that protection measures should be established to achieve better results with these treatments.

Thus, we consider acupuncture and moxibustion as important complementary methods to improve cancer patients' HRQoL.

References

Banning, A., Sjeugren, P., & Henreksen, H. (1991). Pain causes in 200 patients referred to a multidisciplinary cancer pain clinic. *Pain, 45*, 45–48.

Brabo, E. P., Paschoal, E. M., Biasoli, I., Nogueira, F. E., Gomes, M. C. B., Martins, L. C., et al. (2006). Brazilian version of the QLQ-LC13 lung cancer module of the european organization for research and treatment of cancer; preliminary reliability and validity report. *Quality of Life Research, 15*, 1519–1524.

Capodice, J. L. (2010). Acupuncture in the oncology setting: Clinical trial update. *Current Treatment Options in Oncology, 11*, 87–94.

Dean-Clower, E., Doherty-Gilman, A. M., Keshaviah, A., Baker, F., Kaw, C, Lu, W., et al. (2010). Acupuncture as palliative therapy for physical symptoms and quality of life for advanced cancer patients. *Integrative Cancer Therapies, 9*, 158–167.

Ernst, E. (2009). Acupuncture: What does the most reliable evidence tell us? *Journal of Pain Symptom Management, 37*, 709–714.

Ezzo, J., Richardson, M. A., Vickers, A., Allen, C., Dibble, S. L., Issell, B., Lao, L., et al. (2009). Acupuncture-point stimulation for chemotherapy-induced nausea or vomiting. *Cochrane Database of Systematic Reviews, 12*, CD002285.

Fayers, P. M., & Machin, D. (2000). *Quality of life-the assessment, analysis and interpretation of patient-reported outcomes*. Chichester: Wiley.
Fayers, P. M., & Machin, D. (2007). *Quality of life-the assessment, analysis and interpretation of patient-reported outcomes* (2ed ed.). Chichester: Wiley.
Ferrans, C., & Varrichio, C. (2010). Introduction. *Seminars in Oncology Nursing, 26*, 1
Han, J. S., Xie, G. X., Zhou, Z. F., Folkesson, R., & Terenius, L. (1984). Acupuncture mechanisms in rabbits studied with microinjection of antibodies against beta-endorphin, enkephalin and substance P. *Neuropharmacology, 23*, 1–5.
Johnstone, P. A., Niemtzov, R. C., & Riffenburg, R. H. (2002). Acupuncture for xerostomia: Clinical update. *Cancer, 94*, 1151–1156.
Jones, E., Isom, S., Kemper, K. J., & McLean, T. W. (2008). Acupressure for chemotherapy-associated nausea and vomiting in children. *Journal of the Society for Integrative Oncology, 6*, 141–145.
Kim, S.-Y., Chae, Y., Lee, S.M., Lee, H., Park, H.-J. (2011). The effectiveness of moxibustion: an overview during 10 years. *Evidence-Based Complementary and Alternative Medicine, 2011*, 306515.
Lee, A., & Fan L. T. Y. (2004). Stimulation of the wrist acupuncture point P6 for preventing postoperative nausea and vomiting. *The Cochrane Database of Systematic Reviews, 12*, CD003281.
Lee, E. J., & Franzier, S. K. (2011). The efficacy of acupressure for symptom management: A systematic Review. *Journal of Pain and Symptom Management, 1*, 1–15.
Lee, S. M., Choi, T. Y., Kang, J. W., Lee, B. J., & Ernst, E. (2010). Moxibustion for treating pain: A systematic review. *The American Journal of Chinese Medicine, 38*, 829–838.
Lu, W., Matulonis, U. A., Doherty- Gilman, A., Lee, H., Dean-Clower, E., Rosulek, A., et al. (2009a). Acupuncture for chemotherapy–induced neutropenia in patients with gynecologic malignancies: A pilot randomized, sham–controlled clinical trial. *Journal of Alternative and Complementary Medicine, 15*, 745–753.
Lu, W, Dean-Clower, E., Doherty-Gilamn, A., & Rosenthal, D. S. (2009b). The value of acupuncture in cancer care. *Hematology/Oncology Clinics of North America, 1*, 1–15.
Macdonald, A. R. J., & Coates, T. W. (1995). The discovery of transcutaneous spinal electroanalgesia and its relief of chronic pain. *Psysiotherapy, 81*, 653–660.
Melchart, D., Weidenhammer, W., & Streng, A. (2004). Prospective investigation of adverse effects of acupuncture in 97733 patients. *Archives of Internal Medicine, 164*, 104–105.
Meneses, K., & Benz, K. (2010). Quality of life in cancer survivorship: 20 years later. *Seminars in Oncology Nursing, 26*, 36–46.
Meneses, K., McNess, P., Azuero, A., Loerzel, V. W., Su, X., & Hassey, L. A. (2009). Preliminary evaluation of psychoeducational support interventions on quality of life in rural breast cancer survivors after primary treatment. *Cancer Nursing, 32*, 385–397.
Mishel, M. H., Germino, B. B., Gill, K. M., Belyea, M., Laney, I. C., & Stewart, J. P. (2005). Benefits from an uncertainty management intervention for African-American and caucasian older long-term breast cancer survivors. *Psychooncology, 14*, 962–978.
Molassiotis, A., Sylt, P., & Diggins, H. (2007). The management of cancer-related fatigue after chemotherapy with acupuncture and acupressure: A randomized controlled trial. *Complementary Therapies in Medicine, 15*, 228–237.
Park, J., Lee, S., Lee, M. S., Choi, S., & Ernest, E. (2010). Adverse events of moxibustion: A systematic review. *Complementary Therapies in Medicine, 18*, 215–223.
Pearce, N. J., Sanson-Fisher, R., & Campbell, H. S. (2008). Measuring quality of life in cancer survivors: A methodological review of existing scales. *Psychooncologym, 17*, 629–640.
Portenoy, R. K., Foley, K. M., & Inturist, C. E. (1990). The nature of opioid responsiveness and its implications for neuropathic pain: New hypotheses derived from studies of opioid infusion. *Pain, 43*, 273–286.
Reagan, D., & Filshie, J. (2010). Acupuncture and cancer. *Autonomic Neuroscience: Basic clinical, 157*, 96–100.

Robb, K., Oxberry, S. G., Bennett, M., Johson, M. I., Simpson, K. H., & Searle, R. D. (2009). A Cochrane systematic Review of transcutaneous electrical nerve stimulation for cancer pain. *Journal of Pain and Symptom Management, 37*, 746–752.

Sawada, N. O., Zago, M. M. F., Galvão, C. M., Cardozo, F. M. C., Zandonai, A. P., Okino, L., et al. (2010). The outcomes of visualization and acupuncture on the quality of life of adult cancer patients receiving chemotherapy. *Cancer Nursing, 33*, 21–28.

Shen, J., Wenger, N., Glaspy, J., Hays, R. D., Albert, P. S., Choi, C., et al. (2000). Electroacupuncture for control of myeloablative chemotherapy-induced emesis: A randomized controlled trial. *The Journal of the American Medical Association, 284*, 2755–2761.

Stabler, F. (2009). The daily use of moxibustion to treat chemotherapy-induced bone marrow depression—A practical evaluation based on 20 years of clinical experience. *Journal of Chinese Medicine, 90,* 65–71.

Stone, J. A. M., & Johnstone, P. A. S. (2010). Mechanisms of action for acupuncture in the oncology setting. *Current Treatment Options in Oncology, 11*, 118–127.

Valois, B. A., Young, T. E., & Melsome, E. (2012). Assessing the feasibility of using acupuncture and moxibustion to improve quality of life for cancer survivors with upper body lymphoedema. *European Journal of Oncology Nursing, 16,* 301–309.

Veith, I. (1973). Acupuncture in Traditional Chinese Medicine—An historical review. *California Medicine, 118,* 70–79.

Walker, E. M., Rodriguez, A. I., Kohn, B., Ball, R. M., Peggy, J., Pocock, R. N., et al. (2010). Acupuncture versus venlafaxine for the management of vasomotor symptoms in patients with hormone receptor-positive breast cancer: A randomized controlled trial. *Journal of Clinical Oncology, 28*, 634–640.

Wang, T., Zhang, Q., Xue, X., & Yeung, A. (2008). A systematic review of acupuncture and moxibustion treatment for chronic fatigue syndrome in china. *The American Journal of Chinese Medicine, 36*, 1–24.

Wheeler, J., Coppock, B., & Chen, C. (2009). Does the burning of moxa (Artemisia vulgaris) in traditional chinese medicine constitute a health hazard? *Acupuncture in Medicine, 27,* 16–20.

Wong R, & Sagar S (2006). Acupuncture treatment for chemotherapy-induced peripheral neuropathy-a case series. *Acupuncture in Medicine, 24*, 87–91.

World Health Organization. (2007). Western Pacific region: WHO international standard terminologies on traditional medicine in the Western Pacific Region Manila.

Wu, S., Liang, J., Zhu, X., Liu, X., & Miao, D. (2011). Comparing the treatment effectiveness of body acupuncture and auricular acupuncture in preoperative anxiety treatment. *Journal of Research in Medical Sciences, 16*, 39–42.

Chapter 10
Acupuncture and Moxibustion for Palliative and Supportive Cancer Care

Steven K. H. Aung, Darcy L. Dennis and Jan T. W. Lim

Abstract Systematic reviews have identified acupoint stimulation as one of the most promising strategies currently being investigated in oncology. Cancer patients require support to cope with the disease, its symptoms, and the side effects of treatment with surgery, radiation therapy and chemotherapy. Supportive care becomes paramount in a palliative setting when curative options are no longer available. Acupuncture and moxibustion are useful when conventional therapy fails to fully support the patient, or becomes intolerable due to attendant side effects. Traditional Chinese Medicine forms the theoretical basis for these modalities, and has an accumulated wealth of experience for dealing with the symptoms experienced by cancer patients. Many acupoint prescriptions have been found helpful for centuries but remain untested in the rigorous analytical studies of modern clinical trials. Following the National Institutes of Health Consensus Statement in 1997, there has been sustained interest in the investigation of acupuncture and moxibustion for cancer-related symptoms. This has resulted in good quality research for a few symptoms and provided objective documentation of the benefits of these modalities. In the main, larger well-designed studies are required to confirm the benefits of these modalities for most symptoms, as small non-randomized studies are open to bias and have reported conflicting results. However, positive results from a number of pilot and retrospective studies suggest beneficial effects of acupuncture and moxibustion.

J. T. W. Lim (✉)
Department of Radiation Oncology, Faculty of Surgery, University of British Columbia,
Vancouver Island Cancer Centre, BC Cancer Agency, 2410 Lee Avenue, Victoria,
BC V8R 6V5, Canada
e-mail: jlim@bccancer.bc.ca

S. K. H. Aung
Department of Medicine and Family Medicine, Faculty of Medicine and Dentistry,
University of Alberta, 9904 106 Street NW, Edmonton, Alberta, AL T5K 1C4, Canada

D. L. Dennis
Department of Clinical Research, Vancouver Island Cancer Centre,
BC Cancer Agency, 2410 Lee Avenue, Victoria, BC V8R 6V5, Canada

W. C. S. Cho (ed.), *Acupuncture and Moxibustion as an Evidence-based Therapy for Cancer*, Evidence-based Anticancer Complementary and Alternative Medicine 3,
DOI 10.1007/978-94-007-4833-0_10, © Springer Science+Business Media Dordrecht 2012

10.1 Introduction

The use of complementary and alternative medicine (CAM) by cancer patients has increased globally in recent years (Tough et al. 2002; Chrystal et al. 2003; Molassiotis et al. 2005; Gerson-Cwilich et al. 2006; Montazeri et al. 2007). The National Center for Complementary and Alternative Medicine in the United States has organized such therapies into five categories: mind-body medicine, energy therapies, manipulative body therapies, natural products, and whole medical systems (Aung 1997; Liu et al. 2011). Traditional Chinese Medicine (TCM) is a whole medical system, based on ancient Chinese philosophy, focused on the vital energy called Qi, and its meridians, to balance the flow of energetic effects from superficial to deep levels of energy systems (Peterson 1998; Bai et al. 2011; Zhou et al. 2011). TCM conceptualizes cancer according to Zangfu organ theory, and Zheng syndrome differentiation of disease, based upon the overarching principles of yin and yang imbalance (Zhou 2009). In the context of palliative and supportive care, acupuncture and related techniques are intended to improve quality of life, by addressing the dysfunction of Zangfu organs, strengthening the patients' constitutions, and enhancing immune system functioning, through identification and treatment of ongoing morbidity (Ferriera and Lopes 2011).

Systematic reviews have identified acupoint stimulation as one of the most promising CAM strategies currently being investigated in oncology (Ernst et al. 2007). A MEDLINE index search of acupuncture for treatment of palliative conditions found that 1,020 controlled and uncontrolled trials were conducted between 1999 and 2007, 3.14 times the number of trials conducted between 1990 and 1998 (Standish et al. 2008). Despite this expanding interest in acupuncture and moxibustion, application of these strategies is limited by the quality and span of the current evidence base (Lu et al. 2008). For example, 85% of 27 controlled trials indexed between 1986 and 2007 reported statistically significant improvements in symptoms such as nausea, pain, and xerostomia with acupuncture (Standish 2008). Much of the current quasi-experimental, qualitative description and controlled research has focused on use of acupuncture and moxibustion as non-curative treatments aimed at improving quality of life, an indication often referred to as supportive or palliative care.

10.1.1 What is Palliative or Supportive Cancer Care?

To discuss the utility of acupuncture and moxibustion in palliative and supportive cancer care, we must first consider the meaning of these terms. The World Health Organization defines 'palliative care' as "an approach that improves the quality of life of patients and their families facing the problems associated with life-threatening illness, through the prevention and relief of suffering by means of early identification and impeccable assessment and treatment of pain and other problems, physical, psychosocial and spiritual" (http://www.who.int/cancer/palliative/definition/en/). From this definition, palliative strategies could be considered at any point in the cancer care continuum, from diagnosis onwards, and could be used for both those undergoing curative (radical) treatment, and those who no longer have curative options. In this sense 'palliative care' is not easily differentiated from 'supportive care'. However, popular opinion often places the term 'palliative care' later in the disease trajectory, and associates it with end of life or hospice care (Fadul et al. 2009). Regardless of the definitions, when used in an oncological setting, both forms of care deal primarily with strategies for symptom and side effect relief, stemming both from the treatments, and the cancer itself.

This chapter will focus its discussion on the use of acupuncture and moxibustion for patients with no curative treatment options, often referred to as palliative rather than radical course of treatment. However, as stated above, supportive and palliative care may also refer to potentially curable cases. Furthermore, palliative patients experience many of the same symptoms and side effects as those undergoing radical treatment. Although some pilot stage research has emerged that focuses on palliative and advanced cancer patients (Nystrom et al. 2008; Perkins and Vowler 2008; Dean-Clower et al. 2010; Lim et al. 2011), often they are not clearly distinguished from curative patients in the research. For these reasons, evidence from trials of all cancer populations will be discussed, with emphasis on the symptom and side effect concerns most applicable to non-curative care.

10.1.2 Advantages of Acupuncture and Moxibustion for Palliative and Supportive Care

There are several potential advantages and arguments for the use of acupuncture and moxibustion in palliative and supportive care. First, these strategies may be useful for symptoms that are not readily controlled by conventional therapies; for example, patients who do not get the desired pain relief from analgesics (O'Regan and Filshie 2010), or advanced cancer patients whose breathlessness cannot be managed using steroids, bronchodilators, and oxygen (Filshie et al. 1996). A second advantage is the relative absence of interactions observed with these strategies, so that they might be used in combination with conventional treatment. For instance, one randomized study found electroacupuncture and anti-emetic medication more effective than anti-emetic medication alone in controlling chemotherapy induced vomiting (Shen et al. 2000). Although less of a concern for patients who have completed treatment, acupuncture and moxibustion may also be used without interaction in primary cancer therapies, such as chemotherapy and radiation therapy (RT) (Cohen et al. 2005). For example, moxibustion at Shenque (CV8) point has been used to reduce toxicities in nasopharyngeal carcinoma patients receiving chemotherapy and RT (Chen et al. 2000).

Acupoint stimulation may also have lower side effect profiles than pharmacological treatments, allowing for reduction of symptoms with fewer adverse reactions, and without the need for long-term medications (O'Regan and Filshie 2010). In a 2010 randomized controlled trial (RCT) of venlafaxine *vs* acupuncture for breast cancer vasomotor symptoms, the venlafaxine group reported nausea, dry mouth, anxiety and dizziness, whereas acupuncture appeared to be just as effective but without these side effects (Walker et al. 2010). In addition, the clinically-based diagnostic procedures that accompany acupoint stimulation therapies allow for the on-going, non-invasive assessment of disease progression, according to consistently applied TCM principles (Ferreira and Lopes 2011). Finally, acupuncture and moxibustion are holistic in nature and may provide secondary benefits, beyond the primary symptoms being treated. For instance, in the above mentioned venlafaxine trial, participants in the acupuncture arm also reported increased sex drive, energy, clarity of thought, and sense of well-being (Walker et al. 2010).

10.1.3 Review of Symptoms and Side Effects

This chapter will provide an overview for the evidence-based integration of acupuncture and moxibustion into palliative and supportive cancer care. Currently, acupuncture and moxibustion is integrated in palliative settings in the United Kingdom (Standish et al. 2008). A review of the oncology literatures provides evidence that stimulation of acupoints, whether by acupuncture, moxibustion, or related strategies, can provide relief for cancer related pain, nausea and emesis, xerostomia and dysphagia, and vasomotor symptoms. Preliminary data is also emerging of potential benefits for fatigue, dyspnea, insomnia, depression, anxiety, and reduced immunological function in cancer populations. In considering the needs of non-curative patients, focus will be placed on prevalent symptoms that are not always controlled by allopathic therapies. These include nausea, vomiting, pain, fatigue, dyspnea, insomnia, depression and anxiety.

In the evidence-based context, research concerning acupuncture and moxibustion is in the early stages. However, consensus regarding the efficacy of specific points has proceeded in a TCM context for centuries. With this in mind, for each symptom, the current evidence base will be complemented by a clinical perspective of suggested acupoints based on TCM theory (Aung and Chen 2007). These suggested acupoints are intended to provide both practical considerations for practitioners, and research considerations for researchers outside of the current TCM context.

10.1.4 Introduction to Relevant TCM Concepts

In TCM, Zangfu organ theory pinpoints the location of malfunctioning Qi throughout the organ systems of the body, with five hollow yin organs (liver, kidney, heart, lung and spleen) having particular significance for cancer etiology (Yeh et al. 2006). Blood stagnation is the primary pathogenesis of cancer, and each of the yin organs is responsible for a separate aspect of circulatory functioning. The liver stores and purifies the blood, the kidney controls its level of dilution, the heart propels the blood, the lung controls the arterial vasculature, and the spleen promotes smooth circulation (Aung and Chen 2007). The TCM concept of cancer is apparent in the etymology of the Chinese character for cancer, "Ai" (Fig. 10.1). The radical "chuang"

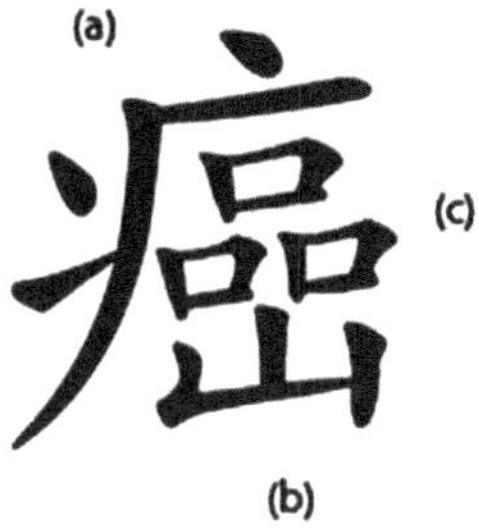

Fig. 10.1 Ai: the Chinese character for cancer

(a) represents severe pathology or illness, while the other characters represent the force of a mountain "shan" (b) pushing upward upon masses, represented by three mouths "pin" (c), and producing stagnant, negative energy, cancer, as a result of the disease radical. Together, (b) and (c) form the character "yan", meaning a cliff, or the action of soaring, as in soaring off of a cliff, indicating consideration of the irreversibility of cancer, as well as indicating the nature of cancer as a disease with proliferating negative cells and negativity (Aung 2006).

According to Zangfu theory, the five primary Fu (hollow) organs exist in complementary pairings with the five primary Zang (solid) organs, functioning together as yin and yang (Zhou 2009). The Zangfu pairings are significant in determining acupuncture treatments, because acute cases require treating Zang acupoints, and chronic cases require treating Fu acupoints (Aung and Chen 2007). Thus, the Zangfu pairings (in Zangfu order) consist of the liver and gallbladder, the kidney and bladder, the heart and small intestine, the lung and large intestine, and the spleen and stomach (Zhou 2009). These ten primary organs, with the addition of the two secondary Zangfu organs, the pericardium and the triple energizer, and the addition of the governor and conception vessels, comprise the basis of the 14 meridian system used in acupuncture and moxibustion.

The clinical perspective of Zheng syndrome differentiation is employed to address dysfunction in treating the whole trajectory of the disease (Li et al. 2011). Thus, in TCM, cancer is treated according to ongoing syndrome differentiation of dysplasia, characterized by deficiency or excess (quantity), the interior or exterior (depth), and the cold or heat (nature) qualities of the physiopathology (Mei 2011; Shen et al. 2011). Each of the 14 acupuncture meridians has its own tonification and sedation acupoints, which can be used to refine the targeting of TCM treatment (Aung and Chen 2007; Dorsher 2008). Tonification and sedation refer to the endogenous sensations of stimulation and relaxation in the body that, when produced, signal for the modification of bodily functions (Andersson and Lundeberg 1995; Sagar 2008). Acupuncture and moxibustion are both very useful for tonification of the patient, but moxibustion is the more powerful tonification technique. Cupping techniques enhance sedation, and are useful when patients experience excessive internal heat as a result of chemotherapy and RT (Aung and Chen 2007).

Evidence-based research can be difficult to implement in the TCM context, but current randomized controlled trials, quasi-experimental designs, qualitative description studies, and clinically-based experience demonstrate the value of TCM as a CAM therapy (Sagar 2008). While results of case descriptions and quasi-experimental designs cannot be generalized, evidence from them can be used to design research questions for testing in feasibility studies and subsequent randomized trials. Moreover, the extension of the evidence-base must consider acupuncture and moxibustion as a multi-component whole system of medicine, and design controlled trials with a view to the coherence of mechanisms developed apart from the Western biomedical tradition (Langevin et al. 2011).

10.2 Nausea and Vomiting

Gastrointestinal symptoms are very common after chemotherapy, abdominal RT and the use of anesthesia in surgical interventions. One of the most prevalent gastrointestinal symptoms is nausea and vomiting. The anti-emetic application of acupuncture for symptoms of nausea and vomiting can be traced through 4,000 years of TCM practice (Bai et al. 2011). Furthermore, anti-emetic acupoint therapies have the largest evidence base of all the symptoms to be discussed.

10.2.1 Evidence Base

Following the National Institutes of Health consensus statement in 1997 (Acupuncture NIH 1997), there has been greater acceptance of the efficacy of acupuncture in cancer nausea and vomiting. This consensus pointed to promising results for the use of acupuncture in treating post-operative and chemotherapy-induced nausea and vomiting (CINV). Since this consensus, there have been a number of randomized trials supporting the efficacy of acupuncture and related strategies, as well as several systematic reviews. Currently, varying levels of evidence exist for applications of acupuncture, acupressure, and moxibustion.

In 2010, Ernst and Lee published a systematic review for acupuncture in palliative and supportive care. They concluded that CINV was the only cancer-related indication supported by good evidence (Ernst and Lee 2010). Similarly, a review of acupuncture in cancer care found that anti-emetic studies are the most prevalent, and contain the most promising results (Cohen et al. 2005). A Cochrane review, examining the role of acupoint stimulation in CINV, examined data from 11 randomized control trials to demonstrate the benefit over drug therapy, particularly for early nausea and vomiting (Ezzo et al. 2005). Clearly, there is good evidence for the use of acupuncture in reducing vomiting for patients receiving chemotherapy. In addition to CINV, evidence has emerged for the use of acupuncture in the prevention of post-operative nausea and vomiting, as well as emesis in those receiving RT to the abdomen or pelvis (Gan et al. 2004; Enblom et al. 2011).

Some trials have considered acupuncture as an adjuvant to current pharmacological therapies. For example, a RCT comparing conventional anti-emetics alone, with either electroacupuncture, or minimal acupuncture plus anti-emetics, demonstrated that the electroacupuncture and anti-emetics arm was the most effective for preventing nausea and vomiting, as associated with high-dose chemotherapy (Shen et al. 2000). However, another study found that acupuncture had no additional effect in preventing acute nausea and vomiting in patients receiving intravenous ondansetron during high-dose chemotherapy (Streitberger et al. 2003). Since ondansetron and other anti-emetics can cause significant side effects, more studies comparing acupuncture with anti-emetics for patients with unmanageable symptoms are needed (Lu et al. 2008; Ernst and Lee 2010).

Evidence for the use of non-needle techniques, such as acupressure, is also accumulating. Acupressure techniques are appealing due to their less invasive basis, and potential for self-administration. One multicenter RCT from the United States found that using an acupressure wrist device at Neiguan (PC6) significantly reduced vomiting and intensity of nausea in women with breast cancer, when compared to placebo acupressure, or usual care (Dibble et al. 2007). Similar results were found in a RCT testing acupressure wristbands in breast cancer patients in the United Kingdom (Molassiotis et al. 2007b). Conversely, at least one earlier study of PC6 wristbands was unable to show significant differences between wristband users and controls (Roscoe et al. 2003).

Moxibustion, another non-needle TCM technique, has a limited Western biomedical evidence base for use in cancer care. A recent systematic review and meta-analysis examined RCTs involving moxibustion as adjuvant cancer treatment (Lee et al. 2010). Only five Chinese trials were included, and only two of these trials assessed the frequency of CINV. Meta-analysis of data from these trials showed that nausea and vomiting were significantly reduced in the moxibustion plus chemotherapy groups, *vs* chemotherapy alone ($p = 0.0005$). However, the authors concluded that the trials were of insufficient quality, and further research was needed to draw meaningful conclusions (Lee et al. 2010).

There is strong evidence to support the use of acupuncture for chemotherapy induced nausea and vomiting, and evidence is beginning to build for the use of non-needling procedures such as acupressure and moxibustion. Consensus is emerging over the use of certain acupoints, in particular PC6 (Ezzo et al. 2005; Lu et al. 2008; O'Regan and Filshie 2010). Continued research is necessary to establish evidence based guidelines for appropriate point selection. Research is also needed to determine the appropriate length and frequency of treatment, as well as to determine the comparative utility of acupuncture *vs* acupressure or other non-needling techniques. Furthermore, future trials should focus on integration of these strategies with current pharmaceutical anti-emetics to determine optimal combination and scheduling of these modalities.

10.2.2 Clinical Perspective

According to TCM, gastrointestinal symptoms result from rebellion of stomach Qi, due to irritation of the liver, and the subsequent effects of this irritation on the spleen

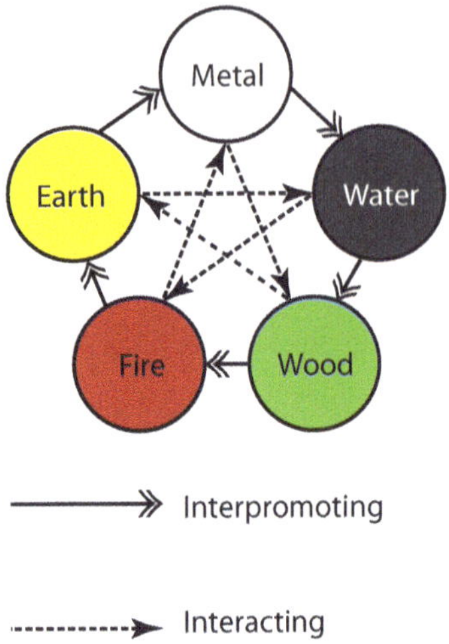

Fig. 10.2 Five elements theory

(Yeh et al. 2006; Aung and Chen 2007). Because the specific function of the liver is to eliminate toxins from the body, chemotherapy, RT and anesthesia may force the liver to overwork, causing damage to its structures and interrupting the smooth flow of Qi to the spleen. This effect is found according to five elements theory (Fig. 10.2) (Yeh et al. 2006), whereby the element of the liver (wood) is no longer bearing the nature of the element of the spleen (earth). The spleen as a hollow yin organ is paired with the stomach as a solid yang organ, according to Zangfu theory (Aung and Chen 2007; Zhou 2009). Thus, in TCM, the treatment of nausea as a gastrointestinal symptom of cancer depends on the progression of syndromes regarding each of these pathological mechanisms (Mei 2011).

In designing a comprehensive acupuncture program for these symptoms, four essential components have to be considered. To prevent the patients' experience of nausea and vomiting, PC6, Liangqiu (ST34) (for acute conditions), Zusanli (ST36), Jiexi (ST41) (for chronic conditions) and Zhongwan (CV12) are used (Aung 1994). Many ancient and modern texts testify to the efficacy of treating patients with PC6 and ST36 (Dundee and McMillan 1991; Lin and Chen 2010; Bai et al. 2011; Johnston et al. 2011). To increase the smooth flow of Qi from the liver to the stomach, through the intervening spleen organ system (Yeh et al. 2006), recommended acupoints include Taichong (LR3) (general), Zhongdu (LR6) (acute) and Ququan (LR8) (chronic) (Johnston et al. 2011). To decrease the excessive heat in the liver, the acupoints are Quchi (LI11), Dazhui (GV14) and Xingjian (LR2), as well as sedation of Ganshu (BL18) by cupping. Finally, to promote liver healing, the acupoints are Zhongshu (GV7), Zhiyang (GV9) and Yanglao (SI6) (Aung and Chen 2007; Chen et al. 2007).

Classical acupuncture is very good for establishing symptom control (Bonta 2002); however, auricular acupuncture will maintain a stable and effective state of this control, and also provide a sense of self-efficacy to the patient, who administers the auricular stimulation to himself or herself (Johnston et al. 2011). The appropriate auricular acupoints are the Shenmen, occiput, lung, liver and stomach points (Josefson and Kreuter 2003).

10.3 Pain

Despite the efficacy and popularity of analgesics in pain control, cancer pain remains a significant issue in palliative cancer care (Lu et al. 2008; O'Regan and Filshie 2010). There is also difficulty in the consideration of pain symptoms, because of the heterogeneity of syndromes (Cohen et al. 2005; Capodice 2010). Cancer related pain syndromes include arthralgia (Mao et al. 2009b; Crew et al. 2010), bone pain (Paley and Johnson 2011), post-surgical pain (Lu et al. 2008; Capodice 2010), neuropathic pain (Lu et al. 2008), spontaneous or movement-related breakthrough pain (Paley et al. 2011a) and metastatic pain (Dean-Clower et al. 2010). Because of barriers to opioid use, such as the levels of medication required, patient resistance and significant side effects (Lu et al. 2008; O'Regan and Filshie 2010; Paley et al. 2011a), acupuncture can present an attractive adjuvant or alternative strategy to pharmacological management.

10.3.1 Evidence Base

The current clinical evidence base for use of acupuncture and related therapies in oncological pain includes both feasibility studies and randomized trials. Several systematic reviews have also been published on the subject. Despite the existence of considerable literature, conclusions are mixed, and depend on the type of pain considered.

Several reviews and discussion papers assessing multiple symptoms have considered the role of acupuncture in cancer pain. A discussion paper in 2005 pointed to promising results from several post-surgical studies and called for further controlled studies (Cohen et al. 2005). Similar conclusions were reached by Lu et al. (2008), who pointed to randomized trials for post-operative pain (Wong et al. 2006; Mehling et al. 2007) as well as neuropathic pain (Alimi et al. 2003). Capodice reviewed three trials: an RCT of breast cancer patients with aromatase inhibitor induced arthralgias (Crew et al. 2010); a pilot, single-armed prospective trial of patients with advanced cancer (Dean-Clower et al. 2010); and a special acupuncture technique after thoracotomy (Deng et al. 2008). She recommended acupuncture as a complementary therapy if pain is poorly controlled, and a primary treatment for cancer-related pain with overall level 1 A evidence (Capodice 2010).

In addition to the above discussion papers, four systematic reviews have considered the use of acupuncture in the management of cancer pain. A review (Lee et al. 2005a) of seven clinical studies involving acupuncture, auricular acupuncture and electroacupuncture concluded that Alimi et al.'s 2003 trial of auricular acupuncture for neuropathic pain was the only high-quality, blinded, controlled study available, and that use of acupuncture as a cancer analgesic was not yet supported. Hopkins Hollis (2010) also reviewed Alimi et al. (2003), as well as Minton and Higginson (2007) on electroacupuncture, and Xia's comparison of acupuncture to conventional cancer treatment (Xia et al. 1986). Contrary to the findings of Capodice (2010), Hopkins Hollis concluded that there was a lack of level 1 evidence for acupuncture in the management of cancer pain. Another systematic review from China identified seven published RCTs comparing acupuncture with placebo, pharmaceuticals or Chinese herbal medications (Peng et al. 2010). As with the earlier reviews, they concluded that Alimi et al. (2003) had provided the only conclusive evidence and that other trials were of poor quality and limited reliability. Finally, a recent Cochrane review of three randomised controlled trials of 204 participants found a high risk of bias in two studies because of low methodological quality, leading to insufficient evidence to judge whether acupuncture is effective in treating adults with cancer pain (Paley et al. 2011b).

Despite multiple published reviews, there appears to be a lack of quality research and little consensus on the evidence base for cancer pain (Lee et al. 2005a; Hopkins Hollis 2010; Peng et al. 2010; Paley et al. 2011b). Clinical evidence is beginning to emerge for the efficacy of acupuncture in neuropathic pain (Alimi et al. 2003), post-operative pain (Wong et al. 2006; Mehling et al. 2007; Deng et al. 2008; Pfister et al. 2010), advanced cancer pain (Dean-Clower et al. 2010; Lim et al. 2011), and aromatase inhibitor-related arthralgia (Mao et al. 2009b; Crew et al. 2010), although further properly controlled trials are necessary to confirm the efficacy of acupuncture in all the above indications. Because analgesics are generally quite effective in relief of cancer pain, future research should focus on acupuncture and related techniques as complementary to pharmaceutical medicine, as well as its use in situations where patients are refractory to conventional treatment.

10.3.2 Clinical Perspective

In TCM, any organ or meridian system that becomes unbalanced or disharmonic will produce pain. When the organ system is disordered, pain is reflected distally through the meridians to the acupoints (Aung 1994; Dorsher 2008). Prompting relief through an analgesic mechanism is not preferred, as balancing and unblocking the patient's Qi, for those organ systems, offers a more long-term approach to relieving pain. There are three different kinds of pain in TCM (Kradahl et al. 1998; Aung and Chen 2007; Mei 2011). The first is the yang type of pain, which corresponds to our Western concept of inflammatory pain. This kind of pain produces feelings of tenderness, distension, throbbing and feverishness. The second type of pain is yin, which is characterized by coolness, deficiency and stabbing sensations, so that touch soothes the patient's pain and feelings of emptiness. The third type of pain is associated with dampness, usually due to phlegm accumulation (Aung and Chen 2007). This kind of pain is usually accompanied by paleness, localized swelling, distension and abnormal temperature. Certain acupoints, known as alarm points (Peterson 1996), become very tender when the organ system is disordered and produce one of the three kinds of pain, which is an indication of the underlying pathology (Mei 2011).

According to Zheng syndrome differentiation, pain is an important factor in determining the ongoing diagnosis and treatment of palliative populations (Ferreira and Lopes 2011; Li et al. 2011; Mei 2011; Shen et al. 2011). Visceral pain can be treated locally, according to its specific location along one of the fourteen meridians (Bonta 2002). Additionally, as per Zangfu theory, pain of a specific tissue system is associated with the energetic physiology of one organ system (Peterson 1996). Thus, the ligaments are associated with the liver, the bones and the nervous system with the kidney, the vascular system with the lung and the muscles with the spleen (Zhou et al. 2011). The heart is associated with stagnant blood, producing stabbing pain (Aung and Chen 2007). Since organs in TCM are thought to be energetic rather than anatomical entities (Peterson 1996), effective acupuncture treatment designs may theorize pain as (a) anatomical, (b) physiological, (c) pathological, and (d) holistic (Aung and Chen 2007).

(a) The anatomical location of pain dictates that treatment should employ the following classical acupoints. Baihui (GV20) should be selected to ease pain experienced in the whole body. Pain in the anterior body should be addressed with CV12, and pain in the posterior body with Jinsuo (GV8) (Aung and Chen 2007). For conjoint pain in both of the upper limbs, GV14 is appropriate for laterally located nociception, while Tanzhong (CV17) is appropriate for medially located nociception. For the individual upper limbs, PC6 is used to treat totally medial, and Sanyangluo (TE8) is used to treat totally lateral, nociceptive pain (Aung and Chen 2007; Lin and Chen 2010). For conjoint pain in both of the lower limbs, Guanyuan (CV4) is appropriate for medial nociception, while Mingmen (GV4) is appropriate for lateral nociception (Aung and Chen 2007). For the individual lower limbs, Sanyinjiao (SP6) is used to treat medial, and Yanglingquan (GB34) is used to treat lateral nociceptive pain (Aung and Chen 2007; Lin and Chen 2010). In post-operative cases, pain above the diaphragm should be treated with Hegu (LI4), as well as Kunlun (BL60). Post-operative abdominal pain should be treated with PC6, Xiangu (ST43), and Neiting (ST44), and post-operative pelvic pain should be treated with PC6, BL60 and ST44 (Aung and Chen 2007; Johnston et al. 2011).

(b) The physiology of cancer pain can be distinguished as acute or chronic, and located in one or a combination of six primary areas of the body, consisting of muscle, bone, neurological, ligament, vascular and visceral tissues. The treatment of acute and chronic pain corresponds to the distinction between yang and yin organs of Zangfu organ theory. Zang solid yang organs are used to treat chronic pain, while Fu hollow yin organs are used to treat acute pain. Each of the aforementioned tissues should be treated with acupoints on the meridian systems corresponding to the organ system which is responsible for its physiology. Muscle pain should be treated with spleen and stomach, bone pain with kidney and bladder, neurological tissue pain with kidney and bladder, vascular tissue pain with lung and large intestine, and visceral tissue pain with liver and the extraordinary meridian of the conception vessel (Table 10.1). Taiyuan (LU9) is also helpful for chronic vascular pain, despite belonging to the Fu hollow yin organ system, due to its being an influential point.

Table 10.1 Zangfu pairings for treatment of acute and chronic physiological pain

Pain	Acute	Chronic
Muscle	Diji (SP8)	Zusanli (ST36)
Bone	Shuiquan (KI5)	Weizhong (BL40)
Neurological	Shuiquan (KI5)	Zutonggu (BL66)
Ligament	Zhongdu (LR6)	Yanglingquan (GB34)
Vascular	Kongzui (LU6)	Quchi (LI11), Taiyuan (LU9)[a]
Visceral	Zhangmen (LR13)	Zhongwan (CV12)

[a]Exception to Zangfu theory due to it being an influential point

(c) The pathology of the patients' pain is very important, and comprises the third aspect of designing appropriate treatment. For instance, nociception of fractures due to spinal metastasis require treatment to address the anatomy of the site, the physiology of bone tissue, and pathology of inflammation (Paley et al. 2011a). Inflammation in any of the meridians can be decreased with GV14 for generalized inflammation and LI11 for localized inflammation (Aung and Chen 2007). Another example is to address the gastric distension that accompanies chemotherapy and RT, as the cause of a patient's abdominal pain. CV12 is useful for generalized Fu organ dysfunction. It may be wise to add PC6 for generalized middle Jiao disorder. Additional points that are helpful include ST34 for acute stomach disorders, ST36 for chronic stomach disorders and Fengshi (GB31) for gastric distension (Aung and Chen 2007; Lin and Chen 2010; Johnston et al. 2011).

(d) Cancer pain is not only physical in nature. There are also holistic considerations that acupuncture can address in order to amplify the effects of the previous three approaches to treatment design (Liu et al. 2011). In addition to treating the physical existence of pain, it is critical to vitally align the patient as a physical, mental and spiritual being (Aung and Chen 2007). Mental pain is associated with the anxiety, tension and depression that accompany cancer. Important acupoints to ease the patients' mental burden are Jueyinshu (BL14), Xinshu (BL15), Quze (PC3), PC6, ST41, Weiguan (TE5) and Shixuan (EX-HN1) (Aung 1994; Johnston et al. 2010). Important acupoints to lift the patient's spirits are Shaohai (HT3), Shenmen (HT7), GV4, GV20, Geshu (BL17), Geguan (BL46), Zulinqi (GB41) and EX-HN1 (Aung 1994; Aung and Chen 2007; Lin and Chen 2010; Zick et al. 2011; Johnston et al. 2011).

Beyond easing the patients' pain, TCM theory is valuable to enhance the healing process through the application of acupuncture. There are certain points which may be applied to directly stimulate healing. LI4 is very good at promoting healing above the neck, while SI6 is useful below the neck, including the extremities and the trunk (Aung and Chen 2007; Lin and Chen 2010). Finally, GV7, GV8 and GV9 are each uniquely important to heal the internal organs (Aung and Chen 2007). GV7 is especially used for treating Zang organs, whereas GV9 is used for Fu organs (Aung and Chen 2007). GV8 is used for the extraordinary Fu organs, the spiritual part of organ healing. By combining these four aspects to design effective acupuncture treatment, the cumulative effects for pain management are enormous.

10.4 Fatigue

Cancer related fatigue is common, often difficult to treat, and is particularly prevalent in people with advanced cancer (O'Regan and Filshie 2010). Fatigue may result from disease progression, tumor burden, complications of cancer (anemia, weight loss), complications of treatment (surgery, chemotherapy and RT), and psycho-spiritual fatigue (depression, anxiety, stress, fear and emotional pollution). Although there are roles for pharmaceutical interventions, consensus on the comparative utility of various drugs has not been reached (Minton et al. 2008). Furthermore, many of these therapies are associated with considerable side effects (Capodice 2010).

10.4.1 Evidence Base

Acupuncture and moxibustion may present an attractive option for fatigue relief, with fewer side effects than pharmaceutical alternatives. Surprisingly, research into their utility in cancer populations is in early stages. Two published studies have examined acupuncture for fatigue in post-chemotherapy populations. A Phase II study in 2004 investigated persistent fatigue in 37 non-anemic patients who had completed cytotoxic chemotherapy. Participants received either 4 weeks of biweekly or 6 weeks of once weekly acupuncture, and reported a mean fatigue score improvement of 31.1% compared to baseline (Vickers et al. 2004). Similarly, a 2007 randomized controlled feasibility trial of 47 Scottish cancer patients found fatigue score improvements of 36% and 19% in those undergoing acupuncture and acupressure, respectively. This was compared to a 0.6% improvement seen in a sham acupressure group (Molassiotis et al. 2007a). Both concluded that future large cohort studies were warranted.

The efficacy of acupuncture has also been considered in RT related fatigue. One single arm feasibility study examined the effects of 12 sessions of acupuncture in 16 non-palliative RT patients (Mao et al. 2009a). Although expected, the study found no statistically significant decline in fatigue or energy level over the course of RT, with the authors suggesting a possible preventative effect of the acupuncture. In a pilot double-blinded, randomized trial of true *vs* sham acupuncture in 27 women receiving RT, improvements were seen in fatigue and fatigue distress in both groups, although differences were not statistically significant, and recruitment was described as poor (Balk et al. 2009).

A recent feasibility study from the United States considered fatigue in breast cancer survivors who had undergone both chemotherapy and RT treatments (Johnston et al. 2011). Thirteen participants were randomized to either of usual-care or self-care education plus eight weekly acupuncture treatments. Fatigue scores did decline significantly in the intervention group when compared to standard care, although several recruitment strategies had to be enlisted in order to achieve the small sample (Johnston et al. 2011).

Most pilot studies have focused on treatment-related cancer fatigue, with only a few reports focusing on palliative settings. However, two recent feasibility studies considering multiple symptoms have provided early evidence for fatigue relief in advanced cancer patients. Self-reported improvements in fatigue were seen in 32 advanced cancer patients in a single armed acupuncture study assessing multiple symptoms and quality of life (Dean-Clower et al. 2010). Likewise, a randomized pilot of 20 incurable cancer patients receiving either acupuncture or nurse-led supportive care found improvements in tiredness and drowsiness in both arms (Lim et al. 2011).

While preliminary research is emerging, the evidence for all forms of cancer related fatigue remains at feasibility level. Evidence of improvement was seen in most studies, although none have been fully powered and some have reported difficulties in recruitment (Balk et al. 2009; Mao et al. 2009a; Johnston et al. 2011; Lim et al. 2011). Continued larger scaled RCTs will be necessary to adequately test the efficacy of acupuncture and related strategies. Furthermore, more studies focusing on fatigue in palliative populations are needed, particularly considering the prevalence and progressive nature of this symptom in patients with advanced cancer.

10.4.2 Clinical Perspective

According to TCM, the proper treatment of fatigue should be based on the underlying cause of the complaint. Treatment with acupuncture and moxibustion can be conducted as follows: to improve general constitution, energy and wellness: CV4, Qihai (CV6), CV17 and GV4 (Aung and Chen 2007; Zick et al. 2011). The following acupoints are for general fatigue: ST36, SP6 and Yingu (KI10) (Aung and Chen 2007; Zick et al. 2011). For specific organ fatigue, such as the liver, treat the liver He Sea point LR8 and the liver tonification point LR3. For anemia and bone marrow stimulation: BL17, Juegu (GB39), LR3, SP6, Xuehai (SP10) and ST36 are recommended (Aung and Chen 2007). For fatigue caused by psycho-spiritual duress: HT7, PC6, TE5, BL14, BL15 and GB41 are helpful (Aung and Chen 2007; Lin and Chen 2010; Johnston et al. 2011; Zick et al. 2011).

Many syndromes of fatigue are associated with different times of the day. Early morning fatigue is usually associated with spleen Qi deficiency. Fatigue from three to seven o'clock in the evening is associated with kidney Qi deficiency. If the fatigue spans the entire day, it is associated with lung Qi deficiency (Lee et al. 2005b). The treatment will be quite different, since according to the meridian clock, the organ system involvement is quite different. Early morning acute conditions should be treated with Diji (SP8) and chronic conditions with Yinlingquan (SP9). Evening acute fatigue should be treated with Shuiquan (KI5) and chronic fatigue with KI10. For fatigue which spans the entire day, acute conditions should be treated with Kongzui (LU6) and chronic conditions with LU9 (Aung and Chen 2007).

Another consideration is the use of highly tonifying moxibustion techniques on the back shu points of the bladder meridian, which are invested with the potential to enhance and improve the energy of the other individual organs. The bladder meridian facilitates the fastest exchange of energy from the inside to the outside, and from the outside to the inside of the body (Aung and Chen 2007; Dorsher 2008). With needles and moxibustion, the tonification effect will increase in intensity. The following bladder meridian points apply to acute and chronic fatigue conditions: treatment of early morning fatigue can be enhanced using Pishu (BL20), evening fatigue with Shenshu (BL23) and entire day fatigue with Feishu (BL13) (Aung and Chen 2007).

It is important to look at fatigue holistically, and to understand whether patients have had any history of unconsciousness, including anesthesia. If so, PC6 should be used to open the inner gate, followed by GV4 and Yintang (EX-HN3), for vital energetic alignment of mind and spirit (Aung 1995; Aung and Chen 2007).

10.5 Breathlessness

Dyspnea, or shortness of breath, is a distressing symptom, and is particularly common in patients with end stage disease (Cohen et al. 2005; Ben-Aharon et al. 2008). Pharmaceutical interventions such as opioids and benzodiadazepines have been proven effective in relieving cancer-related breathlessness, but may be associated with adverse effects (Ben-Aharon et al. 2008). While supplemental oxygen can be beneficial in numerous respiratory conditions, the benefits remain mixed in cancer populations (Ben-Aharon et al. 2008). Acupuncture in the treatment of breathlessness is used to dilate the bronchial passageways, and increase the perfusion of oxygen and carbon dioxide exchange at the alveolar level (Bonta 2002).

10.5.1 Evidence Base

Cancer specific evidence for treatment of breathlessness with acupoint therapies is very limited, with only feasibility level data available. In an early single arm pilot study of breathlessness in 20 cancer patients who had been refractory to medication (Filshie et al. 1996), significant improvements for breathlessness scores occurred in 70% of subjects, although the study was uncontrolled. A more recent pilot considered acupuncture followed by self-administered acupressure in 47 advanced cancer patients (Vickers et al. 2005). Patients were randomized to either true needles and acupressure studs applied at true points, or blunt placebo needles and acupressure studs applied at sham points. Although both groups experienced improvements both immediately and after one week of follow up, no significant differences were observed between the true and sham groups (Vickers et al. 2005). A randomized pilot study of acupuncture for various palliative symptoms found slightly larger improvements in self-scored shortness of breath when compared to controls receiving supportive nursing care, but the study was not powered for significance (Lim et al. 2011).

The current evidence base for acupuncture and moxibustion in cancer dyspnea is insufficient, with only two published pilot studies. However, despite current mixed results, studies of acupoint stimulation for other conditions have shown improvements in dyspnea. These include chronic obstructive pulmonary disease (Wu et al. 2004), bronchiectasis (Maa et al. 2007) and chronic obstructive asthma (Maa et al. 2003). Given this evidence and the potential for relief with fewer side effects than current therapies, the role of acupuncture and related therapies in breathlessness deserves further examination. Phase I and II data is needed to clarify the current body of evidence and justify future fully powered RCTs.

10.5.2 Clinical Perspective

Breathlessness in palliative care is provoked by physical, mental and spiritual disorders, disease and imbalance. It is very important to consider breathlessness according to its specific etiology of syndrome differentiation (Aung and Chen 2007; Mei 2011). Qi initiation and peripheral circulation is controlled by the lungs, which play an important role in breathing. In TCM, the general treatment for breathlessness involves improving the flow of Qi and blood in the patient's body, addressing Qi deficiency in both the lung and the heart, and strengthening the lung with its complementary organ, the kidney. In order to improve the general flow of Qi and blood, LR3 and SP10 are very important points for enhancing recovery (Aung and Chen 2007; Johnston et al. 2011; Zick et al. 2011). Treatment of the lung Qi deficiency involves BL13, Zhongfu (LU1), Lieque (LU7), LU9 and Tanzhing (CV17) (Aung and Chen 2007). To further address lung Qi deficiency, according to the relation of the five elements, it is important to treat the kidney (Yeh et al. 2006). The relationship of the lung to the kidney, according to this theory, is as that of a mother and son; therefore, by strengthening the kidney, it is possible to improve the relative condition of the lung. The acupoints which strengthen the kidney are BL14, BL15, BL23, Taixi (KI3), Fului (KI7) and KI10 (Aung and Chen 2007). To address the Qi deficiency of the heart, important acupoints include BL14, BL15, HT3, HT7 and Juque (CV14) (Bonta 2002; Aung and Chen 2007; Johnston et al. 2011; Zick et al. 2011).

We should not only consider the physical aspects of breathlessness, but also treat the mental aspects of the patient's condition, such as their anxiety, depression and stress. For the mental components of anxiety and stress, acupoints which will be helpful are as follows: PC6 to open the inner gate, TE5 to open the outer gate, BL15, HT7 and EX-HN1 for anxiety. For the mental components of depression, PC6, BL14, ST41, LR3 and Zhangmen (LR13) are beneficial (Aung and Chen 2007).

We should not forget the spiritual aspect of breathlessness, as without the treatment for their spiritual reunion, patients will not complete recovery (Aung and Chen 2007). After undergoing chemotherapy, RT and surgery, the spiritual components of patients' health can be affected. Important acupoints to uplift the spirit of cancer patients are GV7, GV9, GV20, BL17, BL46 and GB41 (Aung and Chen 2007; Johnston et al. 2011).

Finally, it is also vitally important to treat the immune system with regard to breathlessness, in order to prevent infections and disorders. Treating the immune system will improve the quality of life for patients, prevent suffering and pain, as well as improve general well-being. The points associated with improving immune system function are GV14 (generalized), LI11 (localized), SP10 (environmental), ST36 (nutritional) and SP6 (hormonal) (Aung and Chen 2007; Lin and Chen 2010; Johnston et al. 2011; Zick et al. 2011).

10.6 Depression and Anxiety

Psychological distress following cancer diagnosis is common, often due to the patient's legitimate but uncertain feelings about his or her state of health. Studies of cancer populations have indicated incidences of up to 25% for depression and between 10–30% for anxiety. Because both are associated with somatic as well as psychological symptoms, it can be difficult to distinguish the resulting physical complaints from those already seen in advanced cancer (Wein et al. 2010). For this reason, acupuncture and moxibustion may be well suited interventions for depression and anxiety, as they allow for holistic consideration of both psychological complaints, as well as associated symptoms such as fatigue, loss of appetite, breathlessness and insomnia.

10.6.1 Evidence Base

To date there have been no published acupuncture or moxibustion trials focusing specifically on depression or anxiety in people with cancer diagnoses. However, early evidence has surfaced in studies considering multiple cancer symptoms. In a series of 32 advanced ovarian and breast cancer patients, significant improvements in self-reported depression ($p = 0.02$) and anxiety ($p = 0.001$) were found after 4 to 8 weeks of acupuncture (Dean-Clower et al. 2010). Likewise, improvements were reported in the anxiety and depression scores of 20 patients both immediately and 6 weeks after undergoing weekly acupuncture treatments for 4 weeks, although the study was not fully powered (Lim et al. 2011). Finally, a RCT of 138 post-operative cancer patients considered combined massage and acupuncture provided in the first 2 days following surgery. Those receiving the intervention ($n = 93$) reported significant improvements in depressed mood compared to patients receiving usual care only ($n = 45$) (Mehling et al. 2007).

Support for the use of acupuncture to treat depression and anxiety has also been noted as secondary outcomes in studies focused on other symptoms. A 2009 pilot RCT testing the feasibility of RT concurrent acupuncture for cancer-related fatigue found improvements in depression. However, these improvements were seen in both true and sham acupuncture groups, and differences were not significant (Balk et al. 2009). Another pilot study considered acupuncture to points in the sternum and hand for relief of cancer-related breathlessness. In addition to improvements in breathlessness, significant improvements were seen in relaxation ($p < 0.005$) and anxiety

($p < 0.001$) in the 20 participants (Filshie et al. 1996). These results are not surprising, given the association of fatigue and breathlessness with depression and anxiety, respectively, and they highlight the importance of a holistic approach in the consideration of psychological complaints.

Currently, studies considering acupoint therapies for cancer related depression and anxiety have demonstrated feasibility and potential efficacy only. However, evidence for improvements in depression and anxiety has been reported in cancer free populations. Acupuncture and electroacupuncture have been shown to have equal or greater efficacy when compared to several pharmaceutical medications for depression (Roschke et al. 2000; Han et al. 2002). Evidence from non-cancer populations has also emerged for acupressure and auricular acupuncture (Wang and Kain 2001; Kober et al. 2003; Agarwal et al. 2005; Mora et al. 2007) in treating anxiety. Clearly the use of acupoint interventions for psychological issues is an important area of further cancer study, with larger scale trials needed.

10.6.2 Clinical Perspective

The smooth flow of patients' Qi can be disturbed by their psychological reaction to their diagnosis (Aung 1994). PC6 is used to open the inner gates of consciousness to relieve depression, while TE5 allows emotional ventilation of the patients' anxiety. When patients have chemotherapy, RT, and surgical anesthesia, they may recognize that the flow of energy through the liver channel is hindered, by feeling like there is something stuck in their throat, as well as feeling the unease of stagnant energy in the meridian systems (Aung and Chen 2007; Dorsher 2008). Depression and anxiety are considered as part of the progression of syndrome differentiation, and thus occur at different stages over the course of the cancer (Mei 2011; Ferreira and Lopes 2011). Depression is mostly associated with liver Qi stagnation, and disruption of Qi flow in the pericardium, whereas anxiety has to do with energetic disharmony of the heart (Yeh et al. 2006). Short term depression is treated with pericardium acupoints, medium term depression is treated with liver acupoints, and long term depression is treated with liver and kidney acupoints. If the depression is associated with anxiety and stress, heart acupoints should be employed (Aung and Chen 2007). To address depression, acupuncture treatment should harmonize the body, produce smoothly flowing liver Qi, and tonify the energy of the kidney.

Tonification of the kidney is necessary to ensure the long-term viability of the treatment according to five elements theory (Yeh et al. 2006). According to this theory, liver (wood) is complemented by kidney (water), so that the kidney supports the liver function to produce smoothly flowing Qi. In addition to treating the pericardium, liver, kidney and heart, to harmonize the body, the acupuncture treatment should employ the acupoints GV20, EX-HN1 and ST41 (Aung and Chen 2007). The acupoints for smoothly flowing liver Qi are BL18, LR3, LR8, LR13 and Qimen (LR14) (Aung and Chen 2007; Johnston et al. 2011; Zick et al. 2011). In order to tonify the kidney, KI3 is useful for developing the patient's kidney yin, Zhaohai

(KI6) for developing their kidney essence, Fuliu (KI7) for their kidney yang, and KI10 for their kidney Qi (Aung and Chen 2007; Johnston et al. 2011; Zick et al. 2011).

In TCM, the heart controls the body's spiritual essence (Dorsher 2008). Anxiety is thus considered to be an energetic imbalance of the heart, evidenced by excessive syndromes such as a quickened pulse, or an irregular heartbeat (Peterson 1996). Acupuncture treatment for anxiety should harmonize and balance the heart energy. The acupoints for balancing the heart are BL15, CV14, HT3, HT7 and LR3 (Aung and Chen 2007; Lin and Chen 2010; Johnston et al. 2011; Zick et al. 2011).

In addition, herbal medicine, medical qigong and auricular acupuncture are very helpful to control the patients' depression and anxiety (Yeh et al. 2006; Liu et al. 2011). Herbal medicine has been referred to by patients as a "comfortable therapy", in that it involves only mild oral or infused medicines (Liu et al. 2011). Likewise, qigong is mild for patients; akin to acupuncture without needles and herbal medicine without herbs (Yeh et al. 2006; Aung and Chen 2007). Auricular acupoints include Shenmen for relaxation, liver, kidney and heart for the associated organ systems, and occiput for healing disharmony (Aung and Chen 2007; Johnston et al. 2011).

10.7 Insomnia

Cancer patients experience insomnia as a frequent symptom of psychosomatic distress. Patients may be concerned about the physical condition of their cancers, have mental uncertainty about their treatment options, or anxiety about possible side effects they might encounter. Insomnia may also occur as a consequence of discomfort due to treatment side effects such as vasomotor symptoms (Frisk et al. 2011). As a result, sleeplessness is prevalent, and is one of the more significant symptoms in cancer patients (Lu et al. 2008).

10.7.1 Evidence Base

Despite its significance in cancer populations, clinical trials considering acupuncture or moxibustion for insomnia are lacking. However, recent evidence has emerged from a randomized trial of electroacupuncture *vs* hormone treatment for women with breast cancer related hot flashes. The electroacupuncture group experienced improvements from baseline to 12 weeks in the number of hours slept ($p = 0.05$) and the number of times they were awoken per night ($p = 0.01$). These parameters remained significantly improved at 12 months (number hours slept $p = 0.02$; number times awoken $p = 0.003$) (Frisk et al. 2011). While these results are encouraging, improvements in sleep were likely related to decreased hot flashes, so results cannot be generalized to other populations.

The use of acupuncture for insomnia in non-cancer populations is better established, although evidence remains mixed. In 2007, a Cochrane review was conducted of RCTs evaluating a variety of insomnia meridian and acupoint strategies including needle acupuncture, auricular magnetic and transcutaneous electroacupuncture. Although the trials reported some improvements, the combined results suggested that acupoint stimulation was not more effective than controls, and further high quality research was needed to support the use of acupuncture for insomnia (Cheuk et al. 2007). Alternatively, a systematic review of auricular acupuncture for insomnia included evidence from six trials, and found that recovery and improvement rates were higher than those obtained with diazepam ($p < 0.05$) (Chen et al. 2007).

The current evidence base for use of acupoint therapies in insomnia is very limited. Although there may be a role for auricular acupuncture (Chen et al. 2007), evidence from other strategies is mixed (Cheuk et al. 2007). Further research is particularly needed in cancer populations, as current evidence has only been examined in hot flash-related sleeplessness (Frisk et al. 2011).

10.7.2 Clinical Perspective

Sleeplessness among cancer patients is quite prevalent, and there are many kinds of insomnia (Lee et al. 2005b). According to TCM, the most common kinds of insomnia in cancer patients are disharmony of the heart, liver, gallbladder and kidney (Yeh et al. 2006; Aung and Chen 2007; Zhou 2009). Because of disharmony, each affected organ system produces negative mental effects. The heart produces anxiety, the liver produces anger and depression, the gallbladder produces low self-esteem and the kidney produces fear (Aung and Chen 2007; Zhou 2009). In order to soothe the patients, and restore the affected organ systems to their proper balance, the primary technique the acupuncturist should employ is "opening the gates". Opening the gates employs TE5 for ventilation and PC6 for relaxation. Following the application of this technique, the acupuncturist should treat the appropriate organ systems depending on which kind of insomnia the patient experiences (Aung and Chen 2007).

Disharmony of the heart is associated with an inability to fall asleep. Effective acupoints are PC6 (opening the gate), Yinxi (HT6) (for acute conditions), HT3 (for chronic conditions) and HT7 (for sedation and relaxation) (Aung and Chen 2007; Lin and Chen 2010; Johnston et al. 2011; Zick et al. 2011). Sedation points include cupping BL14 and cupping BL15 for this kind of insomnia (Aung and Chen 2007).

Disharmony of the liver is associated with dream-disturbed sleep. It is important to harmonize the liver by using the following acupoints: Xingjuan (LR2), LR3, LR6 (acute), LR8 (chronic) and sedation by cupping BL18 (Aung and Chen 2007). Other acupoints can be incorporated into the treatment as required, particularly kidney acupoints, according to the five elements theory (Yeh et al. 2006; Aung and Chen 2007).

Disharmony of the gallbladder can cause early morning awakening, which in Western typology is associated with depression. Acupoints for this kind of insomnia include Waiqiu (GB36) in acute conditions, GB34 in chronic conditions, and GB41 for spiritual reunion (Aung and Chen 2007; Johnston et al. 2011).

Disharmony of the kidney can cause broken sleep. Patients experience frequent waking states during the sleeping period, and increased nocturnal perspiration and urination. Acupoints to use for this condition are KI3 (yin), KI5 (acute), KI7 and GV4 (yang), KI10 (Qi) and BL23 (Aung and Chen 2007; Johnston et al. 2011).

It is very important to treat the patient with spiritual acupoints, especially in palliative care, to obtain a more effective response. Acupoints for mental stability, balancing of the body systems, and spiritual reconnection are very useful. For mental stability, EX-HN1 is an excellent point to combine with GV20 (Aung and Chen 2007; Johnston et al. 2011). Balancing the body systems can be achieved with Ermen (TE21), Tinggong (SI19), Tinghui (GB2), LI11 and Dabao (SP21). Spiritual reconnection treatment acupoints include Ghiyang (GV9), BL17, BL46, and GB41 (Aung and Chen 2007). Auricular acupuncture is also very helpful in treating insomnia, not only to maintain sleep patterns, but to improve the patients' self-confidence with self-manipulation of ear patches (Johnston et al. 2011). Useful auricular acupoints include Shenmen, heart, tranquility and occiput (Aung and Chen 2007).

10.8 Conclusions

There is growing evidence for the role of acupuncture in palliative and supportive cancer care. Sustained interest in the investigation of acupuncture and moxibustion for cancer related symptoms has resulted in quality research and objective documentation of the benefits of these modalities. Although definitive evidence is not uniformly available for all the symptoms considered, the substantial reports available for nausea and vomiting form the foundation for current and future studies in this patient population. Reports and reviews for pain management are also numerous, but there is a lack of high quality trials available for the various pain syndromes. Integration of acupuncture and moxibustion with current anti-emetic and analgesic pharmaceuticals is an important area of future research for both of these symptoms.

Evidence for fatigue, breathlessness, anxiety, depression and insomnia is emerging, but remains at the feasibility level. Fatigue and breathlessness are particularly common in advanced cancer, and it is imperative that larger adequately powered trials are available to address these concerns as these symptoms are not readily helped by drugs. There is some evidence for the use of acupuncture to treat depression, anxiety, and insomnia in non-cancer populations, but future studies are needed to confirm their beneficial effects in cancer populations.

With the extensive clinical experience available in TCM, the challenge is to design studies that will confirm the benefits of treatment for each symptom, taking into account the holistic approach of these modalities, and adapting them into an analytical format. More importantly, it would also be useful to discover how best to integrate acupuncture and moxibustion with conventional medication, given the different strengths and limitations of each type of treatment. Ideally, the selected acupoints will not only augment the medication in relieving the symptom, but also reduce the side effects that commonly accompany the various modalities of cancer treatment.

References

Acupuncture. (1997). Acupuncture. *NIH Consensus Statement, 15*, 1–34.

Agarwal, A., Ranjan, R., Dhiraaj, S., Lakra, A., Kumar, M., & Singh, U. (2005). Acupressure for prevention of pre-operative anxiety: A prospective, randomised, placebo controlled study. *Anaesthesia, 60*, 978–981.

Alimi, D., Rubino, C., Pichard-Leandri, E., Fermand-Brule, S., Dubreuil-Lemaire, M. L., & Hill, C. (2003). Analgesic effect of auricular acupuncture for cancer pain: A randomized, blinded, controlled trial. *Journal of Clinical Oncology: Official Journal of the American Society of Clinical Oncology, 21*, 4120–4126.

Andersson, S., & Lundeberg, T. (1995). Acupuncture- from empiricism to science: Functional background to acupuncture effects in pain and disease. *Medical Hypotheses, 45*, 271–281.

Aung, S. K. (1994). The clinical use of acupuncture in oncology: Symptom control. *Acupuncture in Medicine, 12*, 37–40.

Aung, S. K. (1995). The "pearls" of medical acupuncture: Six vital energetic (Qi) alignment preocedures. *Le Revue de Médicine Traditionelle Chinoise, 168*, 203–207.

Aung, S. K. (1997). Traditional Chinese medicine and cancer care: An integrated approach. *Canadian Journal of Clinical Medicine, 4*, 2–7.

Aung, S. K. (2006). Traditional medicine in breast cancer management with a focus on the Chinese integrative approach. In C. K. O. Williams, O. I. Olopade, & C. I. Falkson (Eds.), *Breast cancer in women of African descent* (pp. 297–307). Dordrecht: Springer.

Aung, S. K., & Chen, W. P. (2007). *Clinical introduction to medical acupuncture*. New York: Thieme Medical Publishers, Inc.

Bai, L., Yan, H., Li, L., Qin, W., Chen, P., Liu, P., Gong, Q., Liu, Y., & Tian, J. (2010). Neural specificity of acupuncture stimulation at pericardium 6: Evidence from an FMRI Study. *Journal of Magnetic Resonance Imaging, 31*, 71–77.

Balk, J., Day, R., Rosenzweig, M., & Beriwal, S. (2009). Pilot, randomized, modified, double-blind, placebo-controlled trial of acupuncture for cancer-related fatigue. *Journal of the Society for Integrative Oncology, 7*, 4–11.

Ben-Aharon, I., Gafter-Gvili, A., Paul, M., Leibovici, L., & Stemmer, S. M. (2008). Interventions for alleviating cancer-related dyspnea: A systematic review. *Journal of Clinical Oncology, 26*, 2396–2404.

Bonta, I. L. (2002). Acupuncture beyond the endorphin concept? *Medical Hypotheses, 58*, 221–224.

Capodice, J. L. (2010). Acupuncture in the oncology setting: Clinical trial update. *Current Treatment Options in Oncology, 11*, 87–94.

Chen, K., Jiang, Y., & Wen, H. (2000). Clinical study on treatment of nasopharyngeal carcinoma by radio- and chemotherapy with supplementary moxibustion on shenque point. *Zhongguo Zhong Xi Yi Jie He Za Zhi, 20*, 733–735.

Chen, H. Y., Shi, Y., Ng, C. S., Chan, S. M., Yung, K. K., & Zhang, Q. L. (2007). Auricular acupuncture treatment for insomnia: A systematic review. *Journal of Alternative and Complementary Medicine, 13*, 669–676.

Cheuk, D. K., Yeung, W. F., Chung, K. F., & Wong, V. (2007). Acupuncture for insomnia. *Cochrane Database of Systematic Reviews*, CD005472.

Chrystal, K., Allan, S., Forgeson, G., & Isaacs, R. (2003). The use of complementary/alternative medicine by cancer patients in a new zealand regional cancer treatment centre. *The New Zealand Medical Journal, 116*, U296.

Cohen, A. J., Menter, A., & Hale, L. (2005). Acupuncture: Role in comprehensive cancer care—a primer for the oncologist and review of the literature. *Integrative Cancer Therapies, 4*, 131–43.

Crew, K. D., Capodice, J. L., Greenlee, H., Brafman, L., Fuentes, D., Awad, D., et al. (2010). Randomized, blinded, sham-controlled trial of acupuncture for the management of aromatase inhibitor-associated joint symptoms in women with early-stage breast cancer. *Journal of Clinical Oncology, 28*, 1154–1160.

Dean-Clower, E., Doherty-Gilman, A. M., Keshaviah, A., Baker, F., Kaw, C., Lu, W., et al. (2010). Acupuncture as palliative therapy for physical symptoms and quality of life for advanced cancer patients. *Integrative Cancer Therapies, 9*, 158–167.

Deng, G., Rusch, V., Vickers, A., Malhotra, V., Ginex, P., Downey, R., et al. (2008). Randomized controlled trial of a special acupuncture technique for pain after thoracotomy. *The Journal of Thoracic and Cardiovascular Surgery, 136*, 1464–1469.

Dibble, S. L., Luce, J., Cooper, B. A., Israel, J., Cohen, M., Nussey, B., et al. (2007). Acupressure for chemotherapy-induced nausea and vomiting: A randomized clinical trial. *Oncology Nursing Forum, 34*, 813–820.

Dorsher, P. T. (2008). Myofacial referred-pain data provide physiologic evidence of acupuncture meridians. *The Journal of Pain, 10*, 723–731.

Dundee, J. W., & McMillan, C. (1991). Positive evidence for P6 acupuncture antiemesis. *Postgraduate Medical Journal, 67*, 417–422.

Enblom, A., Lekander, M., Hammar, M., Johnsson, A., Onelov, E., Ingvar, M., et al. (2011). Getting the grip on nonspecific treatment effects: Emesis in patients randomized to acupuncture or sham compared to patients receiving standard care. *PLoS One, 6*, e14766.

Ernst, E., Lee, M. S. (2010). Acupuncture for palliative and supportive cancer care: A systematic review of systematic reviews. *Journal of Pain and Symptom Management, 40*, e3–5.

Ernst, E., Pittler, M. H., Wider, B., Boddy, K. (2007). Complementary/alternative medicine for supportive cancer care: Development of the evidence-base. *Supportive Care in Cancer, 15*, 565–568.

Ezzo, J., Vickers, A., Richardson, M. A., Allen, C., Dibble, S. L., Issell, B., et al. (2005). Acupuncture-point stimulation for chemotherapy-induced nausea and vomiting. *Journal of Clinical Oncology, 23*, 7188–7198.

Fadul, N., Elsayem, A., Palmer, J. L., Del Fabbro, E., Swint, K., Li, Z., et al. (2009). Supportive versus palliative care: What's in a name?: A survey of medical oncologists and midlevel providers at a comprehensive cancer center. *Cancer, 115*, 2013–2021.

Ferreira, A. S., & Lopes, A. J. (2011). Chinese medicine pattern differentiation and its implications for clinical practice. *Chinese Journal of Integrated Medicine, 17*, 818–823.

Filshie, J., Penn, K., Ashley, S., & Davis, C. L. (1996). Acupuncture for the relief of cancer-related breathlessness. *Palliative Medicine, 10*, 145–150.

Frisk, J., Kallstrom, A. C., Wall, N., Fredrikson, M., & Hammar, M. (2011). Acupuncture improves health-related quality-of-life (HRQoL) and sleep in women with breast cancer and hot flushes. *Support Care Cancer, 20*, 715–724.

Gan, T. J., Jiao, K. R., Zenn, M., & Georgiade, G. (2004). A randomized controlled comparison of electro-acupoint stimulation or ondansetron versus placebo for the prevention of postoperative nausea and vomiting. *Anesthesia and Analgesia, 99*, 1070–1075.

Gerson-Cwilich, R., Serrano-Olvera, A., & Villalobos-Prieto, A. (2006). Complementary and alternative medicine (CAM) in mexican patients with cancer. *Clinical & Translational Oncology, 8*, 200–207.

Han, C., Li, X. W., & Luo, H. C. (2002). Comparative study of electro-acupuncture and maprotiline in treating depression. *Zhongguo Zhong Xi Yi Jie He Za Zhi, 22*, 512–514, 521.

Hopkins Hollis, A. S. (2010). Acupuncture as a treatment modality for the management of cancer pain: The state of the science. *Oncology Nursing Forum, 37*, E344–348.

Johnston, M. F., Hays, R. D., Subramanian, S. K., Elashoff, R. M., Axe, E. K., Li, J. J. et al. (2011). Patient education integrated with acupuncture for relief of cancer-related fatigue randomized controlled feasibility study. *BMC Complementary and Alternative Medicine, 11*, 49.

Josefson, A., & Kreuter, M. (2003). Acupuncture to reduce nausea during chemotherapy treatment of rheumatic diseases. *Rheumatology, 42,* 1149–1154.

Kober, A., Scheck, T., Schubert, B., Strasser, H., Gustorff, B., Bertalanffy, P., et al. (2003). Auricular acupressure as a treatment for anxiety in prehospital transport settings. *Anesthesiology, 98*:1328–1332.

Langevin, H. M., Wayne, P. M., MacPherson, H., Schnyer, R., Milley, R. M., Napadow, V., Lao, L., Park, J., Harris, R. E., Cohen, M., Sherman, K. J., Haramati, A., & Hammerschlag, R. (2011). Paradoxes in acupuncture research: Strategies for moving forward. Evidence-based Complementary and Alternative Medicine, 1–9.

Lee, H., Schmidt, K., & Ernst, E. (2005a). Acupuncture for the relief of cancer-related pain—a systematic review. *European Journal of Pain, 9,* 437–444.

Lee, M. S., Shin, B., & Jeong, D. (2005b). An exploratory study of the relationship between the midday-mignight law and electrical conduction properties of corresponding acupuncture points. *Acupuncture & Electrotherapeutics Research, 30,* 201–206.

Lee, M. S., Choi, T. Y., Park, J. E., Lee, S. S., & Ernst, E. (2010). Moxibustion for cancer care: A systematic review and meta-analysis. *BMC Cancer, 10,* 130.

Li, J., Wan, H., Zhang, H., & Tian, M. (2011). Current applications of molecular imaging and luminescence-based techniques in traditional Chinese medicine. *Journal of Ethnopharmacology, 137,* 16–26.

Lim, J. T., Wong, E. T., & Aung, S. K. (2011). Is there a role for acupuncture in the symptom management of patients receiving palliative care for cancer? A pilot study of 20 patients comparing acupuncture with nurse-led supportive care. *Acupuncture in Medicine, 29,* 173–179.

Lin, J., & Chen, Y. (2010). Supportive cancer care with acupuncture. In W. C. Cho (Ed.), *Supportive cancer care with chinese medicine* (pp. 39–54). Heidelberg: Springer.

Liu, C. H., Tang, W. R., Wang, H. M., & Lee, K. C. (2011). Cancer patients' experience of combined treatment with conventional and traditional chinese medicine: A biopsychosocial phenomenon. *Cancer Nursing, 34,* 495–502.

Lu, W., Dean-Clower, E., Doherty-Gilman, A., & Rosenthal, D. S. (2008). The value of acupuncture in cancer care. *Hematology/Oncology Clinics of North America, 22,* 631–648, viii.

Maa, S. H., Sun, M. F., Hsu, K. H., Hung, T. J., Chen, H. C., Yu, C. T., et al. (2003). Effect of acupuncture or acupressure on quality of life of patients with chronic obstructive asthma: A pilot study. *Journal of Alternative and Complementary Medicine, 9,* 659–670.

Maa, S. H., Tsou, T. S., Wang, K. Y., Wang, C. H., Lin, H. C., & Huang, Y. H. (2007). Self-administered acupressure reduces the symptoms that limit daily activities in bronchiectasis patients: Pilot study findings. *Journal of Clinical Nursing, 16,* 794–804.

Mao, J. J., Styles, T., Cheville, A., Wolf, J., Fernandes, S., & Farrar, J. T. (2009a). Acupuncture for nonpalliative radiation therapy-related fatigue: Feasibility study. *Journal of the Society for Integrative Oncology, 7,* 52–58.

Mao, J. J., Bruner, D. W., Stricker, C., Farrar, J. T., Xie, S. X., Bowman, M. A., et al. (2009b). Feasibility trial of electroacupuncture for aromatase inhibitor—related arthralgia in breast cancer survivors. *Integrative Cancer Therapies, 8,* 123–129.

Mehling, W. E., Jacobs, B., Acree, M., Wilson, L., Bostrom, A., West, J., et al. (2007). Symptom management with massage and acupuncture in postoperative cancer patients: A randomized controlled trial. *Journal of Pain and Symptom Management, 33,* 258–266.

Mei, M. F. (2011). A systematic analysis of the theory and practice of syndrome differentiation. *Chinese Journal of Integrated Medicine, 17,* 803–810.

Minton, O., & Higginson, I. J. (2007). Electroacupuncture as an adjunctive treatment to control neuropathic pain in patients with cancer. *Journal of Pain and Symptom Management, 33,* 115–117.

Minton, O., Richardson, A., Sharpe, M., Hotopf, M., & Stone, P. (2008). A systematic review and meta-analysis of the pharmacological treatment of cancer-related fatigue. *Journal of the National Cancer Institute, 100,* 1155–1166.

Molassiotis, A., Fernadez-Ortega, P., Pud, D., Ozden, G., Scott, J. A., Panteli, V., et al. (2005). Use of complementary and alternative medicine in cancer patients: A european survey. *Annals of Oncology, 16*:655–663.

Molassiotis, A., Sylt, P., & Diggins, H. (2007a). The management of cancer-related fatigue after chemotherapy with acupuncture and acupressure: A randomised controlled trial. *Complementary Therapies in Medicine, 15*, 228–237.

Molassiotis, A., Helin, A. M., Dabbour, R., & Hummerston, S. (2007b). The effects of P6 acupressure in the prophylaxis of chemotherapy-related nausea and vomiting in breast cancer patients. *Complementary Therapies in Medicine, 15*, 3–12.

Montazeri, A., Sajadian, A., Ebrahimi, M., Haghighat, S., & Harirchi, I. (2007). Factors predicting the use of complementary and alternative therapies among cancer patients in iran. *European Journal of Cancer Care, 16*, 144–149.

Mora, B., Iannuzzi, M., Lang, T., Steinlechner, B., Barker, R., Dobrovits, M., et al. (2007). Auricular acupressure as a treatment for anxiety before extracorporeal shock wave lithotripsy in the elderly. *The Journal of Urology, 178*:160–164.

Nystrom, E., Ridderstrom, G., & Leffler, A. S. (2008). Manual acupuncture as an adjunctive treatment of nausea in patients with cancer in palliative care—a prospective, observational pilot study. *Acupuncture in Medicine, 26*, 27–32.

O'Regan, D., & Filshie, J. (2010). Acupuncture and cancer. *Autonomic Neuroscience: Basic & Clinical, 157*, 96–100.

Paley, C. A., & Johnson, M. I. (2011). Acupuncture for cancer-induced bone pain: A pilot study. *Acupuncture in Medicine, 29*, 71–73.

Paley, C. A., Johnson, M. I., & Bennett, M. I. (2011a). Should physiotherapists use acupuncture for treating patients with cancer-induced bone pain? A discussion paper. *Physiotherapy, 97*, 256–263.

Paley, C. A., Johnson, M. I., Tashani, O. A., & Bagnall, A. M. (2011b). Acupuncture for cancer pain in adults. *Cochrane Database of Systematic Reviews, 19*, CD007753.

Peng, H., Peng, H. D., Xu, L., & Lao, L. X. (2010). Efficacy of acupuncture in treatment of cancer pain: A systematic review. *Zhong Xi Yi Jie He Xue Bao, 8*:501–509.

Perkins, P., & Vowler, S. L. (2008). Does acupressure help reduce nausea and vomiting in palliative care patients? Pilot study. *Palliative Medicine, 22*:193–194.

Peterson, J. R. (1996). Acupuncture in the 1990s: A review for primary care physiscans. *Archives of Family Medicine, 5*, 237–240.

Pfister, D. G., Cassileth, B. R., Deng, G. E., Yeung, K. S., Lee, J. S., Garrity, D., et al. (2010). Acupuncture for pain and dysfunction after neck dissection: Results of a randomized controlled trial. *Journal of Clinical Oncology, 28*, 2565–2570.

Roschke, J., Wolf, C., Muller, M. J., Wagner, P., Mann, K., Grozinger, M., et al. (2000). The benefit from whole body acupuncture in major depression. *Journal of Affective Disorders, 57*, 73–81.

Roscoe, J. A., Morrow, G. R., Hickok, J. T., Bushunow, P., Pierce, H. I., Flynn, P. J., et al. (2003). The efficacy of acupressure and acustimulation wrist bands for the relief of chemotherapy-induced nausea and vomiting. A university of rochester cancer center community clinical oncology program multicenter study. *Journal of Pain and Symptom Management, 26*, 731–742.

Sagar, S. M. (2008). Acupuncture as an evidence-based option for symptom control in cancer patients. *Complementary and Alternative Therapies in Oncology, 9*, 11–126.

Shen, J., Wenger, N., Glaspy, J., Hays, R. D., Albert, P. S., Choi, C., et al. (2000). Electroacupuncture for control of myeloablative chemotherapy-induced emesis: A randomized controlled trial. *JAMA, 284*, 2755–2761.

Shen, S., Hui, J., Yumen, Y., Wang, J., Chen, L., Niu, Y., Peng, N., Tang, Z., & Zhao, Y. (2011). Study on canceration law of gastric mucosal dysplasia based on syndromes of Chinese medicine. *Chinese Journal of Integrated Medicine, 17*, 346–350.

Standish, L., Kozak, L., & Congdon, S. (2008). Acupuncture is underutilized in hospice and palliative medicine. *American Journal of Hospice & Palliative Medicine, 25*, 298–308.

Streitberger, K., Friedrich-Rust, M., Bardenheuer, H., Unnebrink, K., Windeler, J., Goldschmidt, H., et al. (2003). Effect of acupuncture compared with placebo-acupuncture at P6 as additional antiemetic prophylaxis in high-dose chemotherapy and autologous peripheral blood stem cell

transplantation: A randomized controlled single-blind trial. *Clinical Cancer Research, 9*:2538–2544.
Tough, S. C., Johnston, D. W., Verhoef, M. J., Arthur, K., & Bryant, H. (2002). Complementary and alternative medicine use among colorectal cancer patients in Alberta, Canada. *Alternative Therapies in Health and Medicine, 8*, 54–56, 58–60, 62–64.
Vickers, A. J., Straus, D. J., Fearon, B., & Cassileth, B. R. (2004). Acupuncture for postchemotherapy fatigue: A Phase II study. *Journal of Clinical Oncology, 22*, 1731–1735.
Vickers, A. J., Feinstein, M. B., Deng, G. E., & Cassileth, B. R. (2005). Acupuncture for dyspnea in advanced cancer: A randomized, placebo-controlled pilot trial [ISRCTN89462491. *BMC Palliative Care, 4,* 5.
Walker, E. M., Rodriguez, A. I., Kohn, B., Ball, R. M., Pegg, J., Pocock, J. R., et al. (2010). Acupuncture versus venlafaxine for the management of vasomotor symptoms in patients with hormone receptor-positive breast cancer: A randomized controlled trial. *Journal of Clinical Oncology, 28*, 634–640.
Wang, S. M., & Kain, Z. N. (2001). Auricular acupuncture: A potential treatment for anxiety. *Anesthesia and Analgesia, 92*, 548–553.
Wein, S., Sulkes, A., & Stemmer, S. (2010). The oncologist's role in managing depression, anxiety, and demoralization with advanced cancer. *Cancer Journal, 16*, 493–499.
Wong, R. H., Lee, T. W., Sihoe, A. D., Wan, I. Y., Ng, C. S., Chan, S. K., et al. (2006). Analgesic effect of electroacupuncture in postthoracotomy pain: A prospective randomized trial. *The Annals of Thoracic Surgery, 81*, 2031–2036.
Wu, H. S., Wu, S. C., Lin, J. G., & Lin, L. C. (2004). Effectiveness of acupressure in improving dyspnoea in chronic obstructive pulmonary disease. *Journal of Advanced Nursing, 45*, 252–259.
Xia, Y. Q., Zhang, D., Yang, C. X., Xu H. L., Li, Y., & Ma, L. T. (1986). An approach to the effect on tumors of acupuncture in combination with radiotherapy or chemotherapy. *Journal of Traditional Chinese Medicine, 6*:23–26.
Yeh, M., Lee, T., Chen, H., & Chao, T. (2006). The influences of Chan-Chuang qi gong therapy on complete bloodcell counts in breast cancer patients treated with chemotherapy. *Cancer Nursing, 29*, 149–155.
Zhou, J. (2009). New understanding of the basic theory of traditional Chinese medicine. *Chinese Journal of Integrated Medicine, 15*, 7–12.
Zhou, K., Fang, J., Wang, X., Wang, Y., Hong, Y., Liu, J., Wang, L., Xue, C., Wang, P., Liu, B., & Zhu, B. (2011). Characterization of de qi with electroacupuncture at acupoints with different properties. *The Journal of Alternative and Complementary Medicine, 17*, 1007–1013.
Zick, S. M., Alwari, S., Merrel, G., Burris, B., Sen, A., Litzinger, A., & Harris, R. E. (2011). Relaxation acupressure reduces persistent cancer-related fatigue. *Evidence-based Complementary and Alternative Medicine, 2010,* 1–10.

Chapter 11
Is Acupuncture or Moxibustion Better than a Sham or Placebo-Treatment?

Myeong Soo Lee, Tae-Hun Kim and Edzard Ernst

Abstract The objective of this chapter is to provide an overview of the specific effects of acupuncture and moxibustion for cancer-related symptoms. Three databases, MEDLINE, AMED and EMBASE, were searched from their inception through February 2012. The selection of studies, data extraction, and validations were performed independently by two reviewers. The risk of bias was assessed using the guidelines of the Cochrane collaboration. A total of seven randomized controlled trials comparing real acupuncture and sham acupuncture were identified. The majority of the included studies had a low risk of bias. In two studies which assessed hot flash symptoms in breast cancer patients, acupuncture showed specific effects compared with sham acupuncture. In two studies that evaluated the efficacy of acupuncture on radiation therapy-induced xerostomia, acupuncture improved the subjective and objective outcomes of xerostomia significantly more than a sham-treatment. One study that tested the anti-emetic effect of acupuncture demonstrated that the number of patients experiencing nausea did not decrease significantly in the real acupuncture group. In one study that evaluated the efficacy of acupuncture on aromatase inhibitor-induced joint symptoms in breast cancer patients, the Western Ontario and McMaster Universities Osteoarthritis Index pain score was significantly improved in the real acupuncture group. Another study that tested the effect of electroacupuncture treatment on radiation therapy-induced fatigue demonstrated that there was no significant improvement in the real acupuncture group. This chapter concluded that there is currently no conclusive evidence whether acupuncture or moxibustion are better than placebo for treating on various cancer-related symptoms or not.

M. S. Lee (✉) · T.-H. Kim,
Medical Research Division, Korea Institute of Oriental Medicine,
461-24, Jeonmin-dong, Yuseong-gu, Daejeon 305-811, South Korea
e-mail: drmslee@gmail.com

E. Ernst
Complementary Medicine, Peninsula Medical School,
University of Exeter, Exeter, UK

W. C. S. Cho (ed.), *Acupuncture and Moxibustion as an Evidence-based Therapy for Cancer*, Evidence-based Anticancer Complementary and Alternative Medicine 3,
DOI 10.1007/978-94-007-4833-0_11, © Springer Science+Business Media Dordrecht 2012

11.1 Introduction

Acupuncture and moxibustion are interventions from eastern Asian medicine, including traditional Chinese medicine (TCM) and traditional Korean medicine, that are currently popular in various clinical areas, such as rheumatology (Ernst and Lee 2010b; Choi et al. 2011), neurology (Kong et al. 2010), rehabilitation medicine (Wong et al. 2011) and gynecology (Borud and White 2010; Ernst et al. 2011; Kang et al. 2011). Acupuncture and moxibustion are also used as alternative or additive therapies for the symptomatic management cancer (Ernst and Lee 2010a; Chan 2011; Paley et al. 2011). According to recent reports, the prevalence of acupuncture usage among cancer patients has been suggested to be close to 31% (Filshie and Hester 2006; Gansler et al. 2008). Considering that many cancer survivors may experience many kinds of bothersome, chronic symptoms, such as nausea and vomiting, fatigue, and pain, during and after cancer therapy managing such symptoms would be a significant advance. Cancer patients need effective and safe interventions for palliative care, and non-drug therapies such as acupuncture and moxibustion might be good alternatives compared with pharmacological treatments (Cassileth et al. 2007; Wesa et al. 2008).

Yet evidence of the effectiveness of acupuncture and moxibustion in cancer treatment remains uncertain (Vickers 2004). The efficacy of acupuncture and moxibustion needs to be evaluated to determine whether these interventions are superior to placebos.

Thus, the aim of this systematic review is to summarize and critically evaluate all sham-controlled, randomized trials of acupuncture and moxibustion as a symptomatic treatment for cancer.

11.2 Methods

11.2.1 Data Sources

The databases that were searched from their respective inceptions through to February 29, 2012 were MEDLINE, AMED and EMBASE. The search phrase used was "(acupuncture AND cancer) OR (moxibustion AND cancer)". In addition, our own files and relevant journals (FACT—Focus on Alternative and Complementary Therapies) were manually searched. Full papers of all articles were obtained and thoroughly read.

11.2.2 Study Selection

All articles were included that reported a randomized clinical trial (RCT) in which patients with any type of cancer were treated with needle acupuncture with or without electrical stimulation to relieve the symptoms of cancer. Acupuncture was defined as the insertion of needles into the skin and underlying tissues at particular sites, known as acupuncture points, for therapeutic or preventive purposes. Trials testing other forms of acupuncture, such as laser acupuncture or auricular acupuncture without needling, were excluded. To be included, a trial had to compare needle acupuncture with various forms of sham acupuncture in a parallel or cross-over design. Only publications in English were included. Dissertations and abstracts were excluded. Trials in which the sample size was less than ten patients in each arm and trials that used less than 4 weeks treatment were also excluded. Trials evaluated only the outcomes related to immunological or other surrogate endpoints were excluded.

11.2.3 Data Extraction and Risk of Bias Assessment

All articles were read by two independent reviewers (MSL and THK), who extracted data from the articles according to predefined criteria. The risk of bias was assessed using the Cochrane classification for eight criteria: random sequence generation, allocation concealment, patient blinding, assessor blinding, reporting of drop-out or withdrawal, intention-to-treat analysis, selective outcome reporting and other potential biases. Disagreements were resolved by discussion between the two reviewers (MSL and THK), with the opinion of a third reviewer (EE) sought if necessary.

11.2.4 Outcome Measures and Data Synthesis

In the absence of clinical heterogeneity, the results were synthesized in a meta-analysis. The mean change in outcome measures compared with the baseline was used to assess differences between the intervention and the control groups. Weighted mean differences or standardized mean differences and 95% confidence intervals (CIs) were calculated using Cochrane Collaboration's software (Review Manager version 5.0, Copenhagen: The Nordic Cochrane Centre). Where necessary, we contacted the primary authors to acquire or verify data. Differences compared to the sham control were considered relevant. The variance of the change was inferred using a correlation factor of 0.5. Cochrane's Q-test and I^2 were used to assess heterogeneity. Heterogeneity was assumed if the χ^2 test was $p < 0.10$ and the I^2 was greater than 75%. In the case of heterogeneity, we attempted to identify and explain the heterogeneity using subgroup analysis. Subgroup analysis was performed for subsets of studies and symptoms of cancer. Where possible, publication bias was assessed using a funnel plot. *Post hoc* sensitivity analyses were performed to test the robustness of the overall effect.

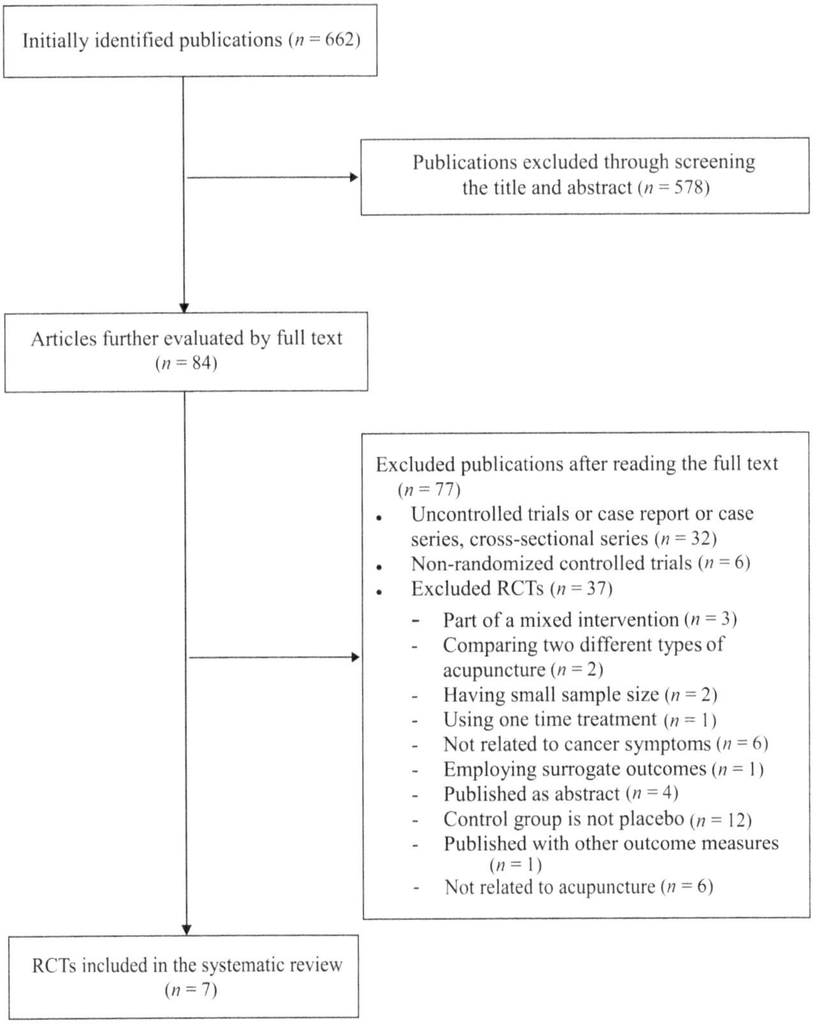

Fig. 11.1 Flow chart of the publication selection process. *RCT* randomized controlled trial

11.3 Results

11.3.1 Study Description

The searches identified 664 potentially relevant articles of which 578 were excluded after screening the abstracts (Fig. 11.1). A total of 84 articles were read by two independent reviewers in full and 76 were excluded: 38 were not RCTs, 39 RCTs were excluded because three were RCTs but tested mixed interventions of treatments, two compared two different types of acupuncture, two had a small sample size, two employed a one-time treatment, six were not related to cancer symptoms, one used surrogate outcomes, four were published as abstracts, one was a publication of the same trial with different outcomes, twelve did not use sham controls and two were not related to acupuncture.

Therefore, 7 RCTs met our inclusion criteria (Blom et al. 1996; Deng et al. 2007; Balk et al 2009; Hervik and Mjaland 2009; Crew et al. 2010; Enblom et al. 2012; Meng et al. 2012) (Table 11.1). These studies targeted a range of different symptoms including radiation-induced nausea (Enblom et al. 2012), hot flashes in breast cancer patients (Deng et al. 2007; Hervik and Mjaland 2009), aromatase inhibitor-induced joint pain (Crew et al. 2010), xerostomia (Blom et al. 1996; Meng et al. 2012) and cancer-related fatigue (Balk et al. 2009). Four studies originated from the US (Deng et al. 2007; Balk et al. 2009; Crew et al. 2010; Meng et al. 2012), two from Sweden (Blom et al. 1996; Enblom et al. 2012) and one from Norway (Hervik and Mjaland 2009).

Specific sensations following acupuncture stimulation, called 'deqi', were mentioned in all of the trials (Table 11.2). Deqi was regarded as the arrival of Qi, which is considered to be essential for clinical efficacy according to ancient acupuncture theory.

11.3.2 Risk of Bias

The majority of the included studies showed a low risk of bias in each domain. Among the seven RCTs, five studies (Deng et al. 2007; Balk et al. 2009; Crew et al. 2010; Enblom et al. 2012; Meng et al. 2012) appropriately conducted sequence generation and allocation concealment (Table 11.3). All of the included studies used sham acupuncture as a control with blind participants. Only three studies (Deng et al. 2007; Crew et al. 2010; Enblom et al. 2012), however, clearly reported the blinding methods of the outcome assessors. Two studies (Blom et al. 1996; Hervik and Mjaland 2009) did not appropriately report drop-out or withdrawal. In one RCT, statistical analysis was conducted on an intention-to-treat basis (Meng et al. 2012). Two studies were suspected of not reporting all the outcomes that had been originally planned to be reported (Deng et al. 2007; Crew et al. 2010).

11.3.3 Outcomes

11.3.3.1 Nausea-related to Radiation Therapy

One RCT tested the effects of acupuncture on nausea related to radiation therapy in patients with various cancers compared to non-penetrating acupuncture (Enblom et al. 2012). There were no differences between five weeks of acupuncture and sham

Table 11.1 Summary of the included studies

First author (year)	Sample size/condition Mean age (years) M/F	Main cancer treatment	The target symptom for the intervention	Intervention group (deqi, needle retention, frequency and duration, measurement time of primary endpoint, number of participants)	Control group (control intervention, number of participants)	Main outcomes	Intergroup differences (MD or RR [95% CI])
Enblom et al. (2012)	215/Cancer of abdomen or pelvic cavity 64 35/180	Radiation therapy	Nausea	(A) Real acupuncture (inducing deqi by twirling and lifting needles, 30 min, 2–3 times/week, 5 weeks, $n = 109$)	(B) Sham acupuncture, (Park sham device at no acupuncture points, $n = 106$)	1) Number of patients experiencing nausea 2) Mean number of days with nausea 3) Patient number of antiemetic consumption at least once	1) RR,1.1 [0.9, 1.4] 2) MD,1.4 [−1.1, 3.9] 3) RR,1.1 [0.8, 1.6]
Hervik (2008)	59/Breast cancer A:54; B:52 0/59	Breast cancer surgery	Hot flashes	(A) Real acupuncture plus estrogen antagonist treatment (inducing deqi manually, 30 min, 1–2 times/week, 10 weeks, $n = 30$)	(B) Sham acupuncture plus estrogen antagonist treatment (minimal penetrating at non-acupuncture points, $n = 29$)	1) Hot flash frequency during day time 2) Hot flash frequency at night 3) Kupperman index	1) MD, −7.0 [−10.4, −3.6] 2) MD, −2.8 [−4.6, −1.1] 3) MD, −4.4 [−6.8, −2.0]
Deng et al. (2007)	72/Breast cancer A:55; B:56 0/72	n.r.	Hot flashes	(A) Real acupuncture (inducing deqi manually, 20 min, 2 times/week, 4 weeks, $n = 42$)	(B) Sham acupuncture (Streitberger sham device at non-acupuncture points, $n = 30$)	Hot flash frequency per day	MD, −2.0 [−4.7, 0.7]

Table 11.1 (continued)

First author (year)	Sample size/condition Mean age (years) M/F	Main cancer treatment	The target symptom for the intervention	Intervention group (deqi, needle retention, frequency and duration, measurement time of primary endpoint, number of participants)	Control group (control intervention, number of participants)	Main outcomes	Intergroup differences (MD or RR, ES [95% CI])
Crew et al. (2010)	43/Breast cancer A:58; B:57 0/43	Aromatase inhibitor	Joint symptoms	(A) Real acupuncture (inducing deqi at body acupuncture points, 30 min, 2 times/week, 6 weeks, $n=23$)	(B) Sham acupuncture (superficial acupuncture at non-acupuncture points, $n=20$)	1) WOMAC (pain) 2) WOMAC (stiffness) 3) WOMAC (function) 4) WOMAC (normalized) 5) BPI-SF (worst pain) 6) FACT-G (physical well-being)	1) MD, −132.0 [−178.5, −85.6] 2) MD, −63.0 [−91.4, −34.58] 3) MD, −304.0 [−485.5, −122.5] 4) MD, −75.0 [−106.5, −43.6] 5) MD, −2.5 [−3.7, −1.3] 6) MD, 4.4 [0.6, 8.2]
Blom et al. (1996)	38/Malignant tumor of the head and neck A:65; B:64 A:14/6; B:12/6	Radiation therapy	Xerostomia	(A) Real acupuncture (inducing deqi manually, 20 min, 2 times/week, 14 weeks, $n=20$)	(B) Sham acupuncture (superficial needling at non-acupuncture points, $n=18$)	1) UWSFR 2) SSFR	1) MD, 0.04 [−0.00, 0.07] 2) MD, 0.24 [0.07, 0.40]

Table 11.1 (continued)

First author (year)	Sample size/condition Mean age (years) M/F	Main cancer treatment	The target symptom for the intervention	Intervention group (deqi, needle retention, frequency and duration, measurement time of primary endpoint, number of participants)	Control group (control intervention, number of participants)	Main outcomes	Intergroup differences (MD or RR, ES [95% CI])
Meng et al. (2012)	22/Nasopharyngeal carcinoma A:46; B:47 A:9/1; B:11/0	Radiation therapy	Xerostomia	(A) Real acupuncture (inducing deqi manually, 20 min, 3 times/week, 6 weeks, $n = 10$)	(B) Sham acupuncture, (Park sham device, $n = 11$)	1) XQ score 2) MDASI-SYM 3) MDASI-INT 4) MDASI-HN 5) UWSFR 6) SSFR	1) MD, −19.3 [−22.0, −15.8] 2) MD, −5.9 [−8.5, −3.3] 3) MD, −3.7 [−5.3, −2.2] 4) MD, −10.9 [−12.9, −8.9] 5) MD, 0.4 [0.3, 0.5] 6) MD, 0.5 [0.3, 0.7]
Balk et al. (2009)	27/Various cancers A:54; B:54 0/27	Radiation therapy	Fatigue	(A) Electrical acupuncture (inducing deqi by electrical stimulation, 30 min, 1–2 times/week, 6 weeks, $n = 16$)	(B) Sham acupuncture with sham electrical acupuncture device (Park sham device at the same points, $n = 11$)	1) FACIT-F 2) CES-D 3) CRFDS	1) MD, 3.0 [−4.3, 10.3] 2) MD, 2.8 [−7.7, 13.4] 3) MD, 5.1 [−25.7, 35.9]

BPI-SF brief pain inventory short form, *CES-D* center for epidemiological studies depression scale, *CRFDS* cancer-related fatigue distress scale, *FACIT-F, G* functional assessment of chronic illness therapy-fatigue, general, *HN* head and neck subscale, *INT* interference subscale, *MD* mean difference, *MDASI* MD Anderson symptom inventory, *n.r.* not reported, *NS* not significant, *PLEK* plasma leucine-enkephalin, *QoL* quality of life, *RR* risk ratio, *SSFR* stimulated salivary flow rates, *SYM* symptom subscale, *UWSFR* unstimulated whole salivary flow rates, *VAS* visual analogue scale, *WOMAC* Western Ontario and McMaster Universities osteoarthritis index, *XQ score* xerostomia questionnaire

Table 11.2 Summary of treatment points and other information related to treatment

First author (Year)	Acupuncture method	Total sessions	Acupuncture points	Rationales	Adverse events
Enblom et al. (2012)	TCM acupuncture (physiologists)	n.r.	Fixed points (2) bilateral: PC6	n.r.	Bleeding (Real: 51) Tiredness (Real: 15; Sham:15) Dizziness (Real:8; Sham:5) Needle scratched the skin (Sham:10)
Hervik (2008)	TCM acupuncture (1 physiotherapist)	15	Fixed points (8) Unilateral: LR3,GB20, LU7, KI3, SP6, CV4, PC7 and LR8	TCM textbooks	n.r.
Deng et al. (2007)	True acupuncture (several licensed acupuncturists)	8	Fixed points (19) Bilateral: GB20, BL13, PC7, HT6, KI7, ST36, SP6, Ear shen men and Ear sympathetic point Unilateral: GV14	Previous reports Expert opinion Standard acupuncture textbook	Very minor adverse effects (slight bleeding or bruising at the needle site) Grade 1 adverse effects:14/560 sessions
Crew et al. (2010)	TCM acupuncture plus National Acupuncture Detoxification Association protocol (1 acupuncturist)	12	Semi-fixed points Body acupuncture points: TE5, GB41, GB34, LI4, ST41 and KI3 Ear acupuncture points: Ear shenmen, Ear kidney, Ear liver, Ear upper lung, and Ear sympathetic points The joint-specific acupuncture points: (1) knee (SP9, SP10, ST34)	Standard acupuncture protocol	Pain (Real:3)

Table 11.2 (continued)

First author (Year)	Acupuncture method	Total sessions	Acupuncture points	Rationales	Adverse events
			(2) fingers (SI5, SI3, ba xie, LI3) (3) lumbar (GV3, GV8, BL23) (4) shoulder (TE15, TE14, SI10) (5) hip (GB30, GB39) (6) wrist (TE4, LI5)		
Blom et al. (1996)	TCM acupuncture	24	Individualized points Body acupuncture (5–8 points): GV20, ST7, ST3, ST6, ST5, SI17, LI18, PC6, HT7, SI3, LI4, LI10, LI11, ST36, LR3, SP3, SP6, SP8, KI4, KI5 and KI 7 Ear acupuncture (2–4 points): Ear shenmen, Ear sympathetic, Ear kidney, Ear mouth, Ear stomach, Ear GI parotis and Ear subcortex	TCM textbooks	A few cases of hematoma at the acupuncture points and tiredness
Meng et al. (2012)	TCM acupuncture (1 acupuncturist)	18	Fixed points (13) Body acupuncture points: CV24, bilateral LU7 and KI6 Ear acupuncture points: bilateral Ear shenmen, Ear point zero, Ear salivary gland 2-prime and Ear larynx	n.r.	None
Balk et al. (2009)	TCM acupuncture (1 acupuncturist)	4–12	Fixed points (10) Bilateral: KI3, SP6, LI6, ST36 and CV6	Expert opinion	None

TCM traditional Chinese medicine, *n.r.* not reported

Table 11.3 Risk of bias assessment[a]

First author (year)	Random sequence generation	Allocation concealment	Patient blinding	Assessor blinding	Reporting drop-out or withdrawal[b]	Intention-to-treat analysis[c]	Selective outcome reporting	Other potential biases
Enblom et al. (2012)	L	L	L	L	L	H	L	L
Hervik (2008)	U	U	L	U	U	U	L	L
Deng et al. (2007)	L	L	L	L	L	H	H	H
Crew et al. (2010)	L	L	L	L	L	H	H	H
Blom et al. (1996)	U	U	L	U	H	H	L	H
Meng et al. (2012)	L	L	L	U	L	L	L	L
Balk et al. (2009)	L	L	L	U	L	U	L	L

H high risk of bias, *L* low risk of bias, *U* unclear (uncertain risk of bias)
[a]Domains of quality assessment based on the Cochrane tools for assessing the risk of bias
[b] Two domains referring to 'incomplete outcome data' in the Cochrane tools for assessing the risk of bias
[c] This study had a baseline imbalance in the subjective outcome values

acupuncture for reducing the number of patients experiencing nausea, the mean number of days with nausea and the amount of anti-emetic consumption.

11.3.3.2 Hot Flashes in Breast Cancer Patients

Two RCTs compared the effects of acupuncture with sham acupuncture in breast cancer patients (Deng et al. 2007; Hervik and Mjaland 2009). One RCT showed favorable effects of acupuncture for reducing hot flash frequency during both the daytime and nighttime compared to minimal penetrating sham acupuncture (Hervik and Mjaland 2009). In contrast, the other RCT failed to show any beneficial effects of acupuncture for hot flash frequency per day during the treatment and after the treatment period compared with non-penetrating sham acupuncture (Deng et al. 2007).

11.3.3.3 Joint Symptoms in Breast Cancer Patients

One RCT tested the effects of acupuncture on aromatase inhibitor-induced joint pain in breast cancer patients compared with sham acupuncture (Crew et al. 2010). The acupuncture group experienced more pain reduction using the Western Ontario and McMaster Universities Osteoarthritis Index (WOMAC) and Brief Pain Inventory Short Form (BPI-SF) indices compared with superficial penetrating acupuncture. Furthermore, this study demonstrated beneficial effects on joint function using the WOMAC and on physical well-being using the Functional Assessment of Chronic Illness Therapy-General scale.

11.3.3.4 Xerostomia-induced by Radiotherapy

Two RCTs compared acupuncture with superficial needling and non-penetrating acupuncture as sham techniques (Blom et al. 1996; Meng et al. 2012). Both of these studies showed no significant intergroup differences regarding unstimulated and stimulated salivary flow rates. One RCT (Meng et al. 2012) showed beneficial effects of acupuncture on subjective symptoms measured by a patient-reported questionnaire, while the other RCT (Blom et al. 1996) failed to do so.

11.3.3.5 Cancer-related Fatigue

One RCT compared the effects of acupuncture for cancer-related fatigue in various cancer patients compared with non-penetrating acupuncture (Balk et al. 2009). The acupuncture group showed improvement in fatigue using the Functional Assessment of Chronic Illness Therapy-Fatigue scale, but there was no significant difference between the two groups.

We had originally intended to submit the above data to a formal meta-analysis. However, the statistical and clinical heterogeneity of the studies prohibited us from doing so.

11.3.3.6 Adverse Events

Six RCTs mentioned adverse events in detail (Blom et al. 1996; Deng et al. 2007; Balk et al. 2009; Crew et al. 2010; Enblom et al. 2012; Meng et al. 2012). One study reported adverse events for both real and sham acupuncture (Enblom et al. 2012). Bleeding was reported only in the real acupuncture group, but the participants of both groups equally reported tiredness and dizziness at the same time. Hematoma at the acupuncture points and mild dizziness were reported in two studies (Blom et al. 1996; Deng et al. 2007). One RCT reported pain at the acupuncture points (Crew et al. 2010). There was no adverse event in two of the studies (Balk et al. 2009; Meng et al. 2012).

11.4 Discussion

This systematic review identified only a few sham-controlled acupuncture RCTs and no sham-controlled moxibustion studies. Their results are contradictory and, in total, fail to provide convincing evidence for the effectiveness of acupuncture in cancer care. Several individual studies suggested a positive effect of real acupuncture on cancer-related conditions, but all of these trials had small sample sizes. Overall, our findings provide no convincing evidence that acupuncture is beneficial beyond a placebo-response.

Our previous overview suggested that there are clinically beneficial effects of acupuncture for chemotherapy-induced nausea and vomiting, while the evidence is mixed for xerostomia and cancer pain (Choi et al. 2012). The results of the present systematic review are similar to the overview. The overview, however, expressed concern regarding the poor methodological quality of the included primary studies (Choi et al. 2012).

No sham-controlled trials of moxibustion met our inclusion criteria. If we assume that the effects of moxibustion could occur by stimulating acupuncture points with heat, sham moxibustion paradigms may include treating outside acupuncture points on non-acupuncture points or preventing heat stimulation on acupuncture points or areas. Two sham moxibustion devices, which are designed to minimize heat transfer, have been described to date (Park et al. 2009; Wang et al. 2009). These methods could help achieve patient and practitioner blinding in future studies.

Several sham acupuncture methods have been developed. These methods range from puncturing the skin outside acupoints, inserting the needle at non-acupoints or superficially puncturing the skin without stimulation. In the present systematic review, no conclusive evidence of the superiority of real acupuncture was found compared with sham acupuncture regardless of the acupuncture technique employed.

Non-penetrating sham acupuncture was reported to be more effective than placebo tablets for subjective pain outcomes (Kaptchuk et al. 2006). This observation may suggest that the effects of needle acupuncture with or without electric stimulation could be non-specific by nature. The effectiveness of acupuncture for hot flashes (Deng et al. 2007; Hervik and Mjaland 2009) and xerostomia (Blom et al. 1996; Meng et al. 2012) are mixed. One trial suggested positive effects of acupuncture in reducing joint symptoms (Crew et al. 2010).The other two studies failed to relieve radiation induced nausea (Enblom et al. 2012) and fatigue (Balk et al. 2009). Most of the studies were too small to generate reliable findings.

The results of this systematic review are consistent with several possible interpretations. Acupuncture might be ineffective, the studies might have been inadequately designed or the treatment had not been optimally administered or sham acupuncture is also an effective treatment. For example, the number of treatment sessions could have been too small to generate a significant effect, treatment could have been suboptimal, or the protocol applied in the acupuncture group might not have been suitable for treating the specific cancer-related symptoms.

The rationale for the selection of acupuncture points was stated in 5 RCTs (Blom et al. 1996; Deng et al. 2007; Balk et al. 2009; Hervik and Mjaland 2009; Crew et al. 2010). The authors quoted expert opinions, standard acupuncture protocols, or previous studies or recommendations from textbooks to justify their point selection. Needle stimulation causing a typical needle sensation has been claimed to be important for reaching the maximum effects of acupuncture on pain. This needle sensation (Deqi) was considered in all of the included RCTs.

One argument for using acupuncture for the management of the symptoms of cancer patients might be that it is safer than other therapeutic options. Six RCTs assessed adverse events of acupuncture treatment (Blom et al. 1996; Deng et al. 2007; Balk et al. 2009; Crew et al. 2010; Enblom et al. 2012; Meng et al. 2012), and one RCT did not (Hervik and Mjaland 2009). Mild adverse effects of acupuncture were noted for both real and sham acupuncture. Relative to those of drug therapies, however, these are mild, infrequent and perhaps even negligible.

The limitation of our systematic review pertain to the potential incompleteness of the evidence reviewed. We aimed to identify all studies on the topic. The distorting effects of publication bias and location bias on systematic reviews are well documented (Ernst and Pittler 1997; Pittler et al. 2000; Rothstein et al. 2005). We restricted our review to RCTs published in English, and only a relatively small number of databases were searched. Therefore, there may be relevant publications which we missed. Further limitations include the paucity and the often suboptimal quality of the primary data.

11.5 Conclusion

The evidence from sham-controlled RCTs of acupuncture or moxibustion for treating several symptoms of cancer is limited by the paucity and poor quality of the primary data. Collectively, the RCTs available to date fail to convincingly demonstrate the effectiveness of acupuncture or moxibustion in cancer care. Further research is required to investigate whether there are specific benefits of these treatments for cancer patients.

Future RCTs of acupuncture or moxibustion should adhere to accepted methodological standards. The reviewed studies have a number of problems, e.g. expertise of practitioners, the pluralism of acupuncture, frequency and duration of treatment, the consideration of point specificity, validated sham intervention methods, employing validated primary outcome measures and adequate statistical tests, and heterogeneous comparison groups. Even though it is difficult to blind practitioner to treatment, employing assessor blinding and allocation concealment are important for reducing bias.

Acknowledgment MSL was supported by the KIOM (K11111 and C12080).

References

Balk, J., Day, R., Rosenzweig, M., & Beriwal S. (2009). Pilot, randomized, modified, double-blind, placebo-controlled trial of acupuncture for cancer-related fatigue. *Journal of the Society for Integrative Oncology, 7,* 4–11.

Blom, M., Dawidson, I., Fernberg, J. O., Johnson, G., & Angmar-Mansson, B. (1996). Acupuncture treatment of patients with radiation-induced xerostomia. *European Journal of Cancer. Part B, Oral Oncology, 32B,* 182–190.

Borud, E., & White, A. (2010). A review of acupuncture for menopausal problems. *Maturitas, 66,* 131–134.

Cassileth, B., Trevisan, C., & Gubili, J. (2007). Complementary therapies for cancer pain. *Current Pain and Headache Reports, 11,* 265–269.

Chan, R. (2011). Cochrane review summary for cancer nursing: drug therapy for the management of cancer-related fatigue. *Cancer Nursing, 34,* 250–251.

Choi, T. Y., Kim, T. H., Kang, J. W., Lee, M. S., & Ernst, E. (2011). Moxibustion for rheumatic conditions: A systematic review and meta-analysis. *Clinical Rheumatology, 30,* 937–945.

Choi, T. Y., Lee, M. S., & Ernst, E. (2012). An overview of acupuncture and moxibustion for cancer care. In: W. C. S. Cho (Ed.), *Acupuncture and/or moxibustion as an evidence-based therapy for cancer* (pp. 1–18). New York: Springer.

Crew, K. D., Capodice, J. L., Greenlee, H., Brafman, L., Fuentes, D., Awad, D., Yann Tsai, W., & Hershman, D. L. (2010). Randomized, blinded, sham-controlled trial of acupuncture for the management of aromatase inhibitor-associated joint symptoms in women with early-stage breast cancer. *Journal of Clinical Oncology, 28,* 1154–1160.

Deng, G., Vickers, A., Yeung, S., D'Andrea, G. M., Xiao, H., Heerdt, A. S., Sugarman, S., Troso-Sandoval, T., Seidman, A. D., Hudis, C. A., & Cassileth, B. (2007). Randomized, controlled trial of acupuncture for the treatment of hot flashes in breast cancer patients. *Journal of Clinical Oncology, 25,* 5584–5590.

Enblom, A., Johnsson, A., Hammar, M., Onelov, E., Steineck, G., & Borjeson, S. (2012). Acupuncture compared with placebo acupuncture in radiotherapy-induced nausea–a randomized controlled study. *Annals of Oncology, 23,* 1353–1361.

Ernst, E., & Lee, M. S. (2010a). Acupuncture for palliative and supportive cancer care: a systematic review of systematic reviews. *Journal of Pain and Symptom Management, 40,* e3–e5.

Ernst, E., & Lee M. S. (2010b). Acupuncture for rheumatic conditions: an overview of systematic reviews. *Rheumatology, 49,* 1957–1961.

Ernst, E., & Pittler, M. H. (1997). Alternative therapy bias. *Nature, 385,* 480.

Ernst, E., Lee, M. S., & Choi, T. Y. (2011). Acupuncture in obstetrics and gynecology: an overview of systematic reviews. *The American Journal of Chinese Medicine, 39,* 423–431.

Filshie, J., & Hester, J. (2006). Guidelines for providing acupuncture treatment for cancer patients–a peer-reviewed sample policy document. *Acupuncture in Medicine, 24,* 172–1782.

Gansler, T., Kaw, C., Crammer, C., & Smith, T. (2008). A population-based study of prevalence of complementary methods use by cancer survivors: A report from the American Cancer Society's studies of cancer survivors. *Cancer, 113,* 1048–1057.

Hervik, J., & Mjaland, O. (2009). Acupuncture for the treatment of hot flashes in breast cancer patients, a randomized, controlled trial. *Breast Cancer Research and Treatment, 116,* 311–316.

Kang, H. S., Jeong, D., Kim, D. I., & Lee, M. S. (2011). The use of acupuncture for managing gynaecologic conditions: An overview of systematic reviews. *Maturitas, 68,* 346–354.

Kaptchuk, T. J., Stason, W. B., Davis, R. B., Legedza, A. R., Schnyer, R. N., Kerr, C. E., Stone, D. A., Nam, B. H., Kirsch, I., & Goldman, R. H. (2006). Sham device v inert pill: Randomised controlled trial of two placebo treatments. *BMJ, 332,* 391–397.

Kong, J. C., Lee, M. S., Shin, B. C., Song, Y. S., & Ernst, E. (2010) Acupuncture for functional recovery after stroke: a systematic review of sham-controlled randomized clinical trials. *Canadian Medical Association Journal, 182,* 1723–1729.

Meng, Z., Kay Garcia, M., Hu, C., Chiang, J., Chambers, M., Rosenthal, D. I., Peng, H., Wu, C., Zhao, Q., Zhao, G., Liu, L., Spelman, A., Lynn Palmer, J., Wei, Q., & Cohen, L. (2012). Sham-controlled, randomised, feasibility trial of acupuncture for prevention of radiation-induced xerostomia among patients with nasopharyngeal carcinoma. *European Journal of Cancer, 48,* 1692–1699.

Paley, C. A., Johnson, M. I., Tashani, O. A., & Bagnall, A. M. (2011). Acupuncture for cancer pain in adults. *Cochrane Database of Systematic Reviews, 19,* CD007753.

Park, J. E., Lee, M. S., & Choi, S. M. (2009). Is it possible to blind subjects using sham moxibustion treatment? *The American Journal of Chinese Medicine, 37,* 407–409.

Pittler, M. H., Abbot, N. C., Harkness, E. F., & Ernst, E. (2000). Location bias in controlled clinical trials of complementary/alternative therapies. *Journal of Clinical Epidemiology, 53,* 485–499.

Rothstein, H. R., Sutton, A. J., & Borenstein, M. (2005). Publication bias in meta-analysis. In: H. R. Rothstein, A. J. Sutton, & M. Borenstein (Eds.), *Publication bias in meta-analysis* (pp. 1–7). Chichester: Wiley.

Vickers, A. (2004). Alternative cancer cures: "Unproven" or "disproven"? *CA: A Cancer Journal for Clinicians, 54,* 110–118.

Wang, L., Zou, W., & Chi, Q. B. (2009). Strengthening innovation in clinical research methodology of acupuncture and moxibustion to promote internationalization process of acupuncture-moxibustion. *Chinese Acupuncture & Moxibustion, 29,* 495–497.

Wesa, K., Gubili, J., & Cassileth, B. (2008). Integrative oncology: Complementary therapies for cancer survivors. *Hematology/Oncology Clinics of North America, 22,* 343–353.

Wong, V., Cheuk, D. K., Lee, S., & Chu, V. (2011). Acupuncture for acute management and rehabilitation of traumatic brain injury. *Cochrane Database of Systematic Reviews*, CD007700.

Chapter 12
Safety and Side Effects of Acupuncture and Moxibustion as a Therapy for Cancer

Stephen M. Sagar and Raimond K. Wong

Abstract Acupuncture and moxibustion are safe treatments if implemented by trained, regulated practitioners with knowledge of human anatomy and potential adverse effects. Major (life-threatening) adverse effects are quite rare. They include pneumothorax, major hemorrhage, infection, septicemia, perforation of the brain stem, spread of blood-borne infections (such as hepatitis and human immunodeficiency virus), vascular damage, perichondritis, organ perforation, cardiac tamponade, bacterial endocarditis, arrhythmias, burns, scarring and allergic reactions. Instant recognition of these complications is required for successful emergent treatment, which may be life-saving. Minor adverse effects include mild skin reactions, dermatitis, local pain, bruising, syncope, and drowsiness. These are usually not problematic unless allowed to cause complications, such as trauma from syncope. Thorough history taking and attention to high practice standards will reduce the complication rate. This chapter covers well-documented adverse effects of acupuncture and provides guidance to avoid complications. In addition, it suggests guidelines for suspecting and dealing with acute emergencies. Cancer patients can be more susceptible to complications such as infection and bleeding. Moxibustion will also be examined, since it is often used as an integral part of cancer treatment in the East. It is important that the acupuncturist works closely with the oncologist to ensure appropriate application of acupuncture/moxibustion and to reduce the incidence of complications and ensure their timely management when they do occur. Risk factors for complications include: inadequate training, bleeding disorders, immunocompromised state, asthma, cachexia, diabetes, open wounds, cardic valve abnormalities and vasovagal sensitivity. There is evidence that increased training and awareness of potential adverse effects will reduce the incidence of adverse effects. Informed patient consent is important. Hospital and clinic practice guidelines and certification of staff will ensure that practice is as safe as possible.

S. M. Sagar (✉) · R. K. Wong
Departments of Oncology and Medicine,
McMaster University; Juravinski Cancer Centre,
699 Concession Street, Hamilton, ON L8V 5C2, Canada
e-mail: sagars@mcmaster.ca

W. C. S. Cho (ed.), *Acupuncture and Moxibustion as an Evidence-based Therapy for Cancer*, Evidence-based Anticancer Complementary and Alternative Medicine 3,
DOI 10.1007/978-94-007-4833-0_12,

12.1 Introduction

12.1.1 Acupuncture

In Traditional Chinese Medicine, acupuncture and moxibustion are integral therapies for the supportive care of cancer patients. They are used together with Chinese medicinal herbs to optimize health and to stabilize or cure the cancer. In Western medicine, acupuncture is mainly recognized for symptom control and alleviating the adverse effects of both the cancer and the cytotoxic treatments. Its utility has been established for specific indications using new data accumulated from clinical trials (Sagar 2008). Systematic reviews for specific indications are emerging and contributing to practice guidelines. For example, the role of acupuncture (or electrical stimulation of acupoints) to treat radiation-induced xerostomia has been critically reviewed (O'Sullivan and Higginson 2010). Although randomized controlled trials of acupuncture are methodologically challenging, they remain the capstone for clinical evidence in Western cancer clinics.

Since acupuncture is an invasive procedure, major concerns as to its safety were raised by Western physicians (Ernst and White 1997). In addition, their skepticism that it had any physical effect beyond placebo led to an initial focus on its potential to do harm. This was well-founded, since there were early reports of major adverse effects, such as the blood-borne transmission of hepatitis, septicemia due to an infected puncture site, and pneumothorax. This led to the eventual establishment of the regulation of acupuncture needles and the establishment of professional standards. For example, early Western acupuncturists would use a personal set of needles that would be autoclaved (with variable effectiveness) between patients. Currently, health regulatory bodies, such as the US Food and Drug Administration (FDA) only allow factory sterilized disposable needles (and these must meet acceptable manufacturing standards). The FDA recognizes and regulates the acupuncture needle as a Class II medical device. The prevention of the spread of infection was bolstered by Western acupuncture training that placed major emphasis on preventing infection through cleaning the skin and using disposable sterile needles. In addition, some contraindications and cautions were taught, such as avoiding lymphoedematous limbs, patients with cardiac valve abnormalities, dermatitis, etc. The new Western acupuncture schools (such as the Acupuncture Foundation of Canada) placed particular emphasis on the knowledge of human anatomy and prior medical training. These concerns were reinforced by new diagnostic imaging techniques that demonstrated the variability in dermal depth, organ positions, and aberrant foramina between different patients (Stark 1985, Chen et al. 2008). Reports of pneumothorax and pithing of the brain stem reduced the credibility of acupuncture. Migrating acupuncture needles were occasionally discovered on imaging and at surgery. However, it should be emphasized that these major adverse effects are currently rare owing to improved training and regulation of acupuncturists that has led to caution when using the riskier acupuncture points. Correct acupuncture technique is mandatory at certain sites, such as placing needles horizontally (rather than deep vertical penetration). Electrical current passed through the acupuncture needle could interfere with a pacemaker or internal defibrillator. Points near the device should be avoided. In addition, caution should be exercised in patients with a history of arrhythmias, especially electrical stimulation across the arms and chest (Fujiwara et al. 1980; Thompson and Cummings 2008).

In addition to adverse effects from errors of commission, inappropriate treatment with acupuncture results in errors of omission. It is important that acupuncturists realize the appropriateness of biomedicine and surgery in specific circumstances. This requires some training in general medicine and excellent communication between the acupuncturist and practitioner. In the West, the primary treatment of cancer would be biomedical, with acupuncture being used in a supportive role.

12.1.2 Moxibustion

Moxibustion is a traditional Chinese method that uses the heat generated by burning herbal preparations containing *Artemisia vulgaris* to stimulate acupuncture points. There are two types of moxibustion. Direct moxibustion is applied directly to the skin surface at an acupuncture point. In indirect moxibustion some insulating materials are placed between the moxa cone and the skin. Sometimes the acupuncture needle is heated with smoldering moxa attached to the head and shaft of the needle (Word Health Organization 2007). Assuming that moxibustion has some action for cancer patients, possible mechanisms of action have been evaluated. Moxa may be absorbed at acupuncture points, as well as direct effects due to acupuncture point stimulation from heat. Mechanisms may be similar to acupuncture, including both fascial and neurological activity. Of course, in models of Asian medicine, its activity will be translated into the flow of Qi along meridians. Moxibustion does influence the multiple cortical, subcortical/limbic, and brainstem areas. This is partly mediated through opioid and monoamimergic neurotransmission (Napadow et al. 2005; Han 2003; Dhond 2007). Another possible mechanism includes an influence on the heat shock proteins and the function of immune cells. It has been shown that moxibustion can up-regulate heat shock protein and decreases the gastric injury and apoptosis of gastric mucosal cells (Yi et al. 2007; Pei 1995). Laboratory work suggests that moxibustion improves the function of immune cells. Moxibustion induces higher cellular immune function and increases the content of β-endorphin in the lymphocytes of the spleen in HAC cancer mice. Moxibustion may modulate immunity through a neurohormonal regulatory mechanism. Moxibustion also inhibits the growth of tumor and enhances cellular immune functions *via* cytokine production (IL-2 or IL-12) and the increase of natural killer cell activity in tumor-bearing mice (Qiu et al. 2004).

In cancer patients, moxibustion is reported to strengthen the mechanisms of host defense through a response to heat-induced local inflammation. It produces immunological responses that include increased numbers of lymphocytes. One study suggests it can help restore immune functions affected by radiation (Hau 1989). In a study of mice, moxibustion at Dazhui (GV14) inhibited the growth of tumors through enhancing cellular immune functions, probably by improvement of the production of cytokines, such as IL-2, and the resulting increased activity of natural killer cells (Jian 1995).

The neurotransmitter, galanin is synthesized in response to moxibustion. It can regulate pain, spasms and neurological disorders such as depression and anxiety (Kashiba et al. 1992). In a laboratory study on rabbits, the equivalent to Zusanli (ST36) was treated with moxibustion, and it was shown that smooth muscle spontaneous bowel movements decreased (Jiqing et al. 1986), suggesting that neurotransmitters were involved. The antispasmodic effect is consistent with what is seen during the clinical treatment of stomach and intestinal spasms with relief of diarrhea.

One of the most frequently mentioned uses of moxibustion in the Chinese literature is to stimulate the immune system. It is not yet known whether moxibustion differs in its effects compared to acupuncture alone. In the elderly, moxa-heated acupuncture needles (using needles and moxa applied for 20 min and daily treatment for 10 days applied to ST36) improved the production of IL-2 (Su 2003). In the system of traditional Chinese medicine, spleen deficiency (a subcategory of Qi deficiency) syndrome is often associated with weakened immune functions. An assessment of the immunological effects of moxibustion in the success or failure rate of cancer treatments was conducted suggesting it was important in reducing symptoms (Huaisheng 1995).

None of the theories of moxibustion therapy are fully established. A systematic review of the effectiveness of moxibustion for supportive cancer care showed that it was only effective for reducing nausea and vomiting (Lee et al. 2010). The review was not limited to the English language literature. However, all studies have a high risk of bias, so effectively there is not enough evidence to draw any conclusion. Further, the role of moxibustion, in our experience, is controversial in most Western medical clinics, although used in traditional Asian clinics. However, experience from Asia suggests that it may have an important role to play with acupuncture, especially in reducing fatigue and pain, as well as improving immunity. Some clinics are restricted by fire regulations and the controversial mistaken identity with marijuana. In addition, the smoke can result in respiratory adverse effects for some patients. Smokeless moxa sticks or a heat lamp can be used as alternative methods for applying heat. When heat sources are used, extreme caution should prevent local skin burns. In some traditions, scarification and scarring with a moxa burn is used as part of the therapy. This is not recommended by these authors.

12.2 Adverse Effects of Acupuncture

Acupuncture is a very safe treatment with a low side effect profile when administered by a trained practitioner who is aware of contraindications and high-risk situations (White et al. 2001). In a study of 98,000 patients, only six reported major adverse events related to the acupuncture (Melchart et al. 2004). These included pneumothorax, vasovagal reaction, hypertensive crisis, an acute asthma attack, and exacerbation of depression. A follow up study of 6,400 patients reported 10%

adverse effects of which only 0.3% were serious (MacPherson et al. 2004). This did not prevent most patients seeking further acupuncture. A prospective study of 34,000 treatments by traditional acupuncturists (nearly 600 practitioners) reported no major life-threatening events, a 15% rate of minor events, and only a 0.3% rate of major events (MacPherson 2001). A prospective study from the Czech Republic surveyed 140,000 acupuncture treatments and found that 7% of patients felt faint and 0.28% actually fainted (Umlauf 1988). The incidence of pneumothorax was rare at only 1/70,000 treatments. In a large prospective study of 74,000 patients, there were approximately 7.5% adverse effects of which only 2% required treatment and this was mainly self administered by the patients themselves (Witt et al. 2011). Assuming there is evidence that the acupuncture treatment is effective for reducing symptoms, the adverse effect rate is less than many drugs that are indicated for supportive care. The relative therapeutic gain should be considered when prescribing treatment options. A systematic review on the safety of acupuncture showed a range of common adverse effects (Ernst and White 2001). In the nine studies reviewed, the most common adverse events found were needle pain (1–45%), tiredness (2–41%), and local bleeding (0.03–38%). The incidence of faintness and syncope ranged from 0 to 3.0%. Feelings of relaxation were reported by 86% of the patients. Pneumothorax was rare, occurring only twice in nearly a quarter of a million treatments.

Proper training in acupuncture and professional standards are essential for safety. An Australian study found that less than 1 year's training resulted in 2.07 adverse events per year; 37–48 months' training reduced this to 1.35 adverse events per year; and 49–60 months' training reduced this further to 0.92 adverse events per year (Bensoussan and Myers 1996).

Adverse effects shall be divided into major or life-threatening, and minor or non-life-threatening. Major adverse effects are relatively rare and include pneumothorax, organ or brain perforation, severe bleeding, systemic infection, and arrhythmia. With adequate training and appropriate precautions, these can mainly be avoided. Minor effects include mild bruising, local pain, syncope, drowsiness, headache, and an atopic reaction. These can be minimized but are not always avoidable. However, with adequate explanation and informed consent, these minor adverse effects do not pose a problem when acupuncture is being used for an appropriate clinical indication.

12.2.1 Major Adverse Effects of Acupuncture

Major adverse effects are potentially life-threatening but quite rare. They are reduced by excellence in training and maintaining professional standards. The practitioner should recognize the worst case scenario when inserting needles or studs into specific acupuncture points. High risk situations and points that are more likely to result in complications should be avoided or the risks minimized by appropriate extra care. The patient should be warned of potential complications and asked to report relevant symptoms. Urgent referral to an emergency specialist for diagnosis and treatment must be made if a serious complication is suspected.

Major adverse effects of acupuncture (in order of frequency of reports, see Appendix for references):

- Pneumothorax
- Hepatitis, human immunodeficiency virus (HIV), and other blood-borne infections
- Retained needle, migrating needle and/or organ perforation
- Brain or spinal cord perforation (pith)
- Bacterial endocarditis
- Perichondritis
- Pericardial effusion or tamponade
- Septicemia
- Major hemorrhage
- Pseudoaneurysm/thromboplebitis
- Compartment syndrome
- Skin infection
- Abscess

Pneumothorax is the most common serious complication that is reported in the literature. Some cases occurred because a blanket was pulled over the patient and pushed the needle further in. Other cases occurred because of the patient falling with a needle in place after developing syncope. Rarely is the pneumothorax a result of direct deep penetration by a well-trained and experienced practitioner. Caution must be practiced for certain points, such as Jianjing (GB21), and horizontal shallow insertion should be used in this situation. In addition, patients with hyperinflated lungs (such as asthma and emphysema) or with thin chest walls (such as cancer cachexia) are at additional risk. Obviously, subjects should not be released with permanent insertions at these high-risk points and should not be doing self-acupuncture. A good practice would be to observe patients for 30 min after treatment, but this does not exclude the later development of a pneumothorax. An early pneumothorax can only be diagnosed with a chest X-ray. A puncture of the pleura can rapidly progress to a tension pneumothorax in which air becomes trapped in the pleural space and the rapidly escalating pressure prevents further inspiration and causes collapse of the cardiac output. At that point, urgent intervention with a chest drainage tube is required. Early suspicious signs can include a dry cough, dyspnoea and chest pain. These signs should indicate a medical emergency.

Perforation of an artery can result in a major hemorrhage. Dilated (varicose) veins can also bleed profusely. The situation is made worse by anticoagulants, inherited coagulation disorders, and platelet aggregating inhibitors (including aspirin). The patient should always have a full drug history taken as well as an inquiry into genetic disorders such as hemophilia. Cardiac tamponade is recorded in the literature. Ectopic sternal foramina may sometimes increase the subject's susceptibility to cardiac perforation. Bleeding into a cavity is usually accompanied by severe pain (pleural, pericardial, or peritoneal irritation) and an obtund patient. Bleeding into a muscle may present simply as an enlarging lump. Again, a high index of suspicion is required, with immediate referral as an emergency if this complication is suspected.

Organ perforation has also been reported with retained or broken needles. A needle count should always be carried out at insertion and removal. If the patient is sent home with semi-permanent studs, careful education of the subject is important, emphasizing that regular self-monitoring is essential. Avoidance of infection by good hygiene is imperative. High risk points must be avoided in these subjects.

The risk of infection is reduced by good hygiene, skin cleaning and the use of sterile needles. Greater caution must be exercised with immune-suppressed subjects. The needle should not be inserted through infected skin since the resultant bacteremia can lead to septicemia (infection of the blood), distant abscesses, and bacterial endocarditis. Staphylococcus poses a major risk of distant abscesses spread *via* the blood. Septicemia can result in shock, renal failure, and death. Needled contaminated skin can introduce "flesh eating disease" or necrotizing fasciitis, a particularly virulent form of group A streptococcal infection of the soft tissues.

The spread of infection through needle contamination with blood and other body fluids should be impossible when using sterile disposable needles. In fact it is law in some jurisdictions that the needles cannot be reused. All acupuncture needles must be sterilized, single use needles. That means that the needles are only used once and then disposed of. This prevents any spread of infections and ensures that every needle is clean and safe to use. It is important that the manufacturing standards and sterilization of these disposable needles are regulated by the importing jurisdiction. Of course, this does not prevent cross-infection from an accidental needle stick injury to the practitioner. It is important that precautions are taken to prevent this by care in needle insertion and removal, protecting the needle with a sheath, and using a sharps box for disposing of used needles. If a needle stick injury does occur, this should be documented, and both patient and practitioner should present for testing for hepatitis and HIV status, and possible prophylaxis. Practitioners should seriously consider hepatitis B vaccination prior to practicing acupuncture.

A needle placed near the craniocervical junction can result in perforation of the medulla oblongata. Pain can be local, in the head, or radiating into the trunk or limbs. A case is well described by Fukaya et al. (2011). The latter case was caused by a broken needle that migrated into the brainstem. The neck must be urgently immobilized to prevent further migration, and neurosurgical extraction carried out. Bleeding into the brainstem can result in sudden death.

Acupuncture in children will require special precautions, especially since the depth of insertion will be less than adults. The safe depth to which the 12 abdominal CV meridian acupoints can be needled was found to increase with age, body weight and waist girth in pediatric patients aged 7–15 years. Practitioners who perform acupuncture in pediatric patients should be aware of the large variations in the safe depth of acupoints to prevent possible complications (Chen et al. 2008).

Retained needles can result in organ perforation and fistulae. Ulloth and Jaines (2007) report a CSF fistula and spine-related headache that resulted after embedded acupuncture needles migrated into the lumbar spinal canal (Fig. 12.1). The patient had undergone a series of low-back acupuncture treatments, the most recent of which had been approximately 14 months prior to the onset of his headache. During his final acupuncture session, several acupuncture needles had been inadvertently driven into

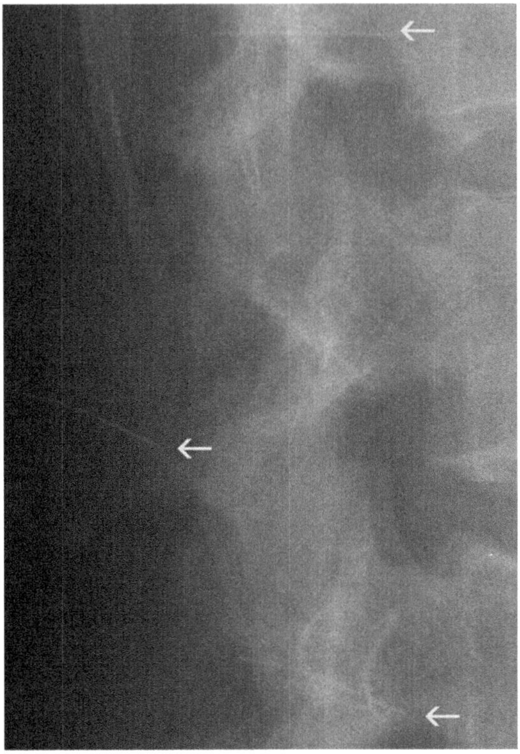

Fig. 12.1 Lateral radiograph of the lumbar spine demonstrating three thin metallic objects (*arrows*) posterior to three lumbar vertebrae

the soft tissues of his lower back. The acupuncturist assured the patient that the retained needles were harmless. The patient underwent surgical removal of the retained needles located at L1, L2, and L3. The L3 needle was noted to have penetrated the lamina and was projecting into the spinal canal. A broken needle can damage tissue, perforate organs, and migrate into body cavities. It is important to check that each withdrawn needle is intact and that a fragment is not left behind. A broken needle may arise from poor quality manufacture, erosion between the shaft and the handle, strong muscle spasm or sudden movement of the patient, incorrect withdrawal of a stuck or bent needle, or the prolonged use of galvanic current. If, during insertion, a needle becomes bent, it should be withdrawn and replaced by another needle. Too much force should not be used when manipulating needles, especially during lifting and thrusting. The junction between the handle and the shaft is the part that is apt to break. Therefore, in inserting the needle, one quarter to one-third of the shaft should always be kept above the skin. If a needle breaks, the patient should be told to keep calm and not to move, so as to prevent the broken part of the needle from going deeper into the tissues. If a part of the broken needle is still above the skin, remove it with forceps. If it is at the same level as the skin, press around the site gently until the broken end is exposed, and then remove it with forceps. If it is completely under the skin, it is probably best to take the patient to an emergency department for surgical intervention. The limb or body part should be immobilized to prevent further migration until emergency surgical treatment can be carried out. It is important not to make the damage worse.

12.2.2 Minor Adverse Effects of Acupuncture

Minor adverse effects are not life-threatening and are more common. Local pain is quite usual and is often described as Deqi in the TCM literature, and is thought to be a prerequisite of effectiveness. This should be differentiated from severe persistent pain, which could suggest a complication. Petechiae and local bruising are common, but can be minimized through avoiding the puncture of veins. A study in pediatric cancer patients revealed minimal complications in the setting of an academic cancer centre with highly trained and experienced acupuncturists (Ladas et al. 2010). This was a retrospective case series that provided descriptive data on the safety of acupuncture using Japanese J-type Seirin needles, with mild manual stimulation administered at 0.5-cun depth in patients with cancer with and without thrombocytopenia. Of 237 acupuncture sessions, 20%, 8% and 19% of the sessions were administered to patients with severe, moderate, and mild thrombocytopenia, respectively. No bleeding side effects were observed. The study suggests that acupuncture is safe even in the setting of platelet counts below 50,000/μL. Seirin needles are particularly sharp and may reduce tissue tearing.

Minor adverse effects of acupuncture (in order of frequency of reports, see Appendix for references):

- Dermatitis
- Pain (at site of insertion or beyond)
- Bruising
- Syncope
- Fatigue and/or drowsiness
- Cutaneous herpes
- Argyria pigmentation
- Worsening symptoms
- Headache
- Stiffness
- Agitation

After insertion, the practitioner may find it difficult to withdraw the needle. This is due to muscle spasm, rotation of the needle with too wide an amplitude, or rotation in only one direction causing the muscle fibers to tangle around and grip the shaft. The patient should be asked to relax. If the cause is excessive rotation in one direction, the condition will be relieved when the needle is rotated in the opposite direction. If the stuck needle is due to muscle spasm, it should be left in place for a while, and then withdrawn by rotating, or massaging around the point, or another needle inserted nearby which often relieves the grip on the needle. If the stuck needle is caused by the patient having changed position, the original posture should be resumed and the needle withdrawn.

Syncope is common, especially after the first treatment. Syncope during acupuncture treatment is a form of vasovagal syncope (also called neurally-mediated or neurocardiogenic syncope), which causes a sudden decrease in or brief cessation of cerebral flow caused by hypotension from inhibition of the sympathetic nervous system and activation of the parasympathetic nervous system (Chen et al. 1990; Abbound 1993). Acupuncture is known to modulate the sympathetic to parasympathetic activities and this is demonstrated by the technique of heart rate variability measurement (Alraek and Tan 2011). The patients often complain of not feeling well and/or fear of blackouts. This is followed by pallor, weakness, lightheadedness, yawning, nausea, diaphoresis, hyperventilation, and subsequently blurred vision. Despite recovering spontaneously in most cases, some patients may lose consciousness, especially if they are not managed immediately (Chen et al. 1990, Norheim and Fønnebø 1996). Convulsive syncope, characterized by irregular clonic-tonic movement, has been reported (Cole et al. 2002). The episode occurred immediately after the insertion of acupuncture needles into the bilateral ST36 acupuncture points. Causes could include oxygen depletion of the brain and/or afferent neurogenic-induced seizure. Transient hypoglycemia is another possibility. Needle phobia and anxiety have been documented as causes of actual syncope, as well as convulsive syncope. In one study, several subjects who experienced convulsive syncope while donating blood had previous histories of convulsive syncope during phlebotomy (Lin 1982). The possibility of needle anxiety in first time acupuncture patients should be anticipated and discussed with each subject. By orienting new patients to the acupuncture process and, in particular, by acquainting them with the needles themselves and the sensations they may produce, anxiety can be reduced or eliminated, thus lessening the risk of convulsive syncope during acupuncture. Convulsive syncope can result in secondary complications, such as a broken needle, organ perforation, pneumothorax, or moxa burns. If a patient becomes syncopal, ensure he is lying flat with his head below the level of his legs. Unless the patient has chronic bronchitis (risking suppression of ventilation from high dose oxygen), 40% oxygen inhalation may be given (ensuring there is no burning moxa around). Although syncope is most common and usually reversible without harm, chest pain and/or shortness of breath could suggest a myocardial infarction, pneumothorax or cardiac tamponade. Persistent unconsciousness or convulsions could suggest hypoglycemia or a cerebrovascular event. The practitioner should carefully attend to the patient's past medical history (including cardiopulmonary disease, type 1 diabetes mellitus and primary seizures), as well as noting the needle insertion points. Measurement of blood pressure (lying flat) and the checking of pulse rate and heart rhythm and determining whether the patient is cyanosed should be done and recorded. This should help to discriminate a straight forward syncope (from which the patient will recover in the recumbent position) from other more serious disorders requiring urgent medical attention. A vasovagal syncope is usually manifest by a slow regular pulse, pale skin color, and hypotension that recover when the subject lies flat. If warning symptoms appear, remove the needles immediately and make the patient lie flat with his head down and his legs raised, since the symptoms are probably due to a transient, insufficient blood supply to the brain. Offer warm sweet drinks. The symptoms usually disappear after a short rest. In severe cases, first aid should be given and, when the patient is medically stable, the most appropriate of the following treatments may be applied: Press or acupuncture Shuigou (GV26), Zhongchong (PC9), Suliao (GV25), Neiguan (PC6) and ST36. If the symptoms persist, emergency medical assistance will be necessary.

Drowsiness may also occur. The sleepiness can be due to release of serotonin and endorphins in the brain and systemically (Yoshimoto et al. 2006, Han 2004). Patients should be warned about driving and operating machinery for a few hours if they should develop these symptoms. Relaxation of muscles can increase the risk of musculoskeletal or neurological injury at an injured site if patients are not warned to be cautious. Observation during and after the first session and charting the patient's symptoms will help to reduce mishaps in future sessions.

12.3 Adverse Effects of Moxibustion

Adverse effects of moxibustion are summarized below (in order of frequency of reports, see Appendix for references):

- Burns
- Scarring
- Allergic reactions
- Respiratory symptoms.

Moxibustion has several kinds of potential adverse events such as allergy, burns and infection. Currently, the incidence of such events is not really known, which may be because it is widely used in Asia (where adverse events reporting has been rare until recently), but to the best of our knowledge, is not used so much in N. America and Europe in medical clinics. A Japanese audit of 65,000 treatments of both acupuncture and moxibustion revealed seven burn injuries of which one deep burn took 2 years to recover. Five cases were indirect burns from a moxa stick, one was from an infra red lamp, and the other from a hot pack (Yamashita et al. 1999). A systematic review revealed the most common effects were allergic reactions, burns, and infections such as cellulitis and hepatitis C (Park et al. 2010). Allergic reactions were reported in six case reports (four case reports related to infections and two related to burns). The other articles from this systematic review included case reports of xerophthalmia, xeroderma, hyperpigmented macules, ptosis and eversion of the eyelids. In clinical trials, various adverse events such as rubefaction, blistering, itching sensations, discomfort due to smoke, general fatigue, stomach upsets, flare-ups, headaches, and burns have been reported. The odor may be deemed unpleasant and cause nausea and dry throat and breathing problems. Other adverse effects have included abdominal pain, premature birth, premature rupture of the membrane and bleeding due to excess pressure from moxa trays on an anterior placenta in pregnant women.

In Chinese medicine, the main contraindication for moxibustion is the presence of a heat syndrome. Theoretically, it could cause the disease to worsen.

Moxa is considered inappropriate for a deficiency heat syndrome (one based on yin deficiency) and it must be used cautiously in cases where there is local dryness. Other contraindications for moxibustion involve the sensitive areas of the body, such as the face (due to potential risks of scarring from burns, and also because the smoke can irritate the eyes or nose), the nipples, and the genitals. Ancient texts specify certain points on the head as being contraindicated for moxibustion, such as Shangxing (GV23), Chengqi (ST1), Sibai (ST2), Touwei (ST8), Jingming (BL1), Cuanzhu (BL2), Sizhukong (TB23), Heliao (LI19) and Yingxiang (LI20). Concerns have also been raised for using moxa during pregnancy in the region of the abdomen and lower back (O'Connor and Bensky 1981).

12.4 Precautions and Guidelines

Risks, precautions and guidelines to prevent complications are summarized below:

12.4.1 Risk Factors for Complications

1. Inadequate training
2. Bleeding
    a. Hemophilia and other coagulation disorders
    b. Extreme thrombocytopenia ($<20{,}000/\mu L$)
    c. Advanced liver disease reduces clotting factors
    d. Anticoagulants and anti-platelet drugs
3. Infection
    a. Immunocompromised patients
        i. High dose steroids
        ii. Transplant immunosuppression
        iii. HIV
        iv. Chronic lymphocytic leukemia
    b. Diabetics
    c. Open wounds
    d. Cardiac valve abnormalities
4. Fainting
    a. Hypoglycemia
    b. Anxiety
    c. Vasovagal sensitivity

12.4.2 *Precautions*

1. Avoid directly needling the tumor.
2. Avoid deep perpendicular penetration of points on thoracic and lumbar regions due to risk of perforating internal organs.
3. Avoid deep penetration of points at base of skull inferior to the occiput, in order to reduce risking perforation of the brainstem (points at risk: Fengchi (GB20); Fengfu (GV16); Tainzhu (BL10)).
4. Avoid deep penetration of Naohu (GV17), to reduce risk of cardiac tamponade.
5. Use extreme caution with GB21, since this risks pneumothorax.
6. Avoid deep and perpendicular penetration over a full stomach or bladder.
7. Points close to the orbit require experience and skill in angling the needle and delivering the correct depth of penetration (ST1, Tongziliao (GB1), BL1). Do not manipulate needle.
8. Avoid points on scalp in infants with open fontanelles.
9. Avoid points in pregnant women that can induce labor (Hegu (LI4), Sanyinjiao (SP6), Kunlun (BL60), Zhiyin (BL67)).

12.4.3 *Guidelines: Acupuncture for Cancer Patients (with Permission and Acknowledgments, Filshie and Hester 2006)*

12.4.3.1 Roles and Responsibilities

It is the responsibility of the doctor/practitioner in charge of the service to ensure that:

a. Doctors receive appropriate training to practice acupuncture safely and competently.
b. Allied health professionals are appropriately trained to practice acupuncture safely and competently.
c. Doctors and nurses and other allied health professionals are aware of the hospital or clinic's policies and guidelines for the safe practice and treatment of patients receiving acupuncture.

12.4.3.2 Criteria for Acupuncture Practice

a. Training and competence.
b. Regulated health professionals who practice acupuncture will commence treatment only after an orthodox medical diagnosis which comprises history, examination and any further investigations as necessary.
c. They must be aware of the diagnosis and stage of cancer in a given patient.

d. All acupuncturists should be a member of a regulated health care professional body and comply with their standards and codes of conduct. Regulation will vary according to the practitioner's primary specialty. For example, a practitioner would be registered under a legislated college or council for general medicine. Regulation may also be mandatory for primary acupuncturists. For example, some states in the USA require registration by a body that is recognized by the Federation of Acupuncture and Oriental Medicine Regulatory Agencies. Similar regulations apply to some provinces within Canada. The practitioners should receive training from an accredited school to a level specified by the regulatory body. In the USA, they should have attended an ACCAOM accredited school and passed the National Certification Commission for Acupuncture and Oriental Medicine (NCCAOM) examination. Practitioners should also be trained by appropriate institutions, such as schools recognized by the American Association of Medical Acupuncture, the British Medical Acupuncture Society, or the Acupuncture Foundation of Canada.

12.4.3.3 Patients Who Should Be Considered for Acupuncture

a. Patients who fail to respond to conventional analgesic approaches and remain in pain.
b. Patients who experience unacceptable side effects with conventional medication such as excessive sedation.
c. Patients who wish to reduce existing medication.
d. Patients who have pain that is likely to respond to acupuncture.
e. Patients who do not wish to have conventional analgesia or other medications for symptom control.

12.4.3.4 Contraindications and Cautions

a. Contraindicated
    i. Needle phobia
    ii. Severe clotting dysfunction or platelets less than 20,000/μL
    iii. Semi-permanent needles (studs) in patients with vascular heart disease (risk of sub-acute bacterial endocarditis) or neutropenic patients or post-splenectomy (risk of infection)
    iv. Electroacupuncture in patients with an intracardiac defibrillator
    v. No needling a tumor nodule or area of ulceration
    vi. Avoid lymphoedematous limbs
    vii. Mainly avoid a limb that has received a groin or axillary node dissection (increased risk of infection and further obliteration of lymphatic vessels)
    viii. Regions of spinal instability (potential for cord or root compression due to acupuncture's muscle-relaxing properties)

ix. Into a breast prosthesis (leading to leakage)
x. Over intracranial skull or vertebral deficits, following neuro-surgery (could inadvertently penetrate spinal cord or brain)

b. Cautions

i. Patient may be very sensitive to acupuncture, especially the vaso-vagal response and drowsiness. Patient should be observed after initial treatments and warned not to drive. Syncope after initial treatments is quite common.
ii. Extreme care not to needle too deeply over the chest wall, especially in cachectic patients (to avoid pneumothorax).
iii. Patients prone to keloid
iv. Pregnancy
v. Epilepsy
vi. Confused patients
vii. Electroacupuncture if pacemaker present

12.4.3.5 Acupuncture Treatment

a. Pre-treatment

i. Critically decide whether the patient is suitable for acupuncture.
ii. Discuss the use of acupuncture, its relative effectiveness, and potential risk of adverse effects, including post-treatment drowsiness, the possibility of exacerbation of symptoms and minor bruising or pain at needle sites.
iii. Obtain the patient's verbal (or written) consent.

b. Acupuncture equipment and handling

i. Use single use disposable needles and clean skin at site of insertion.
ii. After insertion, the introducers will be counted twice and the number recorded, and/or the needles are counted.
iii. When the needles are removed, they will be counted twice and formally checked against the earlier record that the same number are removed as inserted.
iv. Used needles will be disposed of directly into a sharps box.

c. First treatment

i. Patients should be treated lying down in case of vaso-vagal reactions; initial treatment should be gentle.
ii. The patient should be observed during first treatment.
iii. The patient should be followed up at least once per week to gauge response and adverse effects. Usually six treatments is considered an adequate clinical trial.

12.4.3.6 Audit

a. Adverse effects should be carefully documented along with treatment response.
b. Unexpected adverse effects should be reviewed by clinical teams and efforts made to reduce these as far as possible.

They are further discussed by Cummings and Reid (2004). Electrical stimulation is potentially harmful. It is contraindicated: in pregnancy; if the patient has a pacemaker; if there is lack of skin sensation; and in cases of impaired circulation, severe arterial disease, undiagnosed fever or severe skin lesions. Careful monitoring of the electrical stimulation is recommended to prevent neural injury. Galvanic current should be used for only a very short period of time.

12.4.4 Guidelines for Moxibustion in Cancer Patients

Acupoints to be avoided or those requiring special skill are listed below:

1. Explain the slight risks of burns and obtain informed consent.
2. Do not leave the patient alone with burning moxa.
3. Contraindications for moxibustion involve the sensitive areas of the body, such as the face (due to potential risks of scarring from burns, and also because the smoke can irritate the the eyes or nose), the nipples, and the genitals. Ancient texts specify certain points on the head as being contraindicated for moxibustion, such as GV23, ST1, ST2, ST8, BL1, BL2, TB23, LI19, and LI20.
4. To avoid the smoke of regular moxibustion, use other methods of heating that allow constant heat output and control over the heat. These can include smokeless moxa or an infra red heat lamp. In many situations, acupuncture can replace moxa.
5. When using herb-slice or cake interposed moxibustion, punch holes in the material to allow the heat to penetrate. The thickness of the slice should be just 0.2–0.3 cm; thicker slices may prevent adequate heating. For practical purposes, ginger slices may be most convenient.
6. For an effective moxibustion, it should cause significant local heating and an inflammatory response, and should be done for a prolonged period, such as 10–20 min. Specific points for moxa heating should be selected from TCM theory to stimulate the immune system or to alter internal organ functions. Warming a broader region is an acceptable treatment for relaxing tension and moderating pain at the site. Chinese medicine practitioners typically administer moxa daily for several treatments or more. They may be alternated with acupuncture.
7. The most frequently mentioned applications of moxa are for cancer, gastrointestinal disorders, asthma, breech pregnancy, organ prolapse, bi-syndromes, and herpes zoster. In particular, herpes zoster is emphasized as a case where moxibustion is effective.
8. The risks of exposure to moxa smoke are probably similar to that for any other smoke, and total exposure time, particularly when it involves prolonged exposure,

is the key concern. Venting or filtering the room is important when moxa is done regularly. There is no evidence that moxa smoke contains any unusually harmful substances, but the long-term outcome data are incomplete. Standard commercial moxa materials do not contain arsenic, but this toxic substance is found in some preparations from China and should be avoided.

9. Specific acupoints are relatively convenient to treat with moxa, and are well accepted by most patients. Most of the points are on the conception and governing vessels, plus ST36 and Yongquan (KI1), and the Shu points on the back.

Although female patients are unlikely to be pregnant during anti-cancer treatment, they may well become pregnant during follow up. In those cases, certain acupuncture points can result in uterine contractions and should be avoided.

12.4.5 Acupoints to Be Avoided or Only Used by Experienced Specialists for Both Acupuncture and Moxibustion

Contraindicated acupuncture points are summarized below:

1. Risk of neurological damage:

   - Yamen (GV15), GV16, may puncture medulla oblongata

2. Risk of organ damage:

   - BL1, ST1, located close to the eyeball
   - Tiantu (CV22), in front of the trachea
   - Renying (ST9), near the carotid artery
   - Jimen (SP11), Chongmen (SP12), near the femoral artery
   - Taiyuan (LU9), on the radial artery
   - GB21, apply caution in thin patients, to prevent pneumothorax
     - Avoid if pregnant
   - First trimester: points on lower abdomen and lumbosacral region
   - Second trimester onwards: upper abdomen and lumbosacral
   - Throughout pregnancy: strong sensation points, ear acupuncture labor points, SP6, LI4

Further guidelines on acupuncture and moxibustion safety have been issued by the World Health Organization (WHO 1999).

12.5 Conclusion

The rate of complications is very low and most complications are transient, lasting 2 weeks at most. Adverse effects occur in 10–15% of patients and are usually quite minor and do not deter patients from further treatment. Major adverse effects, that can be life-threatening, occur in less than 0.3% of treatments. Practitioners must be well aware of potentially fatal progression when patients report shortness of breath, pleuritic chest pain, severe bruising, an enlarging tissue mass, abdominal and chest pain, persistent syncope, or a fever after receiving acupuncture treatment. A third degree burn from moxibustion can result in severe infection and non-healing. All of these situations require urgent referral to an appropriate specialist.

The conclusion that acupuncture is a very safe intervention in the hands of a competent practitioner is justified on the evidence available (Leung and Zhang 2008). In considering the dangers of orthodox treatments, the proven efficacy of the optional treatments must be considered. Clinical trials in Chinese medicine have improved and there is some encouraging evidence that acupuncture is effective for many chronic conditions and in the supportive care of cancer patients (Sagar 2008; Wong and Sagar 2010). The considerable risks of hospital treatment are becoming more apparent, along with the rates of adverse drug reactions or prescribing errors. Whereas the risks of acupuncture cannot be discounted, it seems that in skilled hands it is one of the safer forms of medical intervention. The balance of risk and benefit is the key for patients and for those regulating or funding health care. Importantly, the surveys and reports of adverse events for acupuncture and moxibustion represent an effort by acupuncture practitioners to address the issue of patient safety. As with all medical interventions, it is important to continuously evaluate efficacy, risks, likely mechanisms, acceptability, and cost effectiveness (Vincent 2001).

Acknowledgments Joel E. Ulloth and Stephen J. Haines, Department of Neurosurgery, University of Minnesota, Minneapolis, Minnesota, USA (Ulloth and Haines 2007).

Appendix

Table 12.1 References for major adverse effects of acupuncture

Adverse effect	Reports
Major hemorrhage	Sakaguchi and Nishimura 1990; Keane et al. 1993; Choo and Yu 2000
Septicemia	Pierik 1982; Carron et al. 1974; Doutscu et al. 1986; Izatt and Fairman 1977
Skin infection	MacPherson et al. 2004
Abscess	Garcia and Venkataramani 1994
Bacterial endocarditis	Cheng 1983; Cheng et al. 1985; Jeffreys et al. 1983; Lee and McIlwain 1985; Scheel et al. 1992
Retained needle, migrating needle and/or organ perforation	Benscholen 1986; Southworth and Hartwig 1990; Chiu and Austin 1995; Keller et al. 1972; Yuzawa et al. 1991; Abumi et al. 1996; Hama and Kaji 2004; Miyamoto et al. 2010; MacPherson et al. 2004
Brain or spinal cord perforation (pith)	Isu et al. 1985; Kida et al. 1988; Kishikawa et al. 1990; Abumi et al. 1996; Gi et al. 1994; Kondo et al. 1979; Sasaki et al. 1984; Shiraishi et al. 1979; Fukaya et al. 2011
Pneumothorax	Gray et al. 1991; Stack 1975; Wright et al. 1991; Hasegawa et al. 1991; Bodner et al. 1983; Corbett and Sinclair 1974; Goldberg 1973; Lewis-Driver 1973; Ritter and Tarala 1978; Valenta and Hengesh 1980; Waldman 1974; Gee 1984; Kuiper 1974; Mazal et al. 1980; Vilke and Wulfert 1997; Carette et al. 1984; Olusanya and Mansuri 1997; Carron et al. 1974; Guerin et al. 1987; Henneghien et al. 1984; Huet et al. 1990; Kropp and Hasler 1983; Morrone et al. 1990; Schneider and Salzberg 1984; Takishma 1983
Hepatitis, human immunodeficiency virus and other blood-borne infections	Alexander et al. 1974; Conn 1988; Kent et al. 1988; Kiyosawa et al. 1987; Phoon et al. 1988; Slater et al. 1988; Stryker et al. 1986; Vittecoq et al. 1989; Castro et al. 1988; Boxall 1978; Hussain 1974; Shimoyama et al. 1993
Perichondritis	Allison and Kravitz 1975; Davis and Powell 1985; Warwick-Brown and Richards 1986
Pericardial effusion or tamponade	Cheng 1991; Halverson et al. 1995; Hasegawa et al. 1991; Kataoka 1997; Nieda et al. 1973
Compartment syndrome	Smith and Walzczyk 1986
Psueudoaneurysm/thromboplebitis	Fujiwara et al. 1994; Lord and Schwarz 1996; Blanchard 1991

Table 12.2 References for minor adverse effects of acupuncture

Adverse effect	Reports
Petechiae/bruising	MacPherson et al. 2004
Dermatitis	Castelain et al. 1987; Dung 1987; Koizumi et al. 1988; Newman 1990; Buchta 1972
Cutaneous herpes	Chang 1974
Pain (at site of insertion or beyond)	Lapeer 1988; MacPherson et al. 2004
Argyria pigmentation	Tanita et al. 1985
Syncope	Zhenlong 1992; MacPherson et al. 2004
Fatigue and/or drowsiness	MacPherson et al. 2004
Worsening symptoms	MacPherson et al. 2004
Headache	MacPherson et al. 2004
Stiffness	MacPherson et al. 2004
Agitation	MacPherson et al. 2004

Table 12.3 References for adverse effects of moxibustion

Adverse effect	Reports
Scarring	Hung and Mines 1991; Park et al. 2010
Burns	MacPherson et al. 2004; Park et al. 2010; Yamashita et al. 1999
Allergic reactions	Park et al. 2010
Respiratory	Park et al. 2010

References

Abboud, F. M. (1993). Neurocardiogenic syncope. *The New England Journal of Medicine, 328,* 1117–1120.

Abumi, K., Anbo, H., Kaneda, K. (1996). Migration of an acupuncture needle into the medulla oblongata. *European Spine Journal, 5,* 137–139.

Alexander, P., Fairley, G. H., Smithers, D. W. (1974). Repeated acupunctures and serum hepatitis (letter). *British Medical Journal, 3,* 466.

Allison, G., Kravitz, E. (1975). Auricular chondritis secondary to acupuncture (letter). *The New England Journal of Medicine, 293,* 780.

Alraek, T., & Tan, C. O. (2011). Acupuncture and heart rate variability. *Acupuncture in Medicine, 29,* 7–8.

Benscholen, M. (1986). On the retention of acupuncture needles. *American Journal of Acupuncture, 14,* 163–164.

Bensoussan, A., Myers, S. P. (1996). *Towards a safer choice. The practice of traditional Chinese medicine in Australia.* Sydney: Macarthur.

Blanchard, B. (1991). Deep vein thrombophlebitis after acupuncture. *Annals of Internal Medicine, 115,* 748.

Bodner, G., Topilsky, M., Greif, J. (1983). Pneumothorax as a complication of acupuncture in the treatment of bronchial asthma. *Annals of Allergy, Asthma and Immunology, 51,* 401–403.

Boxall, E. H. (1978). Acupuncture hepatitis in the West Midlands. *Journal of Medical Virology, 2,* 377–379.

Buchta, R. M. (1972). An unusual cause of petechiae. *American Journal of Diseases of Children, 123,* 613.

Carette, M., Mayaud, C., Houacine, S., Milleron, B., Toty, L., Akoun, G. (1984). Treatment of an asthmatic crisis by acupuncture: Probable role in the onset of pneumothorax with development to status asthmaticus. *Revue de Pneumologie Clinique, 40,* 69–70.
Carron, H., Epstein, B. S., Grand, B. (1974). Complications of Acupuncture. *JAMA, 228,* 1552–1554.
Castelain, M., Castelain, P. Y., Ricciardi, R. (1987). Contact dermatitis to acupuncture needles. *Contact Dermatitis, 1,* 44.
Castro, K. G., Lifson, A. R., White, Cr. (1988). Investigation of AIDS patients with no previous identified risk factors. *Journal of American Medical Association, 259,* 1338–1342.
Chang, T. (1974). Activation of cutaneous herpes by acupuncture (letter). *The New England Journal of Medicine, 291,* 1310.
Chen, F. P., Hwang, S. J., Lee, H. P., Yang, H. Y., Chung, C. (1990). Clinical study of syncope during acupuncture treatment. *Acupuncture and Electro-Therapeutics Research, 15,* 107–119.
Chen, H.-N., Lin, J.-G., Yang, A. D., Chang, S.-K. (2008). Safe depth of abdominal acupoints in pediatric patients. *Complementary Therapies in Medicine, 16,* 331–335.
Cheng, T. O. (1983). Acupuncture needles as a cause of bacterial endocarditis. *BMJ, 287,* 689.
Cheng, T., Lee, R. J., Mcllwain, J. C. (1985). Subacute bacterial endocarditis following ear acupuncture (letter). *International Journal of Cardiology, 8,* 97.
Cheng, T. O. (1991). Pericardial effusion from self-inserted needle in the heart. *European Heart Journal, 12,* 958.
Chiu, E. S., Austin, J. H. (1995). Images in clinical medicine: Acupuncture-needle fragments. *The New England Journal of Medicine, 332,* 304.
Choo, D. C., Yue, G. (2000). Acute intracranial hemorrhage caused by acupuncture. *Headache, 40,* 397–398.
Cole, M., Shen, J., Hommer, D. (2002). Convulsive syncope associated with acupuncture. *The American Journal of the Medical Sciences, 324,* 288–289.
Conn, H. (1988). Acupuncture in epidemic HBV hepatitis in China too? *Hepatology, 8,* 1176–1177.
Corbett, M., Sinclair, M. (1974). Acu- and pleuro-puncture. *The New England Journal of Medicine, 290,* 167–168.
Cummings, M., Reid, F. (2004). BMAS policy statements in some controversial areas of acupuncture practice. *Acupunture in Medicine, 22,* 134–136.
Davis, O., Powell, W. (1985). Auricular perichondritis secondary to acupuncture. *Archives of Otolaryngology, 111,* 770–771.
Dhond, R. P., Kettner, N., Napadow, V. (2007). Neuroimaging acupuncture effects in the human brain. *Journal of Alternative and Complementary Medicine, 13,* 603–616.
Doutscu, Y., Tao, Y., Sasayama, K. (1986). A case of staphylococcus aureus septicemia after acupuncture therapy. *Kansenshogaku Zasshi, 60,* 911–916.
Dung. H. C. (1987). An immediate atopic erythroid reaction induced by acupuncture needles on the skin of the posterior thoracic wall. *Alternative Medicine, 2,* 209–214.
Ernst, E., White, A. (1997). Life-threatening adverse reactions after acupuncture? A systematic review. *Pain, 71,* 123–126.
Ernst, E., White, A. R. (2001). Prospective studies of the safety of acupuncture: A systematic review. *The American Journal of Medicine, 110,* 481–485.
Filshie, J., Hester, J. (2006). Guidelines for providing acupuncture treatment for cancer patients: A peer reviewed sample policy document. *Acupuncture in Medicine, 24,* 172–182.
Fukaya, S., Kimura Sora, S., Morita, A. (2011). Medulla oblongata injury caused by an acupuncture needle; warning for serious complications due to a common method of alternative medicine. *Journal of Neurology, 258,* 2093–2094.
Fujiwara, H., Taniguchi, K., Ikezono, E. (1980). The influence of low frequency acupuncture on a demand pacemaker. *Chest, 78,* 96–97.
Garcia, A. A., Venkataramani, A. (1994). Bilateral psoas abscesses following acupuncture. *The Western Journal of Medicine, 161,* 90.
Gee, D. (1984). Fatal pneumothorax due to acupuncture. *BMJ, 288,* 114.

Gi, H., Takahashi, J., Kanamoto, H., Matsubayashi, K., Mikuni, N., Okamoto, S. (1994). Spinal cord stab injury by acupuncture needle: a case report (in Japanese). *No Shinkei Geka, 22,* 151–154.
Gray, R., Maharajh, G. S., Hyland, R. (1991). Pneumothorax resulting from acupuncture. *Candian Association of Radiologists Journal, 42,* 139–140.
Goldberg, I. (1973). Pneumothorax associated with acupuncture. *The Medical Journal of Australia, 2,* 942–946.
Guerin, J. M., Tibourtine, O., Lhote, F., Segrestaa, J. M. (1987). Two cases of pneumothorax following acupuncture. *La Revue de Medecine Interne, 8,* 71.
Halvorsen, T. B., Anda, S. S., Naess, A. B., Levang, O. W. (1995). Fatal cardiac tamponade after acupuncture through congenital sternal foramen. *Lancet, 345,* 1175.
Hama, Y., Kaji, T. (2004). A migrated acupuncture needle in themedulla oblongata. *Archives of Neurology, 61,* 1608.
Han, J. S. (2003). Acupuncture: Neuropeptide release produced by electrical stimulation of different frequencies. *Trends in Neuroscience, 26,* 17–22.
Han, J. S. (2004). Acupuncture and endorphins. *Neuroscience Letters, 361,* 258–261.
Hau, D. M. (1989). Effects of moxibustion on cellular immunocompetence of γ-irradiated mice. *American Journal of Chinese Medicine, 17,* 157–163.
Hasegawa, J., Nogushi, N., Yamasaki, J. (1991). Delayed cardiac tamponade and hemithorax induced by an acupuncture needle. *Cardiology, 78,* 58–63.
Henneghien, C., Bruart, J., Remacle, P. (1984). A new iatrogenic pathology: Pneumothorax after acupuncture. *Revue de Pneumologie Clinique, 40,* 197–199.
Huaisheng, S. (1995). Ginger-partitioned moxibustion on Sifeng point (extra-29) in treating children's asthenia and its effects on cellular immune functions. *ChiAcu Moxibust, 6,* 9–10.
Huet, R., Renard, E., Blotman, M. J., Jaffiol, C. (1990). Unrecognised pmeumothorax after acupuncture in a female patient with anorexia nervosa. *Presse Médicale, 19,* 1415.
Hung, V. C., Mines, J. S. (1991). Eschars and scarring from hot needle acupuncture. *Journal of the American Academy of Dermatology, 24,* 148–149.
Hussain, K. K. (1974). Serum hepatitis associated with repeated acupuncture. *British Medical Journal, 3,* 41–42.
Isu, T., Iwasaki, Y., Sasaki, H., Abe, H. (1985). Spinal cord and root injuries due to glass fragments and acupuncture needles. *Surgical Neurology, 23,* 255–260.
Izatt, E., & Fairman, M. (1977). Staphylococcal septicaemia with DIC associated with acupuncture. *Postgraduate Medical Journal, 53,* 285–286.
Jeffreys, D. B., Smith, S., Brennand-Roper, D. A., Curry, P. V. L. (1983). Acupuncture needles as a cause of bacterial endocarditis. *British Medical Journal, 287,* 326–327.
Jian, P. (1995). Effect of moxibustion of dazhui (GV-14) on cellular immune function in tumor-bearing mice. *Internatonal Journal of Oriental Medicine, 2,* 72–76.
Jiqing, M., Deshan, W., Yanbin, Q. (1986). Effects on the interdigestive myoelectric complex of small intestine by zusanli moxibustion. *Journal of Traditional Chinese Medicine, 16,* 213–215.
Kashiba, H., Nishigori, A., Useda, Y. (1992). Expression of galanin in rat primary sensory afferents after moxibustion to the skin. *The American Journal of Chinese Medicine, 20,* 103–114.
Kataoka, H. J. (1997). Cardiac tamponade caused by penetration of an acupuncture needle into the right ventricle. *The Thoracic and Cardiovascular Surgeon, 114,* 674–676.
Keane, J., Ahmadi, J., Gruen, P. (1993). Spinal epidural hematoma with subarachnoid hemorrhage caused by acupuncture. *American Journal of Neuroradiology, 14,* 365–366.
Keller, W. J., Parker, S. G., Garvin, J. P. (1972). Possible renal complications of acupuncture. *JAMA, 222,* 1559.
Kent, G. P., Brondum, J., Keenlyside, R. A., LaFazia, L. M., Scott, H. D. (1988). A large outbreak of acupuncture-associated hepatitis B. *American Journal of Epidemiology, 127,* 591–598.
Kida, Y., Naritomi, H., Sawada, T., Kuriyama, Y., Ogawa, M., Miyamoto, S. (1988). Cervical spinal cord injury caused by acupuncture. *Archives of Neurology, 45,* 831.

Kishikawa, K., Nakae, Y., Fujiwara, S., Namiki, A., Mori, T. (1990). A spinal cord injury caused by acupuncture needles. *Pain Clinical, 3,* 179–184.
Kiyosawa, K., Gibo, Y., Sodeyama, T., Furuta, K., Imai, H., Yoda, H., Koike, Y., et al. (1987). Possible infectious causes in 651 patients with acute viral hepatitis during a 10-year period (1976–1985). *Liver, 7,* 163–168.
Koizumi, H., Tomoyori, T., Kumakri, M., Ohkawara, A. (1988). Acupuncture needle dermatitis. *Contact Dermatitis, 21,* 352.
Kondo, A., Koyama, T., Ishikawa, J., Yamasaki, T. (1979). Injury of the spinal cord produced by acupuncture needle. *Surgical Neurology, 11,* 155–156.
Kropp, R., Hassler, R. (1983). Accidental pneumothorax following injections and acupuncture in the thoracic region. *Die Medizinische Welt, 34,* 1143–1144.
Kuiper, J. (1974). Pneumothorax as complication of acupuncture. *JAMA, 229,* 1422.
Ladas, E. J., Rooney, D., Taromina, K., Ndao, D. H., & Kelly, K. M. (2010). The safety of acupuncture in children and adolescents with cancer therapy-related thrombocytopenia. *Support Care Cancer, 18,* 1487–1490.
Lapeer, G. (1988). Pain secondary to acupuncture therapy. *Craniology, 6,* 189–190.
Lee, M. S., Choi, T. Y., Park, J. -E., Lee, S, -S., Ernst, E. (2010) Moxibustion for cancer care: A systematic review and meta-analysis. *BMC Cancer, 10,* 130.
Lee, R. J. E., McIlwain, J. C. (1985). Subacute bacterial endocarditis following ear acupuncture. *International Journal of Cardiology, 7,* 62–63.
Leung, P. C., Zhang, L. (2008). Complications and adverse events in Chinese trials of acupuncture. *Acupuncture in Medicine, 26,* 121–122.
Lewis-Driver, D. J. (1973). Pneumothorax associated with acupuncture. *The Medical Journal of Australia, 2,* 296–297.
Lin, J. T. -Y. (1982). Convulsive syncope in blood donors. *Annals of Neurology, 11,* 525–528.
Lord, R., Schwartz, P. (1996). False aneurysm of the popliteal artery complicating acupuncture. *The Australian and New Zealand Journal of Surgery, 66,* 645–647.
MacPherson, H., Thomas, K., Walters, S., Fitter, M. (2001). The York acupuncture safety study: Prospective survey of 34,000 treatments by traditional acupuncturists. *BMJ, 323,* 486–487.
MacPherson, H., Scullion, A., Thomas, K. J., Walters, S. (2004). Patient reports of adverse events associated with acupuncture treatment: A prospective national survey. *Quality and Safety in Health Care, 13,* 349–355.
Mazal, D. A., King, T., Harvey, J., Cohen, J. (1980). Bilateral pneumothorax after acupuncture. *The New England Journal of Medicine, 302,* 1365–1366.
Melchart, D., Weidenhammer, W., Streng, A., Reitmayr, S., Hoppe, A., Ernst, E., et al. (2004). Prospective investigation of adverse effects of acupuncture in 97,733 patients. *Archives of Internal Medicine, 164,* 105.
Miyamoto, S., Ide, T., Takemura, N. (2010). Risks and causes of cervical cord and medulla oblongata injuries due to acupuncture. *World Neurosurgery, 73,* 735–741.
Morrone, N., Freire, J. A., Ferreira, A. K., Dourada, A. M. (1990). Iatrogenic pneumothorax caused by acupuncture. *Revista Paulista de Medicina, 108,* 189–191.
Napadow, V., Makris, N., Liu, J., Kettner, N. W., Kwong, K. K., Hui, K. K. (2005). Effects of electroacupuncture versus manual acupuncture on the human brain as measured by fMRI. *Human Brain Mapping, 24,* 193–205.
Newman, T. R. (1990). Microscopic needle damage: A potential source of microtrauma. *British Journal of Acupuncture, 13,* 7–9.
Nieda, S., Abe, T., Kuribayashi, R., Sato, M., Abe, S. (1973). Cardiac trauma as complication of acupuncture treatment: A case report of cardiac tamponade resulting from a broken needle. *Japanese Journal of Thoraxic Surgery, 293,* 780.
Norheim, A. J., Fønnebø, V. (1996). Acupuncture adverse effects are more than occasional case reports: Results from questionnaires among 1,135 randomly selected doctors, and 197 acupuncturists. *Complementary Therapies in Medicine, 4,* 8–13.

Olusanya, O., Mansuri, I. (1997). Pneumothorax following acupuncture. *The Journal of the American Board of Family Practice, 10,* 296–297.
O'Sullivan, E. M., Higginson, I. J. (2010). Clinical effectiveness and safety of acupuncture in the treatment of irradiation-induced xerostomia in patients with head and neck cancer: A systematic review. *Acupuncture in Medicine, 28,* 191–199.
O'Connor, J., & Bensky, D. (1981). *Acupuncture: A comprehensive text.* Seattle: Eastland
Park, J. E., Lee, S. S., Lee, M. S., Choi, S. M., Ernst, E. (2010). Adverse events of moxibustion: A systematic review. *Complementary Therapies in Medicine, 18,* 215–223.
Pei, J. (1995). Effect of moxibustion of dazhui (GV-14) on cellular immune function in tumor-bearing mice. *International Journal of Oriental Medicine, 20,* 72–76.
Phoon, W. O., Fong, N. P., Lee, J. (1988). History of blood transfusion, tattooing, acupuncture and risk of hepatitis B surface antigenaemia among Chinese men in Singapore. *American Journal of Public Health, 78,* 958–960.
Pierik, M. G. (1982). Fatal staphylococcal septicemia following acupuncture: Report of two cases. Occurrence of staphylococcal septicemia following acupuncture emphasizes need for thorough medical evaluation before such procedures. *Rhode Island Medical Journal, 65,* 251–253.
Qiu, X., Chen, K., Tong, L., Shu, X., Lu, X., Wen, H., Deng, C. (2004). Effects of moxibustion at shenque (CV 8) on serum IL-12 level and NK cell activities in mice with transplanted tumor. *Journal of Traditional Chinese Medicine, 24,* 56–58.
Ritter, H. G., Tarala, R. (1978). Pneumothorax after acupuncture. *BMJ, 26,* 602–603.
Sagar, S. M. (2008). Acupuncture as an evidence-based option for symptom control in cancer patients. *Current Treatment Options in Oncology, 9,* 117–126.
Sakaguchi, M., Nishimura, S. (1990). Subarachnoid hemorrhage and spinal root injury caused by acupuncture needle-case report. *Neurologica Medico Chirurgica, 30,* 956–959.
Sasaki, H., Abe, H., Iwasaki, Y., Tsuru, M., Itoh, T. (1984). Direct spinal cord and root injury caused by acupuncture (in Japanese). *No Shinkei Geka, 12,* 1219–1223.
Scheel, O., Sundsjford, A., Lunde, P., Andersen, B. M. (1992). Endocarditis after acupuncture and injection treatment by a natural healer. *Journal of American Medical Association, 267,* 56.
Schneider, L. B., Salzberg, M. R. (1984). Bilateral pneumothorax following acupuncture. *Annals of Emergency Medicine, 13,* 643.
Huaisheng, S. (1995). Ginger-partitioned moxibustion on sifeng point (extra-29) in treating children's asthenia and its effects on cellular immune functions. *Chinese Acupuncture Moxibustion, 6,* 9–10.
Shimoyama, R., Sekiguchi, S., Suga, M., Subamoto, S., Yachi, A. (1993). The epidemiology and infection route of asymptomatic HCV carriers detected through blood donations. *Gastroenterology Japan, 28,* 1–5.
Shiraishi, S., Goto, I., Kuroiwa, Y., Nishio, S., Kinoshita, K. (1979). Spinal cord injury as a complication of an acupuncture. *Neurology, 29,* 1180–1182.
Slater, P., Ben-Ishai, P., Leventhal, A., Zahgar, D., Bashary, A., Moses, A., et al. (1988). An acupuncture associated outbreak of hepatitis B in Jerusalem. *European Journal of Epidemiology, 4,* 322–325.
Smith, D. L., Walczyk, M. H., Campbell, S. (1986). Acupuncture: Needle-induced compartment syndrome. *The Western Journal of Medicine, 144,* 478–479.
Southworth, S. R., Hartwig, R. H. (1990). Foreign body in the median nerve: A complication of acupuncture. *Journal of Hand Surgery, 15,* 111–112.
Stack, B. H. (1975). Pneumothorax associated with acupuncture. *British Medical Journal, 1,* 96.
Stark, P. (1985). Midline sternal foramen: CT demonstration. *Journal of Computer Assisted Tomography, 9,* 489–490.
Stryker, W. S., Gunn, R. A., Francis, D. P. (1986). Outbreak of hepatitis B associated with acupuncture. *The Journal of Family Practice, 22,* 155–158.
Su, L. (2003). Effects of warm needling at zusanli (ST-36) on nitrous oxide and IL-2 levels in middle-aged and old people. *Journal of Traditional Chinese Medicine, 23,* 127–128.

Takishma, T. (1983). Pneumothorax as a complication of acupuncture in the treatment of bronchial asthma. *Annals in Allergy, 51,* 402–403.

Tanita, Y., Kato, T., Hanada, K., Tagami, H. (1985). Blue macules of localized argyria caused by implanted acupuncture needles: Electron microscopy and roentgenographic microanalysis of deposited metal. *Archives of Dermatology, 121,* 1550–1552.

Thompson, J. W., Cummings, M. (2008.) Investigating the safety of electroacupuncture with a picoscope. *Acupuncture in Medicine, 26,* 133–139.

Ulloth, J. E., & Haines, S. J. (2007). Acupuncture needles causing lumbar cerebrospinal fluid Fistula. *Journal of Neurosurgery in Spine, 6,* 567–569.

Umlauf, R. (1988). Analysis of the main results of the activity of the acupuncture department of the faculty hospital. *Acupuncture in Medicine, 5,* 16–8.

Valenta, L. J., Hengesh, J. W. (1980). Pneumothorax caused by acupuncture. *Lancet, 330,* 322.

Vilke, G., Wulfert, E. (1997). Case reports of two patients with pneumothorax following acupuncture. *The Journal of Emergency Medicine, 15,* 155–157.

Vincent, C. (2001). The safety of acupuncture. *BMJ, 323,* 467–468.

Vittecoq, D., Mettetal, J. F., Rouzioux, C., Bach, J. F., Bouchon, J. P. (1989). Acute HIV infection after acupuncture treatments (letter). *The New England Journal of Medicine, 320,* 250–251.

Waldman, I. (1974). Pneumothorax from acupuncture. *The New England Journal of Medicine, 290,* 633.

Warwick-Brown, N. P., Richards, A. E. (1986). Perichondritis of the ear following acupuncture. *The Journal of Laryngology and Otology, 100,* 1177–1179.

White, A., Hayhoe, S., Hart. A., Ernst, E. (2001). Adverse events following acupuncture: Prospective survey of 32,000 consultations with doctors and physiotherapists. *BMJ, 323,* 485–486.

Witt, C. M., Pach, D., Reinhold, T., Wruck, K., Brinkhaus, B., Mank, S., et al. (2011) Treatment of the adverse effects from acupuncture and their economic impact: A prospective study in 73,406 patients with low back or neck pain. *European Journal of Pain, 15,* 193–197.

Wong, R. K., Sagar, S. M. (2010). Supportive cancer care using Chinese medicine. In W. C. Cho (Ed.), *Supportive cancer care with Chinese medicine* (p. 1). New York: Springer.

WHO. (1999). *Guidelines on basic training and safety in acupuncture.* http://apps.who.int/medicinedocs/en/d/Jwhozip56e/4.3.2.html (verified Jan, 2012).

WHO. (2007). WHO International; World Health Organization Western Pacific Region standard terminologies on traditional medicine in the Western Pacific Region (pp. 251–254). Manila: World Health Organization Western Pacific.

Wright, R. S., Kupperman, J. L., Liebhaler, M. I. (1991). Bilateral tension pneumothoraxes after acupuncture. *The Western Journal of Medicine, 154,* 102–103.

Jianwei, X. (1998). Impact of medicated mugwort moxibustion on serum gastrin, d xylose excretion rate, and T-cell subgroup in patients with spleen deficiency syndrome. *Chinese Acupuncture Moxibustion, 1,* 15–16.

Yamashita, H., Tsukayama, H., Tanno, Y., Nishijo, K. (1999). Adverse events in acupuncture and moxibustion treatment: A six-year survey at a national clinic in Japan. *Journal of Alternative Complementary Medicine, 5,* 229–236.

Yi, S. X., Peng, Y., Chang, X. R., Peng, N., Yan, J., Lin, Y. P. (2007). Effect of pre-moxibustion on apoptosis and apoptosis and proliferation of gastric mucosa cells. *World Journal of Gastroenterology, 13,* 2174–2178.

Yoshimoto, K., Fukuda, F., Hori, M., Kato, B., Hattori, H., Tokuda, N., et al. (2006). Acupuncture stimulates the release of Serotonin, but not Dopamine, in the rat nucleus accumbens. *Tohoku Journal of Experimental Medicine, 208,* 321–326.

Yuzawa, M., Hara, Y., Kobayashi, Y. (1991). Foreign body stone of the ureter as a complication of acupuncture: Report of a case history (in Japanese). *Acta Urologica Japonica, 37,* 1323–1327.

Zhenlong, W. (1992). Acupuncture induced fainting: Its prevention and treatment. *British Journal of Acupuncture, 15,* 28.

Chapter 13
Acupuncture and Moxibustion in Animal Models of Cancer

Ruixin Zhang and Lixing Lao

Abstract Recent advances in oncological acupuncture research provide evidence to support the use of acupuncture and moxibustion for symptom management in cancer patients. Studies in tumor-bearing animals demonstrate that acupuncture significantly enhances immune function by decreasing the percentage of $CD4^+$ $CD25^+$ regulatory T cells and increasing natural killer (NK) cell activity. The modality's effect on NK cells has been shown to be mediated by β-endorphins. Acupuncture also has been shown to inhibit spinal interleukin-1β, dynorphin, and substance P to suppress cancer-induced pain, as well as to activate spinal opioids that alleviate chemotherapy-induced pain. Data from animal studies support the use of acupuncture for chemotherapy-induced emesis and suggest that it can improve cancer-induced depression. Moxibustion has also been shown to improve immune cell function by increasing NK cell activity, and it may alleviate cancer-induced pain. Although animal studies do not mimic human studies exactly, they reveal mechanisms by which these complementary therapies improve cancer-related symptoms. Most cancer patients experience multiple symptoms related either to cancer itself or to treatment effects. Since acupuncture and moxibustion alleviate some of these symptoms, use of these modalities has the potential to improve the patients' quality of life.

13.1 Introduction

Acupuncture, an important component of the traditional Chinese system of medicine, has been increasingly used in recent years to control cancer- or cancer therapy-caused symptoms. Potentially, acupuncture can alleviate symptoms and improve quality of life in cancer patients (Cho et al. 2008; Balk et al. 2009; Donald et al. 2011; Feng et al. 2011; Frisk et al. 2012). It is helpful for relieving cancer-related fatigue (Balk et al. 2009; Kirshbaum 2010; O'Regan and Filshie 2010), in which the immune system has been implicated (Lorusso et al 2009), and clinical data indicate that it may be an effective adjunctive treatment for cancer-related pain (Dang and Yang 1998; Paley et al. 2011a). Studies also consistently report that it significantly reduces incidence

R. Zhang (✉) · L. Lao
Center for Integrative Medicine, School of Medicine, University of Maryland, Rm 8-22, MSTF, 685 West Baltimore Street, Baltimore, MD 21201, USA
e-mail: rzhan001@umaryland.edu

W. C. S. Cho (ed.), *Acupuncture and Moxibustion as an Evidence-based Therapy for Cancer*, Evidence-based Anticancer Complementary and Alternative Medicine 3,
DOI 10.1007/978-94-007-4833-0_13,

of chemotherapy-caused vomiting (Dibble et al. 2007; Gardani et al. 2007; Taspinar and Sirin 2010). Taken together, the data suggest that acupuncture can help control and manage cancer- and cancer treatment-induced symptoms. Scattered moxibustion studies showed that this modality may improve immune function and inhibit pain.

Recent animal studies are beginning to reveal the mechanisms by which acupuncture and moxibustion produce their effects. These include studies showing that electroacupuncture enhances endogenous anticancer immune function and inhibits expression of the neurotransmitters and pro-inflammatory cytokines involved in transmission of noxious messages in the nervous system. The following paragraphs summarize studies that are helping to clarify how acupuncture and moxibustion target cancer-related symptoms.

13.2 Effects of Acupuncture on the Immune System

13.2.1 Acupuncture Enhances the Immune Function

Clinical studies suggest that acupuncture has great potential in the management of cancer-related fatigue (Molassiotis et al. 2007; Balk et al. 2009), a difficult symptom to manage that can badly impair patient quality of life. Immune dysfunction, including abnormal activation of T lymphocyte subsets, alteration in cytokine profiles, and decreased function of natural killer (NK) cells, is known to play a role in fatigue (Lorusso et al 2009).

Recent studies demonstrate that acupuncture modulates immune function, an effect that may be related to the modality's relief of fatigue. Compared to control, acupuncture treatment has been shown to significantly increase median leukocyte value and decrease incidence of grade 2–4 leukopenia during chemotherapy in patients with ovarian cancer after adjustment for baseline value (Lu et al. 2009). Further, the modality significantly increased the number of CD3, CD4, CD8 and NK cells in colorectal cancer patients with liver metastasis (Zhao et al. 2010). In an animal study, 20 min of electroacupuncture at 2 Hz, 2 mA, was given to BALB/c mice at acupoints Dazhui (GV14) and left Huantiao (GB30) every other day from days 2–12 after a hypodermic injection of H22 tumor cells. The treatment significantly downregulated the proliferation of cultured splenetic $CD4^+$ $CD25^+$ regulatory T cells, which were significantly increased in the tumor-bearing mice compared to naive control (Liu et al. 2009). Investigators also report that the cytokines interleukin (IL)-2, IL-4, IL-7 and IL-15 maintain the optimal regulatory function of human $CD4^+$ $CD25^+$ T cells (Yates et al. 2007) and that IL-2, IL-4 and IL-15 in *in vitro* regulatory T cell cultures stimulate the proliferation of $CD4^+$ $CD25^+$ T cells from the spleen and lymph nodes of naive C57BL/6 mice (Wang et al. 2008). Interestingly, acupuncture significantly decreased serum IL-4 in rats exhausted from swimming (Zhang et al. 2011a), and electroacupuncture effectively lowered serum tumor necrosis factor-alpha (TNF-α), IL-1 and IL-4 levels in inflammatory pain rats (Wang et al. 2010). These data suggest that acupuncture may suppress IL-4 to subsequently inhibit $CD4^+$ $CD25^+$ regulatory

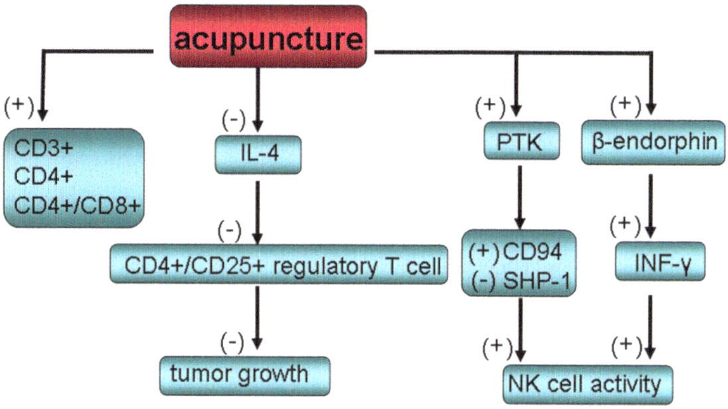

Fig. 13.1 Acupuncture mechanisms on immune function. (+): represents enhancement, (−): represents inhibition, IFN-γ: interferon-γ, IL-4: interleukin-4, PTK: protein tyrosine kinase, SHP-1: Src homology 2 (SH2) domain-containing cytoplasmic phosphatase

T cells. Since the level of $CD4^+$ $CD25^+$ regulatory T cells is positively related to tumor growth in mice (Liyanage et al. 2006), acupuncture may hamper tumor growth. In fact, a study reported that tumor volume in an acupuncture group was significantly less than in control (Liu et al. 1995). Another study reported that, compared to control, electroacupuncture treatment at Zusanli (ST36), Hegu (LI4) and Sanyinjiao (SP6) for 15 min, once a day for 15 days, significantly decreased gross tumor volumes in liver cancer, gastric cancer, and hypodermic tumor rat models produced by implanting the replicated Walker-256 cell strain (Lai et al. 2008b). However, the effect of acupuncture on tumor growth warrants further study.

Clinical data show that acupuncture, concomitant with chemotherapy, effectively maintains CD3, CD4, CD8 and CD4/CD8 values and NK cell activity after a month of treatment (Ye et al. 2002, 2007), indicating that acupuncture increases patients' immune function. In another study, acupuncture significantly increased the percentage of T lymphocyte subsets $CD3^+$ and $CD4^+$ and the $CD4^+/CD8^+$ ratio in patients with malignant tumors compared to control (Wu et al. 1996).

Animal studies produced similar results. In one, mice with transplanted MA-737 mammary cancer cells received a total of eight acupuncture/moxibustion treatments, given alternately every other day at two groups of acupoints: (1) bilateral ST36, Danzhong (CV17) and Dazhui (GV14); and (2) Guanyuan (CV4) and right Wuyi (ST15). Moxibustion was performed only at GV14 and CV4. The data show that acupuncture significantly increases NK cell activity, the T-lymphocyte positive rate of acid alpha-naphthyl acetate esterase and the rate of lymphocyte transformation (Liu et al. 1995). In another study investigating the effect of electroacupuncture at ST36, LI4 and/or SP6 on immune function in post-surgery gastric carcinoma rats, electroacupuncture (2–100 Hz, 1–3 mA) for 30 min, once a day for 7 days, significantly increased $CD4^+$ and $CD4^+/CD8^+$, as well as serum IgG, IgM, IgA, C3 and C4 (Lai et al. 2008a). These data clearly suggest that acupuncture can enhance NK cell activity in cancer patients and tumor-bearing rodents (Fig. 13.1).

13.2.2 Mechanisms of Acupuncture Enhancement of the Immune Function

It has been well demonstrated that acupuncture/electroacupuncture activates the central nervous system to release endogenous opioids into the nervous system and peripheral blood (He 1987; Mayer 2000; Zhao 2008). Electroacupuncture may also induce opioid release from peripheral inflammatory sites (Zhang et al. 2005a) to enhance the immune system. Electroacupuncture treatment at ST36 once a day (30 min) for three successive days significantly enhanced splenic NK cell activity in BALB/c mice and increased levels of splenic β-endorphins and interferon (IFN)-γ. Pretreatment with 10 mg/kg of the opiate antagonist naloxone prior to electroacupuncture blocked electroacupuncture-produced increase of both NK cell activity and IFN-γ levels, and IFN-γ monoclonal antibody abolished electroacupuncture-induced increase of NK cell activity. This leads to the hypothesis that electroacupuncture induces an increase of endogenous β-endorphins and IFN-γ that in turn enhances NK cell activity (Yu et al. 1998). Studies also suggest that granzyme B cytotoxicity-associated molecules are involved in β-endorphin-induced enhancement of NK activity (Wakao et al. 2000). Further, it has been shown that electroacupuncture treatment increases protein tyrosine kinase, CD94, and vascular cell adhesion molecule-1 expression and that it decreases protein tyrosine phosphatase and Src homology 2 domain-containing cytoplasmic phosphatase-1 to enhance NK cell activities (Kim et al. 2005). It seems that electroacupuncture-induced β-endorphin may activate NK cells through multiple pathways.

Rats with β-endorphin-producing cells transplanted into the paraventricular nucleus exhibited a reduction in mammary tumor incidence, growth, malignancy rate, and metastasis compared to cortical cell transplant rats. The former also showed increased peripheral NK cell and macrophage activities. These anti-metastatic effects, along with NK cell and macrophage stimulation, were reversed by treatment with naloxone (Sarkar et al. 2011). Similarly, β-endorphin neuron transplant rats demonstrated remarkable protection against the induction of prostate cancer and showed increased NK cell cytolytic function in spleen and peripheral blood mononuclear cells, elevated levels of IFN-γ, and decreased levels of TNF-α in plasma (Sarkar et al. 2008). Another study shows that intra-cerebroventricular administration of β-endorphin augments *in vivo* NK cell-mediated cytotoxicity (Jonsdottir et al. 1996). The fact that bilateral lesions on the lateral hypothalamic area block electroacupuncture-enhanced NK cell activity suggests that this area is related to the electroacupuncture-induced increase of NK cell activity (Choi et al. 2002). Together, these data suggest that acupuncture exerts its action against tumors by modulating the immune function through the peripheral and central release of β-endorphin (Fig. 13.1).

Table 13.1 Electroacupuncture on cancer- and chemotherapy-induced pain in rats

References	Main outcomes	Pain models
Zhang et al. (2008a)	Electroacupuncture significantly inhibited thermal hyperalgesia and downregulated spinal IL-1β	AT-3.1 prostate cancer cell into tibia
Zhang et al. (2008b)	Electroacupuncture significantly inhibited mechanical and thermal hyperalgesia and downregulated spinal dynorphin	AT-3.1 prostate cancer cell into tibia
Lee et al. (2009b)	Electroacupuncture significantly alleviated mechanical allodynia, downregulated spinal substance P, and increased β-endorphin in blood and brain	S-180 sarcoma cells around the sciatic nerve
Mao-Ying et al. (2006)	Early electroacupuncture starting on day 8 showed analgesia, but late electroacupuncture starting on day 16 showed no analgesia	B16-BL6 melanoma cells into hind paw
Meng et al. (2011)	Electroacupuncture significantly alleviated mechanical hyperalgesia and allodynia through three subtypes of spinal opioid receptors	Paclitaxel-induced peripheral neuropathy

13.3 Acupuncture Alleviation of Pain

13.3.1 Acupuncture Alleviation of Cancer Pain

Cancer-caused pain is the most common physical symptom in cancer patients and is extremely disruptive to patients' lives. Current pain-relief strategies include the use of opioid-based analgesia, bisphosphonates, radiotherapy, and nerve block. Nevertheless, a reported 50% of those with cancer-related pain do not receive adequate pain relief (Strang 1998; Cleary 2000). This severely influenced their physical and psychological welfare and results in a lower quality of life. These interventions can also produce unacceptable side effects that inevitably impair well being.

Acupuncture represents a potentially valuable adjunct to existing strategies for pain relief. Although there is insufficient evidence to judge whether the modality is effective in treating cancer pain in adults (Paley and Johnson 2011; Paley et al. 2011b), scattered case series, clinical studies, and randomized controlled trials (RCTs) suggest its benefits in managing such pain (Zhang and Lao 2010; Wang et al. 2011; Choi et al. 2012).

In support of the scattered clinical data, studies using animal cancer pain models clearly show that acupuncture significantly alleviates cancer pain (Table 13.1). Metastatic bone tumor-caused pain is the most common type of pain in cancer patients (Reale et al. 2001). A rat model established by injecting AT-3.1 prostate cancer cells into the tibia of the adult male Copenhagen rat shows a gradual development of hyperalgesia and closely mimics bone cancer pain caused by prostate cancer-induced skeletal metastasis (Zhang et al. 2005b). This model was treated with 10 Hz/2 mA/0.4 ms pulse electroacupuncture for 30 min a day

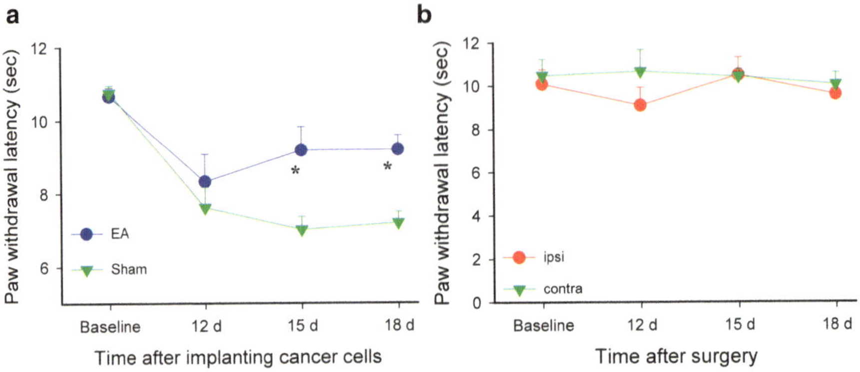

Fig. 13.2 (**a**) Effects of electroacupuncture treatments on bone cancer-induced thermal hyperalgesia. Electroacupuncture (10 Hz, 2 mA, 0.4 ms pulse, 30 min) was given at Huantiao (GB30) on days 14–18 following cancer cell inoculation of the tibia. Electroacupuncture significantly suppressed cancer-induced thermal hyperalgesia in the treated rats ($n = 7$) compared to sham control ($n = 7$). *$p < 0.05$. (**b**) Effects of electroacupuncture on paw withdrawal latency (PWL) in sham cancer rats ($n = 6$). Electroacupuncture did not significantly alter PWL. Ipsi: ipsilateral; contra: contralateral. Reprint with permission. (From Wolters Kluwer Health, Anesthesia and Analgesia 105(5), 2008)

at the equivalent of human acupoint GB30 between day 14 and day 18 after the cancer-cell injection. For sham control, electroacupuncture needles were inserted into GB30 without stimulation. Thermal hyperalgesia, a decrease in paw withdrawal latency to a noxious thermal stimulus, and mechanical hyperalgesia, a decrease in paw withdrawal pressure threshold, were measured at baseline and 20 min after electroacupuncture. The data shows that electroacupuncture significantly attenuated both thermal and mechanical hyperalgesia (Fig. 13.2). Moreover, the treatment inhibited upregulation of preprodynorphin mRNA and dynorphin as well as IL-1β and its mRNA compared to sham control (Figs. 13.3 and 13.4). Intrathecal administration of antiserum against dynorphin A (1–17) and an IL-1 receptor antagonist (0.1 mg/rat) significantly suppressed the cancer-induced hyperalgesia, indicating that electroacupuncture alleviates bone cancer pain at least in part by suppressing spinal dynorphin and IL-1β expression (Zhang et al. 2008a,b). Further, electroacupuncture and 5 mg/kg/d of Celebrex synergistically alleviated mechanical allodia induced by Walker 256 cancer cell inoculation into the tibiae of female rats (Mao-Ying et al. 2008).

Tumors can also press directly on nerves to cause pain. In order to mimic this clinical condition, S-180 sarcoma cells were inoculated around the left sciatic nerve of BALB/c mice to cause mechanical allodynia. Compared to control, electroacupuncture treatment (2 Hz) at ST36 for 30 min once a day for 9 days significantly increased paw withdrawal latency, beginning 5 days, and decreased cumulative lifting duration, beginning 7 days, after the inoculation (Lee et al. 2009b). The electroacupuncture also inhibited over-expression of the pain peptide substance P in the dorsal horn of spinal cord and increased the concentration of β-endorphin in the blood and

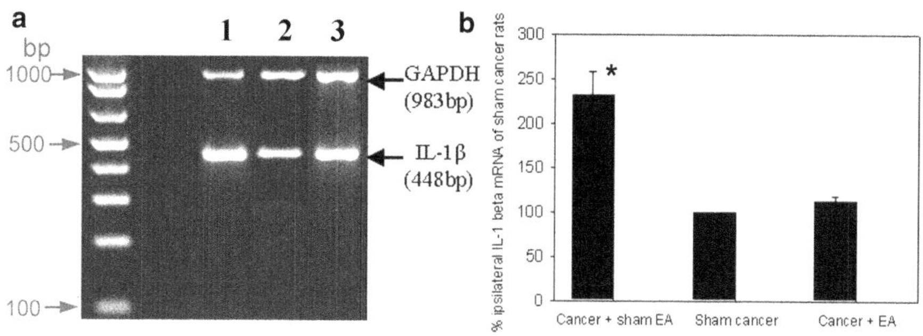

Fig. 13.3 Effect of electroacupuncture treatment on bone cancer-induced IL-1β mRNA transcription in ipsilateral spinal cords ($n = 4$ per group). (**a**) An example of agarose gel electrophoresis of PCR products. GAPDH PCR (a specific 983 bp segment of cDNA) was used as an internal control. GAPDH primers were added after the first 10 cycles of PCR reaction of IL-1β (448 bp). *1*. Cancer + sham electroacupuncture control; *2*. Sham cancer; *3*. Cancer + electroacupuncture treatment. (**b**) Quantification of relative levels of spinal IL-1β mRNA expression in the three groups. Each bar is expressed as a percentage (mean ± SEM) of the levels in sham cancer rats, which is set arbitrarily as 100%. The IL-1β mRNA levels in the cancer plus sham electroacupuncture group were markedly higher than those of sham cancer rats. Electroacupuncture suppressed upregulated IL-1β mRNA compared to sham electroacupuncture. $^{*}p < 0.05$ compared to sham cancer rats and cancer rats given electroacupuncture treatment. Reprint with permission. (From Wolters Kluwer Health, Anesthesia and Analgesia 105(5), 2008)

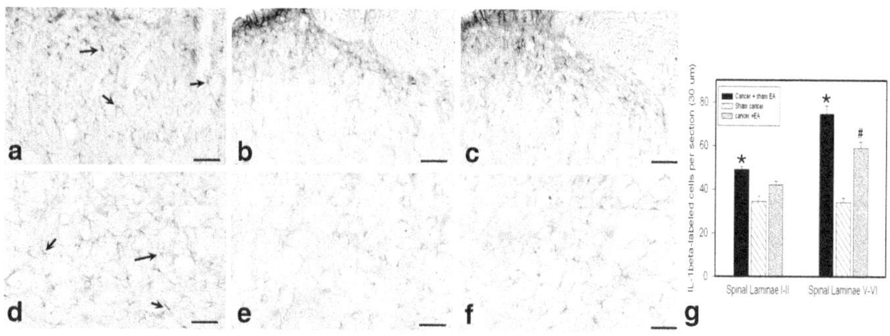

Fig. 13.4 Effect of electroacupuncture treatments on bone cancer-induced IL-1β upregulation in ipsilateral spinal cords ($n = 4$ per group). (**a–c**) Microphotographs of IL-1β-labeled cells (*arrows*) in superficial laminae of the spinal dorsal horn. (**a**) Cancer + sham electroacupuncture control, (**b**) Sham cancer, (**c**) Cancer + electroacupuncture treatment. Cancer induced IL-1β upregulation in superficial laminae (**a**) compared to sham cancer (**b**); electroacupuncture treatment inhibited this upregulation (**c**). (**d–f**) Microphotographs of IL-1β-labeled cells (*arrows*) in laminae V–VI of the spinal dorsal horn. Cancer induced IL-1β upregulation in laminae V–VI (**d**) compared to sham cancer (**e**); electroacupuncture treatment inhibited this upregulation (**f**). (**g**) Quantification of spinal IL-1β in the three groups. Each bar is expressed as mean ± SEM. There were significantly more IL-1β-labeled cells in cancer rats plus sham electroacupuncture than in sham cancer rats. Electroacupuncture treatments slightly inhibited IL-1β upregulation in superficial laminae and significantly suppressed this upregulation in laminae V–VI. $^{*}p < 0.05$ compared to sham cancer rats; $^{\#}p < 0.05$ compared to cancer rats plus sham electroacupuncture. Scale bar = 50 μm. Reprint with permission. (From Wolters Kluwer Health, Anesthesia and Analgesia 105(5), 2008)

brains of mice (Lee et al. 2009b). Taken together, these findings suggest that electroacupuncture treatment can be a complementary therapeutic method for cancer pain that decreases dynorphin, substance P, and IL-1β in the spinal cord and increases central and peripheral β-endorphins (Zhang et al. 2012).

It should be noted that the relative efficacy of electroacupuncture depends on when it is given to the cancer pain animal model. For instance, in a mouse model of cancer pain made using B16-BL6 melanoma cells, a single electroacupuncture treatment given on day 8 after inoculation showed significant analgesia while treatment on day 20 did not. Multiple electroacupuncture treatments given once every other day starting on day 8 showed analgesia at day 20 but did not if started on day 16. These animal studies support the clinical use of electroacupuncture in the treatment of cancer pain, and their results suggest that electroacupuncture exerts anti-hyperalgesic effects on early- but not late-stage cutaneous cancer pain (Mao-Ying et al. 2006).

13.3.2 Acupuncture Alleviation of Chemotherapy-induced Pain

Chemotherapy-induced peripheral neuropathy is a major clinical problem (Bhagra and Rao 2007; Malik and Stillman 2008; Windebank and Grisold 2008; Wolf et al. 2008; Kaley and DeAngelis 2009; Judith 2009; Argyriou et al. 2010; Pachman et al. 2011). It is a dose-limiting side effect of a significant number of anti-neoplastic drugs that adversely affects the administration of planned therapy and impairs patient quality of life. The clinical features of anti-neoplastic drug-induced neuropathy manifest predominantly as sensory symptoms (Peltier and Russell 2002; Quasthoff and Hartung 2002; Hausheer et al. 2006), and pharmacotherapy is the most common treatment. These include antidepressants, anticonvulsants, serotonin and norepinephrine re-uptake inhibitors, topical analgesics, corticosteroids, non-steroidal anti-inflammatory drugs, and opioids (Armstrong et al. 2005; Kaley and DeAngelis 2009; Dworkin et al. 2010), all of which are only partially effective and have significant side effects.

Acupuncture is frequently used in patients with neuropathy, most of which is diabetic-, idiopathic- or paraprotein-associated (Chong and Bajwa 2003; Brunelli and Gorson 2004). It has been reported that 30% of patients with neuropathy have turned to acupuncture due to inadequate control of neuropathic pain (Brunelli and Gorson 2004).

Some clinical studies suggest that acupuncture can be an effective therapy for chemotherapy-induced neuropathy, but the evidence is not conclusive. A five-patient pilot study reported that acupuncture improved the symptoms of this disorder (Wong and Sagar 2006), and a case report also showed that acupuncture relieves pain in patients with the condition (Bao et al. 2011). In another case series, 82% ($n = 14$) of the patients reported an improvement in symptoms after a course of six weekly acupuncture treatments (Donald et al. 2011).

In our basic science study (Meng et al. 2011), an animal model of chemotherapy-induced peripheral neuropathic pain was produced by intraperitoneal (i.p.) injection of 2 mg/kg/ml paclitaxel (Polomano et al. 2001; Flatters and Bennett 2006) given on days 0, 2, 4 and 6. Electroacupuncture (10 or 100 Hz, 2 mA, 0.4 ms pulse width for 30 min) at GB30 was administered by a stimulator (Electro-stimulator 8-C, Pantheon Research Inc.) *via* two electrodes on days 14, 16, 18 and 20. Mechanical allodynia/hyperalgesia was assessed 30 min after each electroacupuncture treatment using von Frey filaments with bending forces of 2, 4, 6 and 15 g. Because previous studies demonstrate that the mechanical threshold of hyperalgesia is 15 g in naive rats (Gong et al. 2010; Chu et al. 2011), we described chemotherapy-induced responses to 15 g of pressure as hyperalgesia-like and chemotherapy-induced responses of <15 g as allodynia-like. Electroacupuncture at 10 Hz significantly ($p < 0.05$) decreased response frequency at 4–15 g compared to sham electroacupuncture; electroacupuncture at 100 Hz only decreased response frequency at 15 g. Compared to sham electroacupuncture plus vehicle, electroacupuncture at 10 Hz plus either a μ, δ or κ opioid receptor antagonist did not significantly decrease mechanical response frequency, indicating that all three antagonists blocked electroacupuncture inhibition of neuropathic pain.

Further investigations into the effects of acupuncture on chemotherapy-induced peripheral neuropathy using rigorous scientific methodology are warranted, and the underlying mechanisms need to be clarified.

13.4 Effects of Acupuncture on Other Symptoms

13.4.1 Effects of Acupuncture on Cancer-caused Depression

Depression is a common psychiatric problem in cancer patients. Studies show that 55% of patients report at least mild symptoms (Salvo et al. 2011) and 22% have moderate to high depression (Mehnert and Koch 2008). The disorder badly impairs quality of life in cancer patients. Antidepressants are efficacious in the treatment of depression occurring in the context of chronic physical health problems (Taylor et al. 2011) but have unwanted side effects (Ferguson 2001).

Acupuncture has been used to treat depression in the clinical setting. However, since both acupuncture and control have resulted in similar improvement of depressive symptoms (Leo and Ligot 2007; Andreescu et al. 2011), well-designed clinical trials with optimal placebo controls are needed.

Several basic studies demonstrate that electroacupuncture exerts antidepressant effects in animal models of depression and that this effect is related, at least in part, to the serotonergic system (Dos Santos et al. 2008). Electroacupuncture at Baihui (GV20) and SP6 for 20 min, once a day for 14 days, upregulated serotonin and acetylcholinesterase (Zhu et al. 2009b) and somatostatin expression (Zhu et al. 2009a) in the hippocampus of rats with chronic, unpredictable, mild, stress-induced depression. Electroacupuncture at GV20, Yintang (EX-HN1), ST36 and

Fenglong (ST40), once every other day for 3 weeks, restored decreased protein kinase (PK) A and PKC expression in the hippocampus of a rat model of depression (Lu et al. 2008). Acupuncture for 5 min at Neiguan (PC6) before i.p. CORT (40 mg/kg) injections, administered once a day for 19 consecutive days, inhibited chronic corticosterone-induced depression-like behavior and increased hypothalamic neuropeptide Y (NPY) expression in rats (Lee et al. 2009a). Acupuncture treatment at Shenmen (HT7), in which the needles were twirled twice a second for 30 sec. and then removed, also significantly alleviated maternal separation-caused depression-like disorder and increased NPY-immunoreactive cells in area CA1 and the dentate gyrus of the hippocampus, while acupuncture at ST36 did not (Lim et al. 2003). Since acupuncture/electroacupuncture has significantly alleviated depression-like behavior in a variety of rat models of depression, its use in patients with cancer-induced depression may be beneficial. Microarray studies show that over 200 genes are down- or upregulated in rats with depression-like behavior compared to control, and those changes were reversed following electroacupuncture treatment (Jiang and Wang 2010). Those data suggest that acupuncture works on depression by regulating neurochemical imbalances.

13.4.2 Effects of Acupuncture on Chemotherapy-caused Emesis

Nausea and vomiting remain problems for patients undergoing cancer chemotherapy despite the availability of anti-emetics (Basch et al. 2011). A large body of evidence, including that from clinical series, uncontrolled trials and RCTs, has consistently reported acupuncture to be effective for chemotherapy-induced nausea and vomiting (Zhang and Lao 2010). However, only a few studies have investigated the acupuncture effect on emesis in animals.

In an animal study using guinea pigs, electroacupuncture at ST36 significantly alleviated intra-stomach infusion of $CuSO_4$-caused vomiting and significantly decreased the amplitude and frequency of gastroenteric electric activity that occurred during vomiting (Len et al. 1991). In a study in cats, electroacupuncture at PC6 significantly decreased the frequency of gastric distention-induced transient lower esophageal sphincter relaxation compared to sham acupoint stimulation. The same treatment also decreased Fos immunoreactivity and nitric oxide synthase reactivity in the solitarius and the dorsal motor nucleus of the vagus. These effects were blocked by pretreatment with cholecystokinin (CCK), L-arginine and naloxone, suggesting that electroacupuncture action is mediated through CCK-A receptor, nitric oxide, and μ opioid receptors (Wang et al. 2007). Moreover, studies also show that oculo-acupuncture at the stomach/spleen region and Zhongjiao region and body acupuncture at Pishu (BL20) and Weishu (BL21) for 20 min significantly ($p<0.05$) inhibit xylazine-induced vomiting in dogs (Liu et al. 2007). Oculo-acupuncture is a new modality of acupuncture therapy. It uses 13 special points on eight parts around the eye's orbit (Liu et al. 2007). Electroacupuncture (5 and 10 Hz) at PC6 for 5 min significantly ($p<0.05$) reduced the number of morphine -induced emetic

Table 13.2 Moxibustion on immunity in tumor-bearing animals

References	Main outcomes	Acupoints
Liu et al. (2009)	Moxibustion downregulated the proliferation of regulatory T cells	Dazhui (GV14)
Wu et al. (2001)	Moxibustion restored the formation rate of altered erythrocytic immunosuppressive factors	Guanyuan (CV4)
Qiu et al. (2004)	Moxibustion elevated serum IL-2 and IL-12 levels and NK cell activity	Shenque (CV8)
Pei et al. (2010)	Moxibustion increased IL-1β and IL-2 and decreased IL-6 in the cerebral cortex	Dazhui (GV14)

episodes and prolonged the onset of emesis in ferrets (Lao et al. 1995). Interestingly, a combination of electroacupuncture and low-dosage ondansetron, droperidol or metoclopramide significantly reduced the number of emetic episodes by 52, 36 and 73%, respectively, as well as the number of early stage emetic episodes compared to a sham acupuncture control. The combinations also significantly prevented emesis compared to electroacupuncture or any of the drugs alone (Lao et al. 2003). These animal studies indicate that electroacupuncture treatment might alleviate emesis with a variety of etiologies and suggest that electroacupuncture treatment may allow drug dosages to be reduced while symptom control is maintained or improved.

13.5 Effects of Moxibustion on Cancer

In moxibustion, herbal preparations containing *Artemisia vulgaris* are burned to heat and stimulate acupuncture points. Although moxibustion reportedly is effective for several conditions, including pain (Lee et al. 2010a) and chemotherapy-induced emesis, the evidence is very limited (Lee et al. 2010b). The possible mechanisms of moxibustion are summarized below.

13.5.1 Moxibustion in Immunity

It has been reported that moxibustion improves immune cell function (Table 13.2). Moxibustion treatment significantly improved gastrointestinal and immune function in post-operative colorectal cancer patients (Zhang and Du 2011) and increased CD3, CD4, CD8 and NK cells in colorectal cancer patients with liver metastasis (Zhao et al. 2010). Moxibustion, applied to GV14 every other day, two cones at each treatment, in BALB/c mice between days 2 and 12 after a hypodermic injection of H22 tumor cells, significantly downregulated the proliferation of regulatory T cells (Liu et al. 2009). The modality restored the formation rate of altered erythrocytic C3b receptor rosettes, the formation rate of erythrocytic immuno-complex rosettes, and activity of the erythrocytic immuno-accelerative and erythrocytic immuno-suppressive factors (Wu et al. 2001), and it significantly elevated serum IL-2 and IL-12 levels and NK cell activity (Qiu et al. 2004) in tumor-bearing mice. Additionally, moxibustion regulated IL-1β, IL-2, IL-6 mRNA and protein expression in the cerebral cortices of tumor-bearing mice (Pei et al. 2010). These preliminary data demonstrate that moxibustion improves immune cell function.

13.5.2 Moxibustion in Pain

Moxibustion has significantly decreased osteoarthritis pain (Cheng et al. 2008; Sun et al. 2008; Zhang and Fu 2010), fibromyalgia syndrome (Zhao and Zhu 2009) and herpes zoster (Li 2007; Zhong et al. 2010) in several clinical trials, and some case series report that the modality effectively suppressed pain in patients with terminal cancer (Zan and Zhang 1999; Qin and Qin 2001). Animal studies have shown similar effects. However, more rigorous studies are needed.

In a mono iodoacetic acid-induced rat model of knee osteoarthritis, indirect moxibustion applied to the lateral aspect of the knee joint every other day for 28 days significantly alleviated the pain, which was antagonized by naloxone pretreatment and assessed by body-bearing differences (Uryu et al. 2007). This result is consistent with a study in which moxibustion significantly increased serum β-endorphin (Zhai et al. 1994). Moxibustion at ST36, in which three moxa cones were burned successively once a day for 9 days beginning 2 days after a complete Freund's adjuvant injection into the synovial cavity of the unilateral knee joint, significantly alleviated pain in an inflammatory pain rat model ($p < 0.05$). It also significantly suppressed the production of nitric oxide and the protein expression of c-Fos and neuronal nitric oxide synthase induced by arthritis in the lumbar spinal cord (Kim et al. 2006). In a rat model of chronic visceral hypersensitivity, bilateral moxibustion at Tianshu (ST25) for 15 min, once a day for 7 days, significantly ($p < 0.05$) increased visceral pain threshold, assessed with abdominal withdrawal reflex scores, and restored serotonin concentrations in the colon (Zhou et al. 2009). Because moxibustion has been shown to be effective for various kinds of pain in patients and animal models, we hypothesize that it can inhibit cancer pain in animal models, thus providing a way to study its mechanisms on such pain.

13.6 Animal Studies *vs* Human Studies

13.6.1 The Species Gap

Despite the usefulness of animal models, a species gap exists between animals and humans. As demonstrated by many drug development studies, drugs that work well in animal models do not always work in human clinical trials. For instance, acupuncture/electroacupuncture has been shown to significantly inhibit pain compared to placebo control in inflammatory (Zhang et al. 2011b), neuropathic (Meng et al.

2011) and cancer (Mao-Ying et al. 2006; Zhang et al. 2008a) pain animal models. However, clinical trials report that verum acupuncture and sham (superficial needling at non-acupuncture points) produce the same effects (Melchart et al. 2005; Diener et al. 2006). It is possible that this kind of sham control is not truly inert; it may stimulate the somatosensory system. Another possibility is that the placebo effect (e.g. patient expectation) masks differences in the effects produced by verum and those produced by sham. These data suggest that a more suitable sham acupuncture control, one that is truly inert, is needed.

13.6.2 Acupoints in Animal Studies

Because of insufficient understanding of the anatomical and physiological nature of acupoints and the meridian system, it can be a challenge to determine animal points that correspond to human points.

The electrical characteristics of acupoints and meridians have been studied (She et al. 2010), and it has been reported that acupoints have lower electrical resistance and meridians have lower electrical impedance and higher capacitance compared to adjacent controls (Ahn et al. 2008). However, the electrical properties of acupoints vary in accordance with physiological and pathological changes in the human body (She et al. 2010). For example, regional cutaneous electric resistance values of acupoints on both sides of the body were found to be significantly lower in encephalomalacia patients than in normal subjects, and the electric resistance of the points changed after operation (Liu et al. 2010). Thus there is insufficient evidence to conclude that electric resistance accurately determines the location of acupoints and meridians (Ahn et al. 2008; She et al. 2010).

The transpositional method, which locates animal acupoints according to the corresponding anatomical sites on humans, is commonly reported in the literature (Han 2003; Lao et al. 2004; Zhao 2008). Taking into account anatomical differences between humans and animals, such as the twelve thoracic, five lumbar, five sacral, and three to six coccygeal vertebrae in humans *vs* the rat's thirteen thoracic, six lumbar, four sacral, and twenty eight coccygeal vertebrae, Yin et al. (2008) mapped 121 commonly used acupoints in the rat.

Since the points are not anatomically visible in humans, their locations are based on the clinical observations of thousands of years. Through experience, Huantiao (GB30) has been shown to successfully alleviate sciatic pain and related symptoms and thus is used to treat lower limb pain and related symptoms. In animal studies, we can only approximate the location of this point because of the species gap. However, the most important factor for determining the accuracy of a point location is effect. For example, if one inserts a needle into an acupoint thought to be appropriate but this produces no effect on pain, either the point is incorrectly located or the quality of the acupuncture is poor. On the other hand, if a point works well in a given animal model, e.g. a rat model of pain, and is anatomically close to the comparable site used in humans, then one may be confident that the right point has been determined.

In basic science, electric resistance measurement, the transpositional method, and outcome assessment should be used together to determine accurate acupoints in laboratory animals with given pathological conditions.

13.6.3 Pros and Cons of Acupuncture Studies in Animal Models

In recent years, the mechanisms of acupuncture have been studied in humans using brain-imaging techniques (Napadow et al. 2005). However, most data on acupuncture mechanisms are derived from animal studies that use invasive procedures (Zhao 2008). For example, medulla opioid-serotonin circuit involvement in acupuncture anti-hyperalgesia can only be revealed using such procedures (Zhang et al. 2011b). Animal models are useful when invasive manipulations are necessary for determining the mechanisms of this therapy.

Understanding the mechanisms and pathways of acupuncture treatment can provide information for formulating optimal acupuncture/drug combinations that maximize treatment effects and minimize side effects by decreasing drug dosages. For example, because adenosine has been shown to mediate acupuncture analgesia, interventions that hamper the degradation of adenosine might prolong the clinical effects of acupuncture and potentially decrease pain medication dosages (Goldman et al. 2010).

Further, translational animal studies from experimental bench to clinical bed can provide useful information for designing appropriate clinical trials. For example, our animal studies demonstrate that low frequency electroacupuncture produces longer-term anti-hyperalgesic and anti-edema effects than high frequency electroacupuncture does (Lao et al. 2004). Thus we used low frequency in our knee osteoarthritis clinical trial and obtained a prolonged effect lasting 26 weeks (Berman et al. 2004).

13.6.4 Prospective

In a growing body of studies, both acupuncture and moxibustion have been shown to enhance the immune function and inhibit cancer-related pain, but the studies are still very limited in terms of quality and quantity. Studies on immune function are immature, and some, such as those on acupuncture inhibition of tumor growth, need confirmation. RCTs and mechanism investigations of the effects of acupuncture and moxibustion in cancer-related pain are needed. Additionally, several basic studies demonstrate that acupuncture exerts anti-depressive effects in animal models of depression. However, since acupuncture and control resulted in similar improvement in depressive symptoms (Leo and Ligot 2007; Andreescu et al. 2011), well-designed clinical trials with optimal placebo control are warranted.

Acknowledgments We would like to thank Dr Lyn Lowry for her editorial assistance. This work was supported by NIH grant R21AT004113.

References

Ahn, A. C., Colbert, A. P., Anderson, B. J., Martinsen, O. G., Hammerschlag, R., Cina, S., et al. (2008). Electrical properties of acupuncture points and meridians: A systematic review. *Bioelectromagnetics, 29,* 245–256.

Andreescu, C., Glick, R. M. Emeremni, C. A., Houck, P. R., & Mulsant, B. H. (2011). Acupuncture for the treatment of major depressive disorder: A randomized controlled trial. *The Journal of Clinical Psychiatry, 72,* 1129–1135.

Argyriou, A. A., Zolota, V., Kyriakopoulou, O., & Kalofonos, H. P. (2010). Toxic peripheral neuropathy associated with commonly used chemotherapeutic agents. *The Official Journal of Balkan Union of Oncology, 15,* 435–446.

Armstrong, T., Almadrones, L., & Gilbert, M. R. (2005). Chemotherapy-induced peripheral neuropathy. *Oncology Nursing Forum, 32,* 305–311.

Balk, J., Day, R., Rosenzweig, M., & Beriwal, S. (2009). Pilot, randomized, modified, double-blind, placebo-controlled trial of acupuncture for cancer-related fatigue. *Journal of the Society for Integrative Oncology, 7,* 4–11.

Bao, T., Zhang, R. X., Badros, A., & Lao, L. (2011). Acupuncture Treatment for Bortezomib-Induced Peripheral Neuropathy: A Case Report. *Pain Research and Treatment*: doi:10.1155/2011/920807.

Basch, E., Prestrud, A. A. Hesketh, P. J. Kris, M. G., Feyer, P. C., Somerfield, M. R., et al. (2011). Antiemetics: American Society of Clinical Oncology Clinical Practice Guideline Update. *Journal of Clinical Oncology, 29,* 4189–4198.

Berman, B. M., Lao, L., Langenberg, P., Lee, W. L., Gilpin, A. M., & Hochberg, M. C. (2004). Effectiveness of acupuncture as adjunctive therapy in osteoarthritis of the knee: A randomized, controlled trial. *Annals of Internal Medicine, 141,* 901–910.

Bhagra, A., & Rao, R. D. (2007). Chemotherapy-induced neuropathy. *Current Oncology Reports, 9,* 290–299.

Brunelli, B., & Gorson, K. C. (2004). The use of complementary and alternative medicines by patients with peripheral neuropathy. *Journal of the Neurological Sciences, 218,* 59–66.

Cheng, H. L., Han, W., Hu, P. J., & Yang, J. (2008). Selection of objects separated moxibustion dialectic treatment of knee osteoarthritis in primary clinical research *Clinical Journal of Traditional Chinese Medicine, 20,* 114–116.

Cho, J. H., Chung, W. K., Kang, W., Choi, S. M., Cho, C. K., & Son, C. G. (2008). Manual acupuncture improved quality of life in cancer patients with radiation-induced xerostomia. *Journal of Alternative and Complementary Medicine, 14,* 523–526.

Choi, G. S., Oha, S. D., Han, J. B., Bae, H. S., Cho, Y. W., Yun, Y. S., et al. (2002). Modulation of natural killer cell activity affected by electroacupuncture through lateral hypothalamic area in rats. *Neuroscience Letters, 329,* 1–4.

Choi, T. Y., Lee, M. S., Kim, T. H., Zaslawski, C., & Ernst, E. (2012). Acupuncture for the treatment of cancer pain: a systematic review of randomised clinical trials. *Supportive Care in Cancer, 20,* 1147–1158.

Chong, M. S., & Bajwa, Z. H. (2003). Diagnosis and Treatment of Neuropathic Pain. *Journal of Pain and Symptom Management, 25,* S4-S11.

Chu, L. C., Tsaur, M. L., Lin, C. S., Hung, Y. C., Wang, T. Y., Chen, C. C., et al. (2011). Chronic intrathecal infusion of gabapentin prevents nerve ligation-induced pain in rats. *British Journal of Anaesthesia, 106,* 699–705.

Cleary, J. F. (2000). Cancer pain management. *Cancer Control, 7,* 120–131.

Dang, W., & Yang, J. (1998). Clinical study on acupuncture treatment of stomach carcinoma pain. *Journal of Traditional Chinese Medicine, 18,* 31–38.

Dibble, S. L., Luce, J., Cooper, B. A., Israel, J., Cohen, M., Nussey, B., et al. (2007). Acupressure for chemotherapy-induced nausea and vomiting: A randomized clinical trial. *Oncology Nursing Forum, 34,* 813–820.

Diener, H-C., Kronfeld, K., Boewing, G., Lungenhausen, M., Maier, C., Molsberger, A., et al. (2006). Efficacy of acupuncture for the prophylaxis of migraine: A multicentre randomised controlled clinical trial. *Lancet Neurology, 5,* 310–316.

Donald, G. K., Tobin, I., & Stringer, J. (2011). Evaluation of acupuncture in the management of chemotherapy-induced peripheral neuropathy. *Acupuncture in Medicine, 29,* 230–233.

Dos Santos, J. G., Jr., Kawano, F., Nishida, M. M., Yamamura, Y., Mello, L. E., & Tabosa, A. (2008). Antidepressive-like effects of electroacupuncture in rats. *Physiology & Behavior, 93,* 155–159.

Dworkin, R. H., O'Connor, A. B., Audette, J., Baron, R., Gourlay, G. K., Haanpaa, M. L., et al. (2010). Recommendations for the pharmacological management of neuropathic pain: An overview and literature update. *Mayo Clinic Proceedings, 85,* S3–14.

Feng, Y., Wang, X. Y., Li, S. D., Zhang, Y., Wang, H. M., Li, M., et al. (2011). Clinical research of acupuncture on malignant tumor patients for improving depression and sleep quality. *Journal of Traditional Chinese Medicine, 31,* 199–202.

Ferguson, J. (2001). SSRI Antidepressant Medications: Adverse Effects and Tolerability. Prim Care Companion. *The Journal of Clinical Psychiatry, 3,* 22–27.

Flatters, S. J. L., & Bennett, G. J. (2006). Studies of peripheral sensory nerves in paclitaxel-induced painful peripheral neuropathy: Evidence for mitochondrial dysfunction. *Pain, 122,* 245–257.

Frisk, J., Källström, A. C., Wall, N., Fredrikson, M., & Hammar, M. (2012). Acupuncture improves health-related quality-of-life (HRQoL) and sleep in women with breast cancer and hot flushes. *Support Care Cancer, 20,* 715–724.

Gardani, G., Cerrone, R., Biella, C., Galbiati, G., Proserpio, E., Casiraghi, M., et al. (2007). A progress study of 100 cancer patients treated by acupressure for chemotherapy-induced vomiting after failure with the pharmacological approach. *Minerva Medica, 98,* 665–668.

Goldman, N., Chen, M., Fujita, T., Xu, Q., Peng, W., Liu, W., et al. (2010). Adenosine A1 receptors mediate local anti-nociceptive effects of acupuncture. *Nature Neuroscience, 13,* 883–888.

Gong, Q-J., Li, Y-Y., Xin, W-J., Wei, X-H., Cui, Y., Wang, J., et al. (2010). Differential effects of adenosine A1 receptor on pain-related behavior in normal and nerve-injured rats. *Brain Research, 1361,* 23–30.

Han, J. S. (2003). Acupuncture: Neuropeptide release produced by electrical stimulation of different frequencies. *Trends in Neurosciences, 26,* 7–22.

Hausheer, F. H., Schilsky, R. L., Bain, S., Berghorn, E. J., & Lieberman, F. (2006). Diagnosis, management, and evaluation of chemotherapy-induced peripheral neuropathy. *Seminars in Oncology, 33,* 15–49.

He, L. F. (1987). Involvement of endogenous opioid peptides in acupuncture analgesia. *Pain, 31,* 99–121.

Jiang, L. H., & Wang, L. L. (2010). Gene chips-aided analysis on the profiles of hippocampal whole-genome expression in depression rats following electroacupuncture treatment. *Acupuncture Research, 35,* 83–89.

Jonsdottir, I. H., Johansson, C., Asea, A., Hellstrand, K., Thorén, P., & Hoffmann, P. (1996). Chronic intracerebroventricular administration of beta-endorphin augments natural killer cell cytotoxicity in rats. *Regulatory Peptides, 62,* 113–118.

Judith, A. P. (2009). Clinical Challenges: Chemotherapy-Induced Peripheral Neuropathy. *Seminars in Oncology Nursing, 25,* S8-S19.

Kaley, T. J., & DeAngelis, L. M. (2009). Therapy of chemotherapy-induced peripheral neuropathy. *British Journal of Haematology, 145,* 3–14.

Kim, C. K., Choi, G. S., Oh, S. D., Han, J. B., Kim, S. K., Ahn, H. J., et al. (2005). Electroacupuncture up-regulates natural killer cell activity: Identification of genes altering their expressions in electroacupuncture induced up-regulation of natural killer cell activity. *Journal of Neuroimmunology, 168,* 144–153.

Kim, J. H., Kim, H. K., Park, Y. I., Sohn, I. C., Choi, D. O., Kim, M. S., et al. (2006). Moxibustion at ST36 alleviates pain in complete Freund's adjuvant-induced arthritic rats. *The American Journal of Chinese Medicine, 34,* 57–67.

Kirshbaum, M. (2010). Cancer-related fatigue: A review of nursing interventions. *British Journal of Community Nursing, 15,* 214–216.

Lai, M., Wang, S. M., Wang, Y., Tang, C. L., Kong, L. W., & Xu, X. Y. (2008a). Effects of electroacupuncture of "Zusanli" (ST 36), "Hegu" (LI 4) and/or "Sanyinjiao" (SP 9) on immunofunction in gastric carcinectomy rats. *Acupuncture Research, 33,* 245–249.

Lai, M., Wang, S. M., Zhang, W. L., Wang, Y., Huang, S. Q., Dong, W., et al. (2008b). Effects of electroacupuncture on tumor growth and immune function in the Walker-256 model rat. *Zhongguo Zhen Jiu, 28,* 607–609.

Lao, L., Wong, R. H., Berman, B., & Wynn, R. L. (1995). Electroacupuncture reduces morphine-induced emesis in ferrets: A pilot study. *Journal of Alternative and Complementary Medicine, 1,* 257–261.

Lao, L., Zhang, G., Wong, R. H., Carter, A. K., Wynn, R. L., & Berman, B. M. (2003). The effect of electroacupuncture as an adjunct on cyclophosphamide-induced emesis in ferrets. *Pharmacology, Biochemistry, and Behavior, 74,* 691–699.

Lao, L., Zhang, R-X., Zhang, G., Wang, X., Berman, B. M., & Ren, K. (2004). A parametric study of electroacupuncture on persistent hyperalgesia and Fos protein expression in rats. *Brain Research, 1020,* 18–29.

Lee, B., Shim, I., Lee, H. J., Yang, Y., & Hahm, D. H. (2009a). Effects of acupuncture on chronic corticosterone-induced depression-like behavior and expression of neuropeptide Y in the rats. *Neuroscience Letters, 453,* 151–156.

Lee, H. J., Lee, J. H., Lee, E. O., Lee, H. J., Kim, K. H., Lee, K. S., et al. (2009b). Substance P and beta endorphin mediate electroacupuncture induced analgesic activity in mouse cancer pain model. *Acupuncture & Electro-Therapeutics Research, 34,* 27–40.

Lee, M. S., Choi, T., Kang, J. W., Lee, B., & Ernst, E. (2010a). Moxibustion for treating pain: A systematic review. *The American Journal of Chinese Medicine, 38,* 829–838.

Lee, M. S., Choi, T. Y., Park, J. E., Lee, S. S., & Ernst, E. (2010b). Moxibustion for cancer care: A systematic review and meta-analysis. *BMC Cancer, 10,* 130.

Len, J., Xu, G., Liu, W., & Zhang, Q. (1991). The regulating effect of electroacupuncture on gastroenteric electric activity in guinea pigs of peripheral vomiting. *Acupuncture Research, 16,* 69–72.

Leo, R. J., & Ligot, J. S. Jr (2007). A systematic review of randomized controlled trials of acupuncture in the treatment of depression. *Journal of Affective Disorders, 97,* 13–22.

Li, W. G. (2007). Cotton Moxibustion treatment of herpes zoster clinical observation of 30 cases. *Journal of Practical Traditional Chinese Internal Medicine, 21,* 97.

Lim, S., Ryu, Y-H., Kim, S-T., Hong, M-S., & Park, H-J. (2003). Acupuncture increases neuropeptide Y expression in hippocampus of maternally-separated rats. *Neuroscience Letters, 343,* 49–52.

Liu, L. J., Guo, C. J., Jiao, X. M., Liu, L. J., Guo, C. J., & Jiao, X. M. (1995). Effect of acupuncture on immunologic function and histopathology of transplanted mammary cancer in mice. *Chinese Journal of Integrative Traditional Western Medicine, 15,* 615–617.

Liu, J., Lee, Y. T., Lee, S. E., Lee, J. Y., & Kim, D. H. (2007). Anti-emetic effect of oculo-acupuncture on dogs with xylazine induced vomiting. *The American Journal of Chinese Medicine, 35,* 447–453.

Liu, Z. D., Pei, J., Fu, Q. H., Li, H. Y., Yu, Q. W., Zhang, J. Y., et al. (2009). Influence of electroacupuncture and moxibustion and their treated mouse serum on the proliferation of the cultured splenetic CD4+CD25+ regulatory T cells of tumor-bearing mice. *Acupuncture Research, 34,* 219–224.

Liu, L. L., Zhao, B. X., Xie, Z. H., & Fan, Y. P. (2010). Changes of electrical property of the twelve source-points in encephaloma patients before and after surgery. *Acupuncture Research, 35,* 52–55.

Liyanage, U. K., Goedegebuure, P. S., Moore, T. T., Viehl, C. T., Moo-Young, T. A., Larson, J. W., et al. (2006). Increased prevalence of regulatory T cells (Treg) is induced by pancreas adenocarcinoma. *Journal of Immunotherapy, 29,* 416–424.

Lorusso, L. M. S., Capelli, E., Ferrari, D., Ngonga, G. K., & Ricevuti, G. (2009). Immunological aspects of chronic fatigue syndrome. *Autoimmunity Reviews, 8,* 287–291.

Lu, F., Zhu, H. M., Xie, J. J., Zhou, H. H., Chen, Y. L., & Hu, J. Y. (2008). Effects of electroacupuncture on behavior, plasma COR and expressions of PKA and PKC in hippocampus of the depression model rat. *Zhongguo Zhen Jiu, 28,* 214–218.

Lu, W., Matulonis, U. A., Doherty-Gilman, A., Lee, H., Dean-Clower, E., Rosulek, A., et al. (2009). Acupuncture for chemotherapy-induced neutropenia in patients with gynecologic malignancies: A pilot randomized, sham-controlled clinical trial. *Journal of Alternative and Complementary Medicine, 15,* 745–753.

Malik, B., & Stillman, M. (2008). Chemotherapy-induced peripheral neuropathy. *Current Neurology and Neuroscience Reports, 8,* 56–65.

Mao-Ying, Q. L., Cui, K. M., Liu, Q., Dong, Z. Q., Wang, W., Wang, J., et al. (2006). Stage-dependent analgesia of electro-acupuncture in a mouse model of cutaneous cancer pain. *European Journal of Pain, 10,* 689–694.

Mao-Ying, Q. L., Ren, D. H., Mi, W. L., Liu, Q., & Wang, Y. Q. (2008). Analgesic effects of electroacupuncture combined with Celebrex on rats with tibial cancer pain. *Journal of Chinese Integrative Medicine, 6,* 830–835.

Mayer, D. J. (2000). Biological mechanisms of acupuncture. *Progress in Brain Research, 122,* 457–477.

Mehnert, A., & Koch, U. (2008). Psychological comorbidity and health-related quality of life and its association with awareness, utilization, and need for psychosocial support in a cancer register-based sample of long-term breast cancer survivors. *Journal of Psychosomatic Research, 64,* 383–391.

Melchart, D., Streng, A., Hoppe, A., Brinkhaus, B., Witt, C., Wagenpfeil, S., et al. (2005). Acupuncture in patients with tension-type headache: Randomised controlled trial. *British Medical Journal, 331,* 376–382.

Meng, X., Zhang, Y., Li, A., Xin, J., Lao, L., Ren, K., et al. (2011). The effects of opioid receptor antagonists on electroacupuncture-produced anti-allodynia/hyperalgesia in rats with paclitaxel-evoked peripheral neuropathy. *Brain Research, 1414,* 58–65.

Molassiotis, A., Sylt, P., & Diggins, H. (2007). The management of cancer-related fatigue after chemotherapy with acupuncture and acupressure: A randomised controlled trial. *Complementary Therapies in Medicine, 15,* 228–237.

Napadow, V., Makris, N., Liu, J., Kettner, N. W., Kwong, K. K., & Hui, K. K. S. (2005). Effects of electroacupuncture versus manual acupuncture on the human brain as measured by fMRI. *Human Brain Mapping, 24,* 193–205.

O'Regan, D., & Filshie, J. (2010). Acupuncture and cancer. *Autonomic Neuroscience: Basic & Clinical, 157,* 96–100.

Pachman, D. R., Barton, D. L., Watson, J. C., & Loprinzi, C. L. (2011). Chemotherapy-Induced Peripheral Neuropathy: Prevention and Treatment. *Clinical Pharmacology and Therapeutics, 90,* 377–387.

Paley, C. A., & Johnson, M. I. (2011). Acupuncture for cancer-induced bone pain: A pilot study. *Acupuncture in Medicine: Journal of the British Medical Acupuncture Society, 29,* 71–73.

Paley, C. A., Johnson, M. I., & Bennett, M. I. (2011a). Should physiotherapists use acupuncture for treating patients with cancer-induced bone pain? A discussion paper. *Physiotherapy, 97,* 256–263.

Paley, C. A., Johnson, M. I., Tashani, O. A., & Bagnall, A. M. (2011b). Acupuncture for cancer pain in adults. *Cochrane Database of Systematic Reviews, 1,* CD007753.

Pei, J., We, IH., Liu, Z. D., Yu, Y. M., Ni, C. R., & Wu, H. G. (2010). Effects of moxibustion on the expression of IL-1beta, IL-2, IL-6 mRNA and protein in the cerebral cortex in tumor-bearing mice. *Acupuncture Research, 35,* 243–249.

Peltier, A. C., & Russell, J. W. (2002). Recent advances in drug-induced neuropathies. *Current Opinion in Neurology, 15,* 633–638.

Polomano, R. C., Mannes, A. J., Clark, U. S., & Bennett, G. J. (2001). A painful peripheral neuropathy in the rat produced by the chemotherapeutic drug, paclitaxel. *Pain, 94,* 293–304.

Qin, F. H., & Qin, Y. H. (2001). Therapy of pressing and moxibustion in treating 36 cases of pain due to primary liver cancer. *Zhongguo Zhen Jiu, 21,* 540.

Qiu, X., Chen, K., Tong, L., Shu, X., Lü, X., Wen, H., et al. (2004). Effects of moxibustion at shenque (CV 8) on serum IL-12 level and NK cell activities in mice with transplanted tumor. *Journal of Traditional Chinese Medicine, 24,* 56–58.

Quasthoff, S., & Hartung, H. P. (2002). Chemotherapy-induced peripheral neuropathy. *Journal of Neurology, 249,* 9–17.

Reale, C., Turkiewicz, A. M., & Reale, C. A. (2001). Antalgic treatment of pain associated with bone metastases. *Critical Reviews in Oncology/Hematology, 37,* 1–11.

Salvo, N., Zeng, L., Zhang, L., Leung, M., Khan, L., Presutti, R., et al. (2011). Frequency of reporting and predictive factors for anxiety and depression in patients with advanced cancer. *Clinical Oncology (Royal College of Radiologists), 24,* 139–148.

Sarkar, D. K., Boyadjieva, N. I., Chen, C. P., Ortigüela, M., Reuhl, K., Clement, E. M., et al. (2008). Cyclic adenosine monophosphate differentiated beta-endorphin neurons promote immune function and prevent prostate cancer growth. *Proceedings of the National Academy of Sciences of the United States of America, 105,* 9105–9110.

Sarkar, D. K., Zhang, C., Murugan, S., Dokur, M., Boyadjieva, N. I., Ortigüela, M., et al. (2011). Transplantation of β-Endorphin Neurons into the Hypothalamus Promotes Immune Function and Restricts the Growth and Metastasis of Mammary Carcinoma. *Cancer Research, 71,* 6282–6291.

She, Y. F., Qi, C. H., & Zhu, J. (2010). History and progress of study on electrical properties of acupoints at home and abroad. *Zhongguo Zhen Jiu 2010, 30,* 1047–1050.

Strang, P. (1998). Cancer pain–a provoker of emotional, social and existential distress. *Acta Oncologica, 37,* 641–644.

Sun, K., Yang, Y. H., Zhou, Z. L., Yang, J., & Shen, D. K. (2008). Clinical observations on the treatment of primary genual osteoarthritis of liver-kidney depletion type by aconite cake-separated moxibustion. Shanghai *J Acupunct Moxibustion, 27,* 9–10.

Taspinar, A., & Sirin, A. (2010). Effect of acupressure on chemotherapy-induced nausea and vomiting in gynecologic cancer patients in Turkey. *European Journal of Oncology Nursing, 14,* 49–54.

Taylor, D., Meader, N., Bird, V., Pilling, S., Creed, F., Goldberg, D., et al. (2011). Pharmacological interventions for people with depression and chronic physical health problems: Systematic review and meta-analyses of safety and efficacy. *The British Journal of Psychiatry, 198,* 179–188.

Uryu, N., Okada, K., & Kawakita, K. (2007). Analgesic effects of indirect moxibustion on an experimental rat model of osteoarthritis in the knee. *Acupuncture in Medicine, 25,* 175–183.

Wakao, K., Matsuzaki, I., Terao, K., Inoue-Murayama, M., Shimojo, N., & Murayama, Y. (2000). Involvement of granzyme B expression in the enhancement of natural killer activity by beta-endorphin. *Brain, Behavior, and Immunity, 14,* 27–40.

Wang, C., Zhou, D. F., Shuai, X. W., Liu, J. X., & Xie, P. Y. (2007). Effects and mechanisms of electroacupuncture at PC6 on frequency of transient lower esophageal sphincter relaxation in cats. *World Journal of Gastroenterology, 13,* 4873–4880.

Wang, J. Y., Xu, L., Zhang, R. X., & Lao, L. (2011). Traditional Chinese medicine for cancer pain. *Zhong Xi Yi Jie He Xue Bao, 9,* 129–134.

Wang, W. J., Lu, J., Niu, C. S., Huang, Y. R., Ma, Q., A Y. G., et al. (2010). Effects of electroacupuncture of unilateral and bilateral "zusanli" (ST 36) on serum TNF-alpha, IL-1 and IL-4 levels in rats with chronic inflammatory pain. *Acupuncture Research, 35,* 429–432.

Wang, Z. H., Zhu, J. Y., Li, T., & Leng, X. S. (2008). Proliferation of $CD4^{+}$ $CD25^{+}$ regulatory T cells of rat by different cytokines in vitro. *Zhonghua Yi Xue Za Zhi, 88,* 844–847.

Windebank, A. J., & Grisold, W. (2008). Chemotherapy-induced neuropathy. *Journal of the Peripheral Nervous System, 13,* 27–46.

Wolf, S., Barton, D., Kottschade, L., Grothey, A., & Loprinzi, C. (2008). Chemotherapy-induced peripheral neuropathy: Prevention and treatment strategies. *European Journal of Cancer, 44,* 1507–1515.

Wong, R., & Sagar, S. (2006). Acupuncture treatment for chemotherapy-induced peripheral neuropathy–a case series. *Acupuncture in Medicine, 24,* 87–91.

Wu, B., Zhou, R. X., & Zhou, M. S. (1996). Effect of acupuncture on immunomodulation in patients with malignant tumors. *Zhongguo Zhong Xi Yi Jie He Za Zhi, 16,* 139–141.

Wu, P., Cao, Y., & Wu, J. (2001). Effects of moxa-cone moxibustion at Guanyuan on erythrocytic immunity and its regulative function in tumor-bearing mice. *Journal of Traditional Chinese Medicine, 21,* 68–71.

Yates, J., Rovis, F., Mitchell, P., Afzali, B., Tsang, J. Y., Garin, M., et al. (2007). The maintenance of human $CD4^+$ $CD25^+$ regulatory T cell function: IL-2, IL-4, IL-7 and IL-15 preserve optimal suppressive potency in vitro. *International Immunology, 19,* 785–799.

Ye, F., Chen, S., & Liu, W. (2002). Effects of electro-acupuncture on immune function after chemotherapy in 28 cases. *Journal of Traditional Chinese Medicine, 22,* 21–23.

Ye, F., Liu, D., Wang, S., & Xu, L. (2007). Effects of electro-acupuncture on T cell subpopulations, NK activity, humoral immunity and leukocyte count in patients undergoing chemotherapy. *Journal of Traditional Chinese Medicine, 27,* 19–21.

Yin, C. S., Jeong, H. S., Park, H. J., Baik, Y., Yoon, M. H., Choi, C. B., et al. (2008). A proposed transpositional acupoint system in a mouse and rat model. *Research in Veterinary Science, 84,* 159–165.

Yu, Y., Kasahara, T., Sato, T., Asano, K., Yu, G-D., Fang, J-Q., et al. (1998). Role of endogenous interferon-γ on the enhancement of splenic NK cell activity by electroacupuncture stimulation in mice. *Journal of Neuroimmunology, 90,* 176–186.

Zan, H. M., & Zhang, D. C. (1999). Application of acupuncture in relieving pain of terminal cancer. *Hua Bei Mei Tan Yi Xue Yuan Xue Bao, 1,* 586–587.

Zhai, D., Chen, H., Wang, R., Hua, X., Ding, B., & Jiang, Y. (1994). Regulation on beta-END in tumor-bearing mice by moxibustion on Guanyuan point. *Acupuncture Research, 19,* 63–65.

Zhang, G. G., Yu, C., Lee, W., Lao, L., Ren, K., & Berman, B. M. (2005a). Involvement of peripheral opioid mechanisms in electroacupuncture analgesia. *Explore, 1,* 365–371.

Zhang, Q. R., & Fu, W. B. (2010). Osteoarthritis of knee joint treated with acupuncture and moxibustion. *Zhongguo Zhen Jiu, 30,* 375–378.

Zhang, R. X., & Lao, L. (2010). Modern Cancer Research on Chinese Medicine: Acupuncture. In W. C. Cho (Ed.), *Supportive cancer care with Chinese medicine* (pp. 253–270). Heidelberg: Springer.

Zhang, R. X., Li, A., Liu, B., Wang, L., Ren, K., Qiao, J. T., et al. (2008a). Electroacupuncture attenuates bone cancer pain and inhibits spinal interleukin-1 beta expression in a rat model. *Anesthesia and Analgesia, 105,* 1482–1488.

Zhang, R. X., Li, A., Liu, B., Wang, L., Xin, J., Ren, K., et al. (2008b). Electroacupuncture attenuates bone-cancer-induced hyperalgesia and inhibits spinal preprodynorphin expression in a rat model. *European Journal of Pain, 12,* 870–878.

Zhang, R. X., Liu, B., Wang, L., Ren, K., Qiao, J. T., Berman, B. M., et al. (2005b). Spinal glial activation in a new rat model of bone cancer pain produced by prostate cancer cell inoculation of the tibia. *Pain, 118,* 125–136.

Zhang, S. Y., & Du, Y. Q. (2011). Effects of warming needle moxibustion on improvement of gastrointestinal and immune function in patients with postoperation of colorectal cancer. *Zhongguo Zhen Jiu, 31,* 513–517.

Zhang, W., Zhao, G. G., Su, L. Q., Zheng, Li. X., & Zhi-Hong, Y. (2011a). Effect, of acupuncture of different acupoints on immune function in rats with exhausted swimming. *Acupuncture Research, 36,* 181–186.

Zhang, Y., Li, A., Lao, L., Xin, J., Ren, K., Berman, B. M., et al. (2011b). Rostral ventromedial medulla μ but not κ, opioid receptors are involved in electroacupuncture anti-hyperalgesia in an inflammatory pain rat model. *Brain Research, 1395,* 38–45.

Zhang, Z., Wang, C., Gu, G., Li, H., Zhao, H., Wang, K., et al. (2012). The effects of electroacupuncture at the ST36 (Zusanli) acupoint on cancer pain and transient receptor potential vanilloid subfamily 1 expression in Walker 256 tumor-bearing rats. *Anesthesia & Analgesia, 114,* 879–885.

Zhao, C. L., Peng, L. J., Zhang, Z. L., Zhang, T., & Li, H. M. (2010). Effect of acupuncture on the activity of the peripheral blood T lymphocyte subsets and NK cells in patients with colorectal cancer liver metastasis. *Zhongguo Zhen Jiu, 30,* 10–12.

Zhao, R. H., & Zhu, Y. B. (2009). Observation on therapeutic effect of herb-partitioned moxibustion on fibromyalgia syndrome. *Zhongguo Zhen Jiu, 29,* 200–202.

Zhao, Z. (2008). Neural mechanism underlying acupuncture analgesia. *Progress in Neurobiology, 85,* 355–375.

Zhong, J., Lin, C., Fang, G., Li, J. J., & Chen, P. (2010). Observation on therapeutic effect of plum-blossom needle combined with medicated thread moxibustion of traditional zhuang nationality medicine on postherpetic neuralgia. *Zhongguo Zhen Jiu, 30,* 773–776.

Zhou, E. H., Liu, H. R., Wu, H. G., Shi, Y., Wang, X. M., Tan, L. Y., et al. (2009). Suspended moxibustion relieves chronic visceral hyperalgesia via serotonin pathway in the colon. *Neuroscience Letters, 451,* 144–147.

Zhu, Y. B. C., Zhuo, L. S., & Feng, W. Q. (2009a). Influence of electroacupuncture on hippocampal somatostatin (SS) and SS mRNA expression in chronic stress-induced depression rats. *Acupuncture Research, 34,* 175–179.

Zhu, Y., Liu, Q. Y., & Zhuo, L. S. (2009b). Influence of electroacupuncture of "Baihui" (GV 20) and "Sanyinjiao" (SP 6) on hippocampal 5-HT and AChE immuno-activity in chronic depression rats. *Acupuncture Research, 34,* 16–20.

Chapter 14
Integrating Acupuncture with Western Medicine in Cancer Treatment

Jun J. Mao and Malini M. Khanna

Abstract Cancer and its many conventional treatments (e.g. chemotherapy, radiotherapy, surgery, and hormonal therapies) can result in substantial symptom burden and diminished quality of life among cancer patients as well as threaten the long term physical and psychological wellbeing of growing numbers of cancer survivors. Acupuncture, an ancient therapy of traditional Chinese medicine, is increasingly being integrated into conventional cancer treatment and survivorship care. We first described the need for the integration of acupuncture into cancer care by reviewing the burden that cancer places on both society and on individuals. Secondly, we review the use of complementary and alternative medicine by individuals with cancer, highlighting the value for potential integration of acupuncture into conventional care. Thirdly, we summarize the current evidence of acupuncture's effectiveness for specific conditions experienced by cancer patients. Fourthly, we discuss the decision making process employed by patients regarding integration of acupuncture into cancer care. Finally, we provide some insight about how research can inform evidence development and generation. In summary, while research is limited, because of the large unmet needs experienced by cancer patients and limitations of conventional cancer care, acupuncture demonstrates potential as a therapy that can be safely integrated into conventional cancer care to improve symptom management and quality of life for cancer patients.

14.1 A Case Study

Jane Smith (not her real name) is a 56-year old women diagnosed with stage IIB hormone receptor positive breast cancer. She received excellent oncology care, including a unilateral mastectomy with lymph node dissection and chemotherapy followed by a course of radiotherapy. She is currently taking letrozole, an aromatase inhibitor,

J. J. Mao (✉)
Department of Family Medicine and Community Health, Abramson Comprehensive Cancer Center, Perelman School of Medicine, University of Pennsylvania, 3400 Spruce Street/2 Gates, Philadelphia, PA 19104, USA
e-mail: maoj@uphs.upenn.edu

M. M. Khanna
Department of Physical Medicine and Rehabilitation, Perelman School of Medicine, University of Pennsylvania, 3400 Spruce Street/ 5 Gates, Philadelphia, PA 19104, USA

W. C. S. Cho (ed.), *Acupuncture and Moxibustion as an Evidence-based Therapy for Cancer*, Evidence-based Anticancer Complementary and Alternative Medicine 3,
DOI 10.1007/978-94-007-4833-0_14,

which she will continue to take for five years because her tumor is estrogen receptor positive. She feels lucky that her cancer is considered to be cured, but struggles with thoughts of recurrence from time to time. Although Jane had finished her primary cancer treatments at the time that she met Dr Mao, she reported that she did "not feel like my old self." She had gained 7 kg following her cancer diagnosis, and in the 3 months since she had started to take the aromatase inhibitor, she had also begun experiencing some common side effects of the letrozole, including arthralgias and myalgias. Jane began having diffuse achiness in the joints of her hands, fingers, and knees: "I am 56," she said, "but I feel that I am 80 years old. I cannot stand the thought of taking this drug for the next five years." She used to enjoy running but reported that she could not run any more, and, instead, struggled to walk about a mile per day to maintain some level of fitness. She was seriously considering discontinuing her aromatase inhibitor, and thereby increasing her risk for recurrence, all due to the decline in her quality of life caused by this medication.

When she presented to Dr Mao's office, her average pain rating per week was a 7 out of a possible 10. Her fingers were mildly edematous and she did not have any focal erythema or warmth in any of her joints. After four sessions of electroacupuncture (acupuncture combined with 2 Hz electro-stimulation *via* a TENS unit), her pain was reduced to a 2 out of 10 on average. Following three more treatments, her pain was too minimal for her to continue since she had to pay for the visits out-of-pocket. In addition to reported improvement in pain, Jane also reported decreased anxiety and a decrease in her level of fatigue. Jane resumed running and felt more like her old self. Both Jane and her oncologist were happy that her symptoms were reduced and that she felt able to continue with her aromatase inhibitor therapy as originally planned.

14.2 Impact of Cancer on Society and Individuals

Jane is just one example of the millions of individuals affected by cancer each year around the globe. According to the World Health Organization (WHO), cancer has a greater economic impact than any other disease worldwide, with patients and families facing premature death and disability. The top three cancers with the highest economic impact are lung, colorectal, and breast cancers. The projected economic burden in 2008 was US$895 billion, which represented roughly 1.5% of the world's GDP. Additionally, it was calculated that 83 million years of "healthy life" were lost to disability and death associated with these cancers (American Cancer Society 2010).

Despite the tremendous progress that has been made in cancer prevention and treatment over the last 50 years, individuals with cancer continue to experience substantial unmet needs (Barg et al. 2007). As cancer has shifted from an almost universally fatal illness to a curable but more often chronic disease, the needs of cancer patients in various domains have gained increasing recognition in research and clinical care (Rowland and Baker 2005; Hewitt et al. 2006; Feuerstein 2007). Cancer patients experience both physical (e.g. chronic pain, fatigue) and psychological (e.g. depression/anxiety, sleep) problems at higher rates than the general population (Cleeland et al. 1994; Savard and Morin 2001; National Institutes of Health State-of-the-Science Panel 2003) (Mao et al. 2007a). Even after being cured of cancer, a subset of individuals continue to have a high level of fear and uncertainty regarding the potential for recurrence or a secondary cancer (Baker et al. 2005; Roberts et al. 2005; Rowland and Baker 2005). While conventional treatments like surgery, chemotherapy and radiation have significantly reduced cancer-related mortality, these therapies often result in substantial temporary and long-term effects that may negatively impact patients' quality of life and functional status (Ganz et al. 2002; Hewitt et al. 2006).

14.3 Use of Complementary and Alternative Medicine (CAM) by Cancer Patients

The challenges faced by individuals with cancer are numerous and require a thoughtful comprehensive treatment and support system to meet these challenges. CAM represents a group of therapies or health practices that are not routinely taught in Western medical schools or provided in Western hospitals (Eisenberg et al. 1993). However, the use of CAM is extensive among cancer patients and survivors (Ernst and Cassileth 1998; Yates et al. 2005; Boon et al. 2007), exceeding the rates seen in the general population without cancer (Mao et al. 2007a). Most cancer survivors use CAM as an adjunct to (complementary) rather than as a substitute for conventional treatments (alternative) (Burstein et al. 1999). While several demographic characteristics such as younger age, female sex and higher education have been shown to predict CAM use in the Western world (Mao et al. 2007b), the psychosocial factors associated with CAM use among cancer survivors often include symptom and psychological distress, increased perceived risk of dying, fear of recurrence, and gaining control (Burstein et al. 1999; Henderson and Donatelle 2003; Davidson et al. 2005; Rakovitch et al. 2005). Recently, using a population-based database comparing individuals with and without cancer, we found that cancer survivors were likely to use CAM for pain control, immune enhancement, and general wellness and disease prevention (Mao et al. 2010).

Emerging research also suggests patients' unmet needs in current conventional cancer care may drive them to use CAM. Paltiel at al. (2001) found perceived needs unmet by conventional medicine were an important determinant of recent CAM use in a large cohort of Israeli cancer patients. In a qualitative study, prostate cancer patients identified several key limitations of existing conventional cancer care: lack of empathy and support during and after treatment, lack of guidance on lifestyle change such as diet and exercise, and poor continuity of care; therefore, they turned to CAM to address these unmet needs (Evans et al. 2007). Additionally, adult survivors of childhood cancer were found to use CAM to address symptoms related to previous diagnosis and treatment (Mertens et al. 2008). Furthermore, research from our group found that those cancer patients with unmet needs in the domains of emotional, physical, nutritional, financial, informational, treatment-related, employment-related, and daily living activities were more likely to use CAM (Mao et al. 2008). In summary, CAM plays an important role in a comprehensive cancer treatment plan that helps meet cancer patients' diverse needs.

Table 14.1 Acupuncture and cancer information on the web

Organization	Web link
National Cancer Institute	http://www.cancer.gov
National Center for Complementary and Alternative Medicine	http://nccam.nih.gov
American Cancer Society	http://www.cancer.org
Susan G. Komen for the Cure	http://ww5.komen.org
OncoLink	http://www.oncolink.org
Breastcancer.org	http://www.breastcancer.org

14.4 Current Integration of Acupuncture in Cancer Care

Acupuncture, a central element of Traditional Chinese Medicine, originated from China at least 3,500 years ago and has been used by millions of individuals around the world. It is also becoming increasingly popular in developed nations and is seen regularly in the Western world. In the United States alone, acupuncture was used by approximately 2 million adults 18 or older in 2002 (Barnes et al. 2004). This number exceeded 3 million in 2007, representing 50% growth in the past 5 years (Barnes et al. 2009). Among its users, 44% of individuals sought acupuncture care because conventional medical care did not help them with their conditions, while 57% felt that combining acupuncture with conventional medical care would help with their specific conditions. Approximately 25–35% of respondents indicated that conventional medical professionals recommended their acupuncture use. This data suggests that patients are turning to acupuncture to fulfill their needs that remained unaddressed through the current conventional health system. Further, among users, 46% felt acupuncture helped a great deal, 26% felt it somewhat help, and about 28% perceived that it provided very little or no help (Burke et al. 2006).

Using population-based data, we found that 10.2% of US cancer patients have used acupuncture, which is a significantly higher percentage than the 6.2% that is found in the general population (Mao et al. 2010). In a survey study among breast cancer patients in a large urban academic cancer center, the majority of patients are in favor of integrating CAM services, including acupuncture, massage, yoga, or tai chi into the cancer center (Bonner Millar et al. 2010). Many large academic medical centers have begun offering acupuncture services in response to patient demand. In a study examining CAM content on the internet, Brauer et al. (2010) found that 59% of National Cancer Institute Designated Comprehensive Cancer Centers in the United States mentioned acupuncture on their websites as a means for managing symptoms and that this treatment tops the list of CAM and supportive care therapies. To assist in patients' medical decision making, the U.S. government (National Cancer Institute and National Center for Complementary and Alternative Medicine), large, well-established non-profit cancer organizations (American Cancer Society, Susan G. Komen Foundation), and popular online resources (Oncolink, Breastcancer.org) all provide information to educate patients about acupuncture (Table 14.1).

14.5 Current Status of Acupuncture Research

Although acupuncture has been practiced for thousands of years, more research must be conducted to elevate its status from that of a therapy used in a predominantly empirical manner to that of one that is more evidence-based and integrative as part of a comprehensive health system. The field of rigorous acupuncture research is fairly new but exciting and rapidly growing.

14.5.1 Mechanism of Acupuncture Effect

The precise mechanism of action for acupuncture has not been fully elucidated. Based on animal research, the acute analgesic effect of acupuncture is mediated in part by a complex system of CNS endogenous opioid (Han 2004), serotonin (Rho et al. 2008), GABA (Gan et al. 2005), and substance P (Aloe and Manni 2009; Lee et al. 2009). Over the last ten years, research using novel functional neuroimaging techniques, including positron emission tomography (PET) scan (Biella et al. 2001; Lewith et al. 2005; Pariente et al. 2005), single-photon emission computed tomography (SPECT) (Newberg et al. 2005), and functional MRI (Hui et al. 2000; Wu et al. 2002; Fang et al. 2004; Napadow et al. 2005) has provided important perspective about the CNS response to acupuncture. With acupuncture stimulation in both healthy subjects with experimentally induced pain and individuals with clinical pain, complex neural networks involved in cognition, emotion, stress, and pain processing have been modulated, including but not limited to the limbic system (Hui et al. 2000; Hui et al. 2005), hypothalamus and brainstem networks (Napadow et al. 2008). Of great importance, expectancy, a non-specific but powerful agent in clinical medicine, appears to mediate the CNS response to acupuncture (Harris et al. 2009; Kong et al. 2009; Lewith et al. 2005; Pariente et al. 2005). Peripherally, acupuncture can result in local vasodilatation (Boutouyrie et al. 2001; Litscher et al. 2002), connective tissue displacement and transduction (Langevin and Yandow 2002; Langevin et al. 2002, 2004), and inhibition of inflammatory response (Chae et al. 2007). All of these factors may play an important role in local signal transduction and tissue repair. Thus, the mechanism of acupuncture provides biological plausibility for managing cancer-related symptom distress such as pain, nausea, and fatigue. However, the effect is likely to be complex, recruiting both the central and peripheral networks and eliciting both physiological and psychological responses in individuals.

14.5.2 Clinical Research of Acupuncture in Oncology

The research field of acupuncture in oncology is still in its infancy. Before discussing clinical evidence, it is important to acknowledge the challenges of methodology in evaluating acupuncture, particularly the choice of control, an area of active debates

Table 14.2 Emerging areas of evidence for acupuncture integration

Symptoms	Evidence grade
Nausea/vomiting	High
Cancer or treatment-related pain	Intermediate
Xerostomia	Intermediate
Hot flashes	Intermediate
Fatigue	Low

and continued controversies (Park et al. 2008). Each control helps answer a small and specific question about the effects of acupuncture such as specific location, depth of needling and penetration of skin (Vickers 2002; White 2002). However, all of the control results in sensory stimulation which may excite diffuse noxious inhibitory control (Bing et al. 1990), a physiological response that is not inert. Acupuncture research methodologists argue that acupuncture trials ought to be conducted with 3-arms: true acupuncture, placebo/sham control and standard medical care. In this way, the specific efficacy of needling effects and clinical relevance of acupuncture as an entire package of care can be evaluated simultaneously (Langevin et al. 2006). While large and rigorously designed and conducted clinical trials of acupuncture for chronic pain (e.g. low back pain (Cherkin et al. 2009), knee osteoarthritis (Berman B 2004; Witt et al. 2005)) have been conducted in non-oncology patients, trials of acupuncture in oncology settings often have substantial limitations, including small sample size, poor choice of control or no control, inadequate acupuncture protocols (e.g. use one point rather than a comprehensive acupuncture protocol) and problematic population characteristics. Thus, the evidence-base for safe and effective integration of acupuncture is just emerging and far from complete.

14.6 Emerging Areas of Evidence for Integration

There are several areas with emerging evidence based on limited research about acupuncture. These are also areas where the evidence for conventional medicine is either lacking or incomplete so the potential for integration of acupuncture to contribute is great (Table 14.2). Since a detailed review of these specific areas has been provided in other chapters, we will briefly review the evidence coupled with the author's clinical experience as a symptom/palliative care physician and acupuncturist.

14.6.1 Nausea and Vomiting

One of the most challenging side effects of chemotherapy is controlling emesis. Medications such as 5-HT_3 receptor antagonists and dexamethasone have provided patients with some relief of chemotherapy-induced emesis (Campora et al. 1994). However, many patients still experience symptoms which significantly affect their quality of life. In the late 1990s, acupuncture gained popularity with the National Institutes of Health's publication of its 1997 Consensus Statement stating that "promising results have emerged, for example, showing efficacy of acupuncture in adult postoperative and chemotherapy nausea and vomiting... in which acupuncture may be useful as an adjunct treatment or an acceptable alternative or be included in a comprehensive management program" (NIH 1998). Dundee et al. found that the most common point used to control nausea and vomiting is Neiguan (PC6) (Dundee 1998). A study by Shen et al. (2000) demonstrated that adding electroacupuncture was more effective in controlling emesis than minimal needling or using pharmacotherapy alone. Ezzo et al. reviewed data from 1,247 subjects in 11 trials and found that electroacupuncture reduced chemotherapy-induced acute vomiting (Ezzo et al. 2005). Given the effectiveness of current anti-emetic medication, the biggest potential for acupuncture integration is for nausea and vomiting that are refractory to conventional medications as well as for persistent residual nausea post-chemotherapy where existing approaches are very limited.

14.6.2 Cancer Pain

Pain in cancer patients can be caused by pre-existing pathologies (e.g. arthritis), cancer status (progression of the disease or metastasis) or treatment (e.g. surgery, chemotherapy, radiotherapy, hormonal therapy). Analgesic medications do not usually provide adequate pain relief (Caraceni and Portenoy 1999). Acupuncture may provide a treatment that is less sedating with less constipating side effects than conventional treatment. A study by Alimi et al. (2003) found a favorable response to auricular acupuncture using an ear stimulator to guide needle placement *vs* using placebo auricular points. In a recent RCT among patients who had head and neck cancer and status post neck dissection, acupuncture was found to reduce pain, and improve functions and xerostomia when compared to usual care (included physical therapy, analgesia, and/or anti-inflammatory medications) (Pfister et al. 2010). However, due to the paucity of the data, in a Cochrane review published in early 2011, the authors concluded that there is insufficient evidence that acupuncture is effective in treating cancer pain and patients should be aware of the limitations before treatment begins (Paley et al. 2011). In clinical practice, acupuncture should not be used as the first line of treatment in the setting of severe and intractable pain if patient-assisted analgesia is available. In settings where medication is not readily available, acupuncture can be utilized to decrease pain or pain-related anxiety. For moderate to severe pain, acupuncture may be used as an adjunct to existing pharmacological treatment to reduce the need for opioid escalation and lower its associated side effects such as sedation and constipation. In the context of mild to moderate pain or survivorship following primary treatment, acupuncture may be used as an alternative to medications if individuals desire a non-pharmacological approach to their symptom management. While these are all potential areas for acupuncture to be integrated, research is needed to inform evidence-based care.

14.6.3 Arthralgia-related to Aromatase Inhibitors (AIs)

Recent studies have shown that AIs are more effective at treating breast cancer than tamoxifen (Baum et al. 2002; Coombes et al. 2004; Goss et al. 2005). Despite their efficacies, close to 50% of individuals taking AIs develop arthralgia or joint pain using this kind of medications (Mao et al. 2009b, 2011), resulting in substantial premature discontinuation of therapy. Crews et al. (2007, 2010) found that acupuncture reduced pain and stiffness among postmenopausal women undergoing AI treatment after 6 weeks of treatment. Electroacupuncture has also shown promise to reduce pain severity, stiffness, and joint symptom interference in a small preliminary study (Mao et al. 2009a). A larger randomized-placebo controlled trial on this topic is currently being conducted by our group. Given that there are no current conventional therapies that have demonstrated efficacy in this setting, acupuncture appears to be the most promising therapy for this condition.

14.6.4 Xerostomia

Radiation induced xerostomia (dry mouth) drastically reduces the quality of life for patients with head and neck cancer. Patients may suffer from dysphagia, difficulty speaking, and alteration of taste and loss of appetite (Garcia et al. 2009). Saliva substitutes and stimulant agents have been developed, however none have been proven to be clinically efficacious (Chambers et al. 2007). A study by Cho et al. (2008) reported a significant increase in unstimulated salivary production compared to using sham acupuncture points. A single arm pilot study found that acupuncture can improve symptoms of xerostomia and physical well-being (Garcia et al. 2009). In a recent trial, Meng et al. (2012) found that acupuncture prevented the development of xerostomia (both self-reported and measured salivary flow) compared to standard care for head and neck cancer patients undergoing radiation therapy. Cohen et al. are currently conducting two large placebo controlled randomized trial: (1) to prevent radiation induced xerostomia ($n = 300$); and (2) to treat radiation induced xerostomia ($n = 240$) (personal communication with Dr. Lorenzo Cohen at MD Anderson Cancer Center, US). These results will provide more convincing evidence about the potential use of acupuncture to prevent as well as to treat xerostomia.

14.6.5 Hot Flashes

Hot flashes are a common symptom affecting many breast cancer patients. Current medications prescribed to treat vasomotor symptoms include clonidine, progesterone and selective serotonin reuptake inhibitors (SSRIs). Hormone replacement therapy is contraindicated in this population. Additionally, many women refuse to take additional medication due to adverse side effects common to SSRIs (sexual side effect, weight gain). In a RCT by Walker et al. (2010) acupuncture was as effective as taking venlafaxine in decreasing hot flashes with an additional benefit of increased libido in some women. Another study reported reduced hot flash frequency in both the acupuncture and sham group during the 10 week treatment; however results did not last in the sham group at the 12 week follow-up (Hervik and Mjaland 2009). Our group is currently conducting a large randomized controlled trial comparing acupuncture against gabapentin for hot flashes ($n = 124$). Current evidence suggests acupuncture may produce an effect size that is similar to existing non-hormonal based medication, thereby providing a therapeutic option for individuals who do not want to take another medication for their hot flashes.

14.6.6 Fatigue

Cancer-related fatigue is one of the most prominent symptoms patients encounter from cancer treatments with up to 90% of patients receiving chemotherapy and up to 80% of patients receiving radiation reporting this issue (Molassiotis et al. 2007). Fatigue can also persist after therapy has been completed. Acupuncture is a promising complementary therapy for the treatment of fatigue, a condition that is currently one of the top reasons people in the United States visit acupuncturists (Cherkin et al. 2002). Molasisotis et al. (2007) found acupuncture resulted in a 36% improvement in fatigue compared with only 19% improvement in the group using acupressure at those points and 0.6% improvement in the sham acupressure group. A study done at Memorial Sloan-Kettering Cancer Center found the mean improvement of fatigue 2 years post-treatment to be about 31.1% (Vickers et al. 2004). Another study done by our group demonstrated that acupuncture enabled patients' fatigue levels to remain relatively stable during radiation therapy. This suggests that acupuncture may help prevent the development of substantial cancer-related fatigue (Mao et al. 2009c). As fatigue is multi-factorial, combining acupuncture with other behavioral interventions (e.g. exercise, sleep hygiene) may help address this important issue in an oncology setting.

14.7 Evidence-based Decision Making by Cancer Patients to Use Acupuncture

In addressing how best to integrate acupuncture into conventional cancer care, health care providers must assist patients with making decisions that are congruent with their belief systems, but also based on research evidence. In a recent study (Mao et al. 2012), we interviewed 25 breast cancer survivors with hot flashes about their decision making process regarding incorporating acupuncture into their symptom management plan. Many women voiced a desire to use acupuncture because they perceived it to be "natural." They could thereby avoid adding another medication

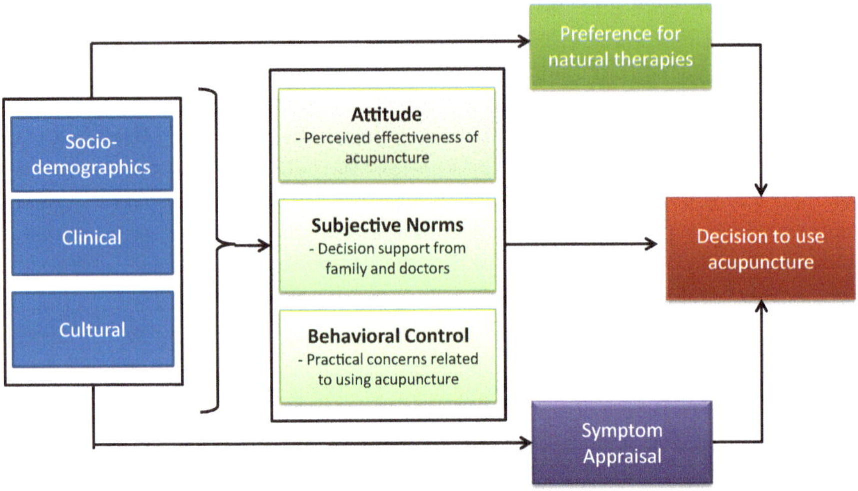

Fig. 14.1 Factors related to decision making about acupuncture

to their already extensive list of drugs. In addition, individuals with a positive expectancy of acupuncture, which is often built on the experiences of their family and friend, want to try acupuncture.

However, a fear/dislike of needles and lack of scientific understanding of acupuncture makes some individuals less inclined to try this treatment. Many barriers ranging from cost/lack of insurance coverage to distance to time commitments to finding qualified acupuncturists prevent some individuals from using acupuncture. Finally, decision support from family members and physicians is important for individuals in choosing one therapy (e.g. acupuncture) *vs* another (e.g. medication). Our study suggests decision making for the use of acupuncture in cancer care is personalized and driven by multiple considerations (Fig. 14.1). Health care professionals must be sensitive to the beliefs and barriers each patient may have and to help support patients in making decisions that ultimately lead to good clinical outcomes.

14.8 Summary and Future Directions

Acupuncture, an ancient traditional Chinese medicine practice, is gradually being integrated into conventional medicine to build a comprehensive and personalized system of care for cancer patients. Despite the longevity of this medical practice, the existing scientific evidence base for acupuncture in oncology is limited. Carefully designed basic science experiments, clinical trials, and outcome studies are needed to expand our understanding of the mechanisms, efficacy, and effectiveness of acupuncture for specific conditions faced by cancer patients. It is important to put acupuncture research in the larger context of cancer care and science (Fig. 14.2).

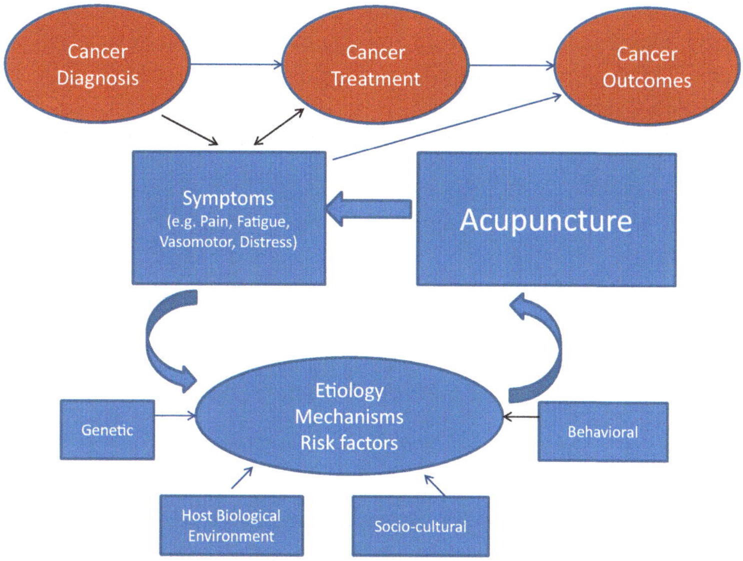

Fig. 14.2 Integrative acupuncture research framework

As cancer diagnosis and treatments result in symptom burden, carefully designed epidemiological research is necessary to investigate the prevalence and progression of these symptoms as well as risk factors for these symptoms. By doing so, it will help inform acupuncture trial design and conduct, so adequately powered randomized controlled clinical trials of acupuncture can be conducted. For example, if a symptom will resolve in six weeks regardless of treatments, doing a six week RCT of acupuncture in that setting will be futile. Basic research will uncover both the mechanisms of symptoms and acupuncture thereby, creating a linkage for symptoms and acupuncture to be paired appropriately for clinical and translational research. Additionally, observational studies and feasibility Phase I studies are needed to discover the optimal treatment design for acupuncture (e.g. electro or non-electroacupuncture, point selection, frequency of treatments, duration of treatments, standardized or manualized treatments). Such studies are necessary for larger trials so that the acupuncture treatment itself is authentic to practice and adequate to produce an expected therapeutic effect. Further, carefully integrated biomarkers and behavioral theories should be applied in acupuncture clinical trials to inform both the mechanism of acupuncture and predictors of treatment response. Lastly, as acupuncture is often used for refractory symptoms or in the setting of palliative and supportive care (e.g. persistent hiccups after radiation for a gastric tumor), large clinical trials for these difficult cases/symptoms may simply never be conducted due to sample size issues and ethical considerations. Quality case studies/series and rigorous qualitative methods can be applied to build the evidence base.

Ultimately, the collective evidence will grow and guide clinicians and patients to make informed medical decisions that both reflect patients' preferences and are based on understood benefits *vs* harms for acupuncture and other available therapies. Taken together, this will lead to evidence-based integration of acupuncture into conventional care, thereby improving the health and wellbeing of millions of individuals who are diagnosed with cancer each year.

References

Alimi, D., Rubino, C., Pichard-Leandri, E., Fermand-Brule, S., Dubreuil-Lemaire, M. L., & Hill, C. (2003). Analgesic effect of auricular acupuncture for cancer pain: A randomized, blinded, controlled trial. *Journal of Clinical Oncology, 21,* 4120–4126.

Aloe, L., & Manni, L. (2009). Low-frequency electro-acupuncture reduces the nociceptive response and the pain mediator enhancement induced by nerve growth factor. *Neuroscience Letters, 449,* 173–177.

Baker, F., Denniston, M., Smith, T., & West, M. M. (2005). Adult cancer survivors: How are they faring? *Cancer, 104,* 2565–2576.

Barg, F. K., Cronholm, P. F., Straton, J. B., Keddem, S., Knott, K., & Grater, J., et al. (2007). Unmet psychosocial needs of Pennsylvanians with cancer: 1986–2005. *Cancer, 110,* 631–639.

Barnes, P. M., Powell-Griner, E., McFann, K., & Nahin, R. L. (2004). Complementary and alternative medicine use among adults: United States. *Advance Data, 343,* 1–19.

Barnes, P. M., Bloom, B., & Nahin, R. L. (2009). Complementary and alternative medicine use among adults and children: United States. *National Health Statistics Reports,* 1–23.

Baum, M., Budzar, A. U., Cuzick, J., Forbes, J., Houghton, J. H., & Klijn, J. G., et al. (2002) Anastrozole alone or in combination with tamoxifen versus tamoxifen alone for adjuvant treatment of postmenopausal women with early breast cancer: First results of the ATAC randomised trial. *Lancet, 359,* 2131–2139.

Berman, B. L. L., Langenberg, P., Lee, W. L., Gilpin, A. M. K. & Hochberg, M. (2004). Effectiveness of acupuncture as adjunctive therapy in osteoarthritis of the knee. *Annals of Internal Medicine, 141,* 901–910.

Biella, G., Sotgiu, M. L., Pellegata, G., Paulesu, E., Castiglioni, I., & Fazio, F. (2001). Acupuncture produces central activations in pain regions. *Neuroimage, 14,* 60–66.

Bing, Z., Villanueva, L., & Le Bars, D. (1990). Acupuncture and diffuse noxious inhibitory controls: Naloxone-reversible depression of activities of trigeminal convergent neurons. *Neuroscience, 37,* 809–818.

Bonner Millar, L. P., Casarett, D., Vapiwala, N., DeMichele, A., Stricker, C., & Velders, L., et al. (2010). Integrating complementary therapies into an academic cancer center: The perspective of breast cancer patients. *Journal of The Society for Integrative Oncology, 8,* 106–113.

Boon, H. S., Olatunde, F., & Zick, S. M. (2007). Trends in complementary/alternative medicine use by breast cancer survivors: Comparing survey data from 1998 and 2005. *BMC Womens Health, 7,* 4.

Boutouyrie, P., Corvisier, R., Azizi, M., Lemoine, D., Laloux, B., & Hallouin, M., et al. (2001). Effects of acupuncture on radial artery hemodynamics: Controlled trials in sensitized and naive subjects. *American Journal of Physiology. Heart and Circulatory Physiology, 280,* H628–633.

Brauer, J. A., El, Sehamy, A., Metz, J. M., & Mao, J. J. (2010). Complementary and alternative medicine and supportive care at leading cancer centers: A systematic analysis of websites. *Journal of Alternative and Complementary Medicine, 16,* 183–186.

Burke, A., Upchurch, D. M., Dye, C., & Chyu, L. (2006). Acupuncture use in the United States: Findings from the National Health Interview Survey. *Journal of Alternative and Complementary Medicine, 12,* 639–648.

Burstein, H. J., Gelber, S., Guadagnoli, E., & Weeks, J. C. (1999). Use of alternative medicine by women with early-stage breast cancer. *New England Journal of Medicine, 340,* 1733–1739.

Campora, E., Giudici, S., Merlini, L., Rubagotti, A., & Rosso, R. (1994). Ondansetron and dexamethasone versus standard combination antiemetic therapy. A randomized trial for the prevention of acute and delayed emesis induced by cyclophosphamide-doxorubicin chemotherapy and maintenance of antiemetic effect at subsequent courses. *American Journal of Clinical Oncology, 17,* 522–526.

Caraceni, A., & Portenoy, R. K. (1999). An international survey of cancer pain characteristics and syndromes. IASP Task Force on Cancer Pain. International Association for the Study of Pain. *Pain, 82,* 263–274.

Chae, Y., Hong, M. S., Kim, G. H., Hahm, D. H., Park, H. J., & Ha, E., et al. (2007). Protein array analysis of cytokine levels on the action of acupuncture in carrageenan-induced inflammation. *Neurological Research, 29*(Suppl 1), S55–58.

Chambers, M. S., Rosenthal, D. I., & Weber, R. S. (2007). Radiation-induced xerostomia. *Head & Neck, 29,* 58–63.

Cherkin, D. C., Deyo, R. A., Sherman, K. J., Hart, L. G., Street, J. H., & Hrbek, A., et al. (2002). Characteristics of visits to licensed acupuncturists, chiropractors, massage therapists, and naturopathic physicians. *The Journal of the American Board of Family Practice, 15,* 463–472.

Cherkin, D. C., Sherman, K. J., Avins, A. L., Erro, J. H., Ichikawa, L., & Barlow, W. E., et al. (2009). A randomized trial comparing acupuncture, simulated acupuncture, and usual care for chronic low back pain. *Archives of Internal Medicine, 169,* 858–866.

Cho, J. H., Chung, W. K., Kang, W., Choi, S. M., Cho, C. K., & Son, C. G. (2008). Manual acupuncture improved quality of life in cancer patients with radiation-induced xerostomia. *Journal of Alternative and Complementary Medicine, 14,* 523–526.

Cleeland, C. S., Gonin, R., Hatfield, A. K., Edmonson, J. H., Blum, R. H., & Stewart, J. A., et al. (1994). Pain and its treatment in outpatients with metastatic cancer. *The New England Journal of Medicine, 330,* 592–596.

Coombes, R. C., Hall, E., Gibson, L. J., Paridaens, R., Jassem, J., & Delozier, T., et al. (2004). A randomized trial of exemestane after two to three years of tamoxifen therapy in postmenopausal women with primary breast cancer. *The New England Journal of Medicine, 350,* 1081–1092.

Crew, K. D., Capodice, J. L., Greenlee, H., Apollo, A., Jacobson, J. S., & Raptis, G., et al. (2007). Pilot study of acupuncture for the treatment of joint symptoms related to adjuvant aromatase inhibitor therapy in postmenopausal breast cancer patients. *Journal of Cancer Survivorship, 1,* 283–291.

Crew, K. D., Capodice, J. L., Greenlee, H., Brafman, L., Fuentes, D., & Awad, D., et al. (2010). Randomized, blinded, sham-controlled trial of acupuncture for the management of aromatase inhibitor-associated joint symptoms in women with early-stage breast cancer. *Journal of Clinical Oncology, 28,* 1154–1160.

Davidson, R., Geoghegan, L., Mc,Laughlin, L., & Woodward, R. (2005). Psychological characteristics of cancer patients who use complementary therapies. *Psychooncology, 14,* 187–195.

Dundee, J. (1998). Acupuncture as an antiemetic: Studies of its use in postoperative vomiting, cancer chemotherapy and sickness of early pregnancy. *Complementary Medicine Research, 3,* 2–14.

Eisenberg, D. M., Kessler, R. C., Foster, C., Norlock, F. E., Calkins, D. R., & Delbanco, T. L. (1993). Unconventional medicine in the United States. Prevalence, costs, and patterns of use. *New England Journal of Medicine, 328,* 246–252.

Ernst, E., & Cassileth, B. R. (1998). The prevalence of complementary/alternative medicine in cancer: a systematic review. *Cancer, 83,* 777–782.

Evans, M., Shaw, A., Thompson, E. A., Falk, S., Turton, P., & Thompson, T., et al. (2007). Decisions to use complementary and alternative medicine (CAM) by male cancer patients: Information-seeking roles and types of evidence used. *BMC Complementary and Alternative Medicine, 7,* 25.

Ezzo, J., Vickers, A., & Richardson, M. A., et al. (2005). Acupuncture-point stimulation for chemotherapy-induced nausea and vomiting. *Journal of Clinical Oncology, 23,* 7188–7198.

Fang, J. L., Krings, T., Weidemann, J., Meister, I. G., & Thron, A. (2004). Functional MRI in healthy subjects during acupuncture: Different effects of needle rotation in real and false acupoints. *Neuroradiology, 46,* 359–362.

Feuerstein, M. (2007). Defining cancer survivorship. *Journal of Cancer Survivorship, 1,* 5–7.

Gan, P., Cheng, J. S., Ng, Y. K., & Ling, E. A. (2005). Role of GABA in electro-acupuncture therapy on cerebral ischemia induced by occlusion of the middle cerebral artery in rats. *Neuroscience Letters, 383,* 317–321.

Ganz, P. A., Desmond, K. A., Leedham, B., Rowland, J. H., Meyerowitz, B. E., & Belin, T. R. (2002). Quality of life in long-term, disease-free survivors of breast cancer: A follow-up study. *Journal of the National Cancer Institute, 94,* 39–49.

Garcia, M. K., Chiang, J. S., Cohen, L., Liu, M., Palmer, J. L., & Rosenthal, D. I., et al. (2009). Acupuncture for radiation-induced xerostomia in patients with cancer: A pilot study. *Head & Neck, 31,* 1360–1368.

Goss, P. E., Ingle, J. N., Martino, S., Robert, N. J., Muss, H. B., & Piccart, M. J., et al. (2005). Randomized trial of letrozole following tamoxifen as extended adjuvant therapy in receptor-positive breast cancer: Updated findings from NCIC CTG MA.17. *Journal of the National Cancer Institute, 97,* 1262–1271.

Han, J. S. (2004). Acupuncture and endorphins. *Neuroscience Letters, 361,* 258–261.

Harris, R. E., Zubieta, J. K., Scott, D. J., Napadow, V., Gracely, R. H., & Clauw, D. J. (2009). Traditional Chinese acupuncture and placebo (sham) acupuncture are differentiated by their effects on mu-opioid receptors (MORs). *Neuroimage, 47,* 1077–1085.

Henderson, J. W., & Donatelle, R. J. (2003). The relationship between cancer locus of control and complementary and alternative medicine use by women diagnosed with breast cancer. *Psycho-oncology, 12,* 59–67.

Hervik, J., & Mjaland, O. (2009). Acupuncture for the treatment of hot flashes in breast cancer patients, a randomized, controlled trial. *Breast Cancer Research and Treatment, 116,* 311–316.

Hewitt, M., Greenfield, S., & Stovall, E., editors (2006). *From Cancer Patient to Cancer Survivor: Lost in Transition.* Washington: National Academies Press.

Hui, K. K., Liu, J., Makris, N., Gollub, R. L., Chen, A. J., & Moore, C. I., et al. (2000). Acupuncture modulates the limbic system and subcortical gray structures of the human brain: Evidence from fMRI studies in normal subjects. *Human Brain Mapping, 9,* 13–25.

Hui, K. K., Liu, J., Marina, O., Napadow, V., Haselgrove, C., & Kwong, K. K., et al. (2005). The integrated response of the human cerebro-cerebellar and limbic systems to acupuncture stimulation at ST 36 as evidenced by fMRI. *Neuroimage, 27,* 479–496.

John, M., & Ross, H. (2010). American Cancer Society. The global economic cost of cancer. http://www.cancer.org/acs/groups/content/@internationalaffairs/documents/document/acspc-026203.pdf. Accessed 9 July 2012.

Kong, J., Kaptchuk, T. J., Polich, G., Kirsch, I., Vangel, M., & Zyloney, C., et al. (2009). Expectancy and treatment interactions: A dissociation between acupuncture analgesia and expectancy evoked placebo analgesia. *Neuroimage, 45,* 940–949.

Langevin, H. M., & Yandow, J. A. (2002). Relationship of acupuncture points and meridians to connective tissue planes. *The Anatomical Record, 269,* 257–265.

Langevin, H. M., Churchill, D. L., Wu, J., Badger, G. J., Yandow, J. A., & Fox, J. R., et al. (2002). Evidence of connective tissue involvement in acupuncture. *The FASEB Journal, 16,* 872–874.

Langevin, H. M., Konofagou, E. E., Badger, G. J., Churchill, D. L., Fox, J. R., & Ophir, J., et al. (2004). Tissue displacements during acupuncture using ultrasound elastography techniques. *Ultrasound In Medicine & Biology, 30,* 1173–1183.

Langevin, H. M., Hammerschlag, R., Lao, L., Napadow, V., Schnyer, R. N., & Sherman, K. J. (2006). Controversies in acupuncture research: Selection of controls and outcome measures in acupuncture clinical trials. *Journal of Alternative and Complementary Medicine, 12,* 943–953.

Lee, H. J., Lee, J. H., Lee, E. O., Lee, H. J., Kim, K. H., & Kim, S. H., et al. (2009). Substance P and beta-endorphin mediate electro-acupuncture induced analgesia in mouse cancer pain model. *Journal of Experimental & Clinical Cancer Research, 28,* 102.

Lewith, G. T., White, P. J., & Pariente, J. (2005). Investigating acupuncture using brain imaging techniques: The current state of play. *Evidence-Based Complementary and Alternative Medicine, 2,* 315–319.

Litscher, G., Wang, L., Huber, E., & Nilsson, G. (2002). Changed skin blood perfusion in the fingertip following acupuncture needle introduction as evaluated by laser Doppler perfusion imaging. *Lasers in Medical Science, 17,* 19–25.

Mao, J., Bowman, M. A., Leed, R., Desai, K., Armstrong, K., & Barg, F. K. (2012). Acupuncture for hot flashes: decision making by breast cancer survivors. *Journal of the American Board of Family Medicine, 25,* 323–332.

Mao, J. J., Armstrong, K., Bowman, M. A., Xie, S. X., Kadakia, R., & Farrar, J. T. (2007a). Symptom burden among cancer survivors: Impact of age and comorbidity. *Journal of the American Board of Family Medicine, 20,* 434–443.

Mao, J. J., Farrar, J. T., Xie, S. X., Bowman, M. A., & Armstrong, K. (2007b). Use of complementary and alternative medicine and prayer among a national sample of cancer survivors compared to other populations without cancer. *Complementary Therapies in Medicine, 15,* 21–29.

Mao, J. J., Palmer, S. C., Straton, J. B., Cronholm, P. F., Keddem, S., & Knott, K., et al. (2008). Cancer survivors with unmet needs were more likely to use complementary and alternative medicine. *Journal of Cancer Survivorship, 2,* 116–124.

Mao, J. J., Bruner, D. W., Stricker, C., Farrar, J. T., Xie, S. X., & Bowman, M. A., et al. (2009a). Feasibility trial of electroacupuncture for aromatase inhibitor–related arthralgia in breast cancer survivors. *Integrative Cancer Therapies, 8,* 123–129.

Mao, J. J., Stricker, C., Bruner, D., Xie, S., Bowman, M. A., & Farrar, J. T., et al. (2009b). Patterns and risk factors associated with aromatase inhibitor-related arthralgia among breast cancer survivors. *Cancer, 115,* 3631–3639.

Mao, J. J., Styles, T., Cheville, A., Wolf, J., Fernandes, S., & Farrar, J. T. (2009c). Acupuncture for nonpalliative radiation therapy-related fatigue: Feasibility study. *Journal of The Society for Integrative Oncology, 7,* 52–58.

Mao, J. J., Palmer, C. S., Healy, K. E., Desai, K., & Amsterdam, J. (2010). Complementary and alternative medicine use among cancer survivors: A population-based study. *Journal of Cancer Survivorship, 5,* 8–17.

Mao, J. J., Su, H. I., Feng, R., Donelson, M. L., Aplenc, R., & Rebbeck, T. R., et al. (2011) Association of functional polymorphisms in CYP19A1 with aromatase inhibitor associated arthralgia in breast cancer survivors. *Breast Cancer Research, 13,* R8.

Meng, Z. M., Garcia, K., Hu, C., Chiang, J., Chambers, M., & Rosenthal, D. I., et al. (2012). Randomized controlled trial of acupuncture for prevention of radiation-Induced xerostomia among patients with nasopharyngeal carcinoma. *Cancer, 118,* 3337–3344.

Mertens, A. C., Sencer, S., Myers, C. D., Recklitis, C., Kadan,-Lottick, N., & Whitton, J., et al. (2008). Complementary and alternative therapy use in adult survivors of childhood cancer: A report from the Childhood Cancer Survivor Study. *Pediatric Blood & Cancer, 50,* 90–97.

Molassiotis, A., Sylt, P., & Diggins, H. (2007). The management of cancer-related fatigue after chemotherapy with acupuncture and acupressure: A randomised controlled trial. *Complementary Therapies in Medicine, 15,* 228–237.

Napadow, V., Makris, N., Liu, J., Kettner, N. W., Kwong, K. K., & Hui, K. K. (2005). Effects of electroacupuncture versus manual acupuncture on the human brain as measured by fMRI. *Human Brain Mapping, 24,* 193–205.

Napadow, V., Ahn, A., Longhurst, J., Lao, L., Stener-Victorin, E., & Harris, R., et al. (2008). The status and future of acupuncture mechanism research. *Journal of Alternative and Complementary Medicine, 14,* 861–869.

NIH Consensus Conference. (1998). Acupuncture. *JAMA, 280,* 1518–1524.

National Institutes of Health State-of-the-Science Panel. (2003). National Institutes of Health State-of-the-Science conference statement: Symptom management in cancer: Pain, depression, and fatigue, July 15–17 2002. *Journal of the National Cancer Institute, 95,* 1110–1117.

Newberg, A. B., Lariccia, P. J., Lee, B. Y., Farrar, J. T., Lee, L., & Alavi, A. (2005). Cerebral blood flow effects of pain and acupuncture: A preliminary single-photon emission computed tomography imaging study. *Journal of Neuroimaging, 15,* 43–49.

Paley, C. A., Johnson, M. I., Tashani, O. A., &Bagnall, A. M. (2011) Acupuncture for cancer pain in adults. *Cochrane Database of Systematic Reviews*: CD007753.

Paltiel, O., Avitzour, M., Peretz, T., Cherny, N., Kaduri, L., & Pfeffer, R. M., et al. (2001). Determinants of the use of complementary therapies by patients with cancer. *Journal of Clinical Oncology, 19,* 2439–2448.

Pariente, J., White, P., Frackowiak, R. S., & Lewith, G. (2005). Expectancy and belief modulate the neuronal substrates of pain treated by acupuncture. *Neuroimage, 25,* 1161–1167.

Park, J., Linde, K., Manheimer, E., Molsberger, A., Sherman, K., & Smith, C., et al. (2008). The status and future of acupuncture clinical research. *Journal of Alternative and Complementary Medicine, 14,* 871–881.

Pfister, D. G., Cassileth, B. R., Deng, G. E., Yeung, K. S., Lee, J. S., & Garrity, D., et al. (2010). Acupuncture for pain and dysfunction after neck dissection: Results of a randomized controlled trial. *Journal of Clinical Oncology, 28,* 2565–2570.

Rakovitch, E., Pignol, J. P., Chartier, C., Ezer, M., Verma, S., & Dranitsaris, G., et al. (2005). Complementary and alternative medicine use is associated with an increased perception of breast cancer risk and death. *Breast Cancer Research and Treatment, 90,* 139–148.

Rho, S. W., Choi, G. S., Ko, E. J., Kim, S. K., Lee, Y. S., & Lee, H. J., et al. (2008). Molecular changes in remote tissues induced by electro-acupuncture stimulation at acupoint ST36. *Molecules and Cells, 25,* 178–183.

Roberts, C. S., Baker, F., Hann, D., Runfola, J., Witt, C., & Mc,Donald, J., et al. (2005). Patient-physician communication regarding use of complementary therapies during cancer treatment. *Journal of Psychosocial Oncology, 23,* 35–60.

Rowland, J. H., & Baker, F. (2005). Introduction: Resilience of cancer survivors across the lifespan. *Cancer, 104,* 2543–2548.

Savard, J., & Morin, C. M. (2001). Insomnia in the context of cancer: A review of a neglected problem. *Journal of Clinical Oncology, 19,* 895–908.

Shen, J., Wenger, N., Glaspy, J., Hays, R. D., Albert, P. S., & Choi, C., et al. (2000). Electroacupuncture for control of myeloablative chemotherapy-induced emesis: A randomized controlled trial. *JAMA, 284,* 2755–2761.

Vickers, A. J. (2002). Placebo controls in randomized trials of acupuncture. *Evaluation & the Health Professions, 25,* 421–435.

Vickers, A. J., Straus, D. J., Fearon, B., & Cassileth, B. R. (2004). Acupuncture for postchemotherapy fatigue: A Phase II study. *Journal of Clinical Oncology, 22,* 1731–1735.

Walker, E. M., Rodriguez, A. I., Kohn, B., Ball, R. M., Pegg, J., & Pocock, J. R., et al. (2010). Acupuncture versus venlafaxine for the management of vasomotor symptoms in patients with hormone receptor-positive breast cancer: A randomized controlled trial. *Journal of Clinical Oncology, 28,* 634–640.

White, A. R. (2002). Acupuncture research methodology. In: G., Lewith, W. B. Jonas, & H. Walach (Eds.), *Clinical research in complementary therapies: Principles, problems and solutions* (pp. 307–323) Vol 1. Edinburgh: Churchill Livingstone.

Witt, C., Brinkhaus, B., Jena, S., Linde, K., Streng, A., & Wagenpfeil, S., et al. (2005). Acupuncture in patients with osteoarthritis of the knee: A randomised trial. *Lancet, 366,* 136–143.

Wu, M. T., Sheen, J. M., Chuang, K. H., Yang, P., Chin, S. L., Tsai, & C. Y., et al. (2002). Neuronal specificity of acupuncture response: A fMRI study with electroacupuncture. *Neuroimage, 16,* 1028–1037.

Yates, J. S., Mustian, K. M., Morrow, G. R., Gillies, L. J., Padmanaban, D., & Atkins, J. N., et al. (2005). Prevalence of complementary and alternative medicine use in cancer patients during treatment. *Support Care Cancer, 13,* 806–811.

Chapter 15
Recent Clinical Trials of Acupuncture for Cancer Patients

Gary Deng, David Seto and Barrie Cassileth

Abstract Acupuncture is one of the most extensively studied complementary medicine modalities. The quality of acupuncture research has become increasingly better, due to refinement of research methodology and its dissemination among the researchers. In recent years, many randomized controlled trials have been reported on the application of acupuncture in cancer care. Here we review the studies deemed of high quality (Jadad scale 3 or above). The studies consist of randomized controlled trials of acupuncture on nausea, vomiting, hot flashes, xerostomia, pain, fatigue, mood-related symptoms and neutropenia. The most solid evidence came from studies of chemotherapy-related nausea and vomiting. Acupuncture has been repeatedly demonstrated to reduce nausea and vomiting in both the post-operative setting and the chemotherapy setting. Less strong evidence with mixed results was demonstrated in trials on hot flashes, xerostomia and post-operative pain, where acupuncture has shown benefit in some but not in other trials. There are insufficient number of trials of reasonable quality to evaluate other indications for acupuncture in cancer care. Serious adverse events are rare or non-existent among those trials. It would help our understanding of acupuncture if future studies take a "whole system" approach, taking into consideration of efficacy and effectiveness questions, and further explore the mechanistic aspect of acupuncture.

15.1 Introduction

Acupuncture is a therapeutic modality in traditional Chinese medicine (TCM), developed over the millennia. Acupuncture treatment involves the placement of needles at selected points on the body, followed by manipulation with physical forces, heat, or, in modern times, electrical stimuli. According to TCM theory, vital energy (Qi or Chi in Chinese) flows throughout the body along channels called meridians. It

G. Deng (✉) · B. Cassileth
Integrative Medicine Service, Memorial Sloan-Kettering Cancer Center,
1429 First Avenue, New York, NY 10021, USA
e-mail: dengg@mskcc.org

D. Seto
Department of Medicine, Weill Cornell Medical College, New York, NY, USA

W. C. S. Cho (ed.), *Acupuncture and Moxibustion as an Evidence-based Therapy for Cancer*, Evidence-based Anticancer Complementary and Alternative Medicine 3,
DOI 10.1007/978-94-007-4833-0_15, © Springer Science+Business Media Dordrecht 2012

was believed that the interruption or obstruction of the energy makes the individual vulnerable to illness. The insertion of needles at specific points along the meridian was thought to regulate the energy flow, which would produce therapeutic benefit.

Although the concepts of Qi and meridians are inconsistent with our current understanding of human anatomy and physiology, research in the past few decades supports the clinical effects of acupuncture. Recent neuroscience research suggests that it appears to work by modulating the nervous system. In large part due to such research, acupuncture has become increasingly integrated into mainstream cancer care in the Western medical practice setting. Most major comprehensive cancer centers and many community hospitals have an integrative medicine component that includes acupuncture treatment as a supportive care measure (Deng et al. 2006; Sagar 2008; Stone and Johnstone 2010).

There is no evidence that acupuncture has direct effects against cancer and it should not be used in efforts to treat the disease. However, clinical research shows that acupuncture can reduce many important physical and emotional symptoms commonly experienced by cancer patients, thereby improving patients' quality of life. In this chapter, we review recent clinical trials that advance understanding of how to best use acupuncture in cancer care.

15.2 Methods

The National Institutes of Health pubmed.gov database was searched using the keywords "acupuncture" and "cancer" and adding the individual indications of "nausea", "vomiting", "hot flashes", "xerostomia", "pain", "fatigue", "neutropenia", "ileus", "lymphedema", "dyspnea", "breath", "breathlessness", "palliative" and "hospice", limited to clinical trials published in the English language for the 5-year period from January 2007 through January 2012).

Methodological quality of trial design was evaluated using the Jadad scale, a widely employed five-item scoring measure for clinical trials (Jadad et al. 1996; Clark et al. 1999). Trials examined and discussed in detail had to be prospective and randomized with at least two experimental arms, and score a minimum of three points on the Jadad scale (trials with only single-blinding of either subjects or investigators were not awarded points for "double-blinding," contrary to the practice of some other reviewers). Trials meeting these criteria were identified. Those that received less than three points or were not randomized were not mentioned. High quality trials that were already reviewed elsewhere were only described briefly. Clinical conditions and specific details of the acupuncture regimens were tabulated using the 2010 Standards for Reporting Interventions in Clinical Trials of Acupuncture (STRICTA), to ensure that reproducibility and theoretically sound rationale for treatment protocols was appropriately documented (MacPherson et al. 2010). All attempts were made to catalogue acupuncture points according to standardized WHO nomenclature (1990).

The majority of recent clinical trials that met the review criteria have focused on managing the complications of chemotherapy surgery or radiation in cancer patients, the most common indications were nausea and vomiting, hot flashes and pain. Other trials focused on xerostomia and various measures of quality of life, including fatigue, depression and insomnia. Other commonly researched cancer-related indications were not examined in any high quality randomized clinical trial in the past 5 years. These included lymphedema, dyspnea, hiccups and post-operative ileus. Overall, the most commonly studied single acupuncture point was Neiguan (PC6), most often for treatment of nausea and vomiting.

15.3 Acupuncture for Nausea and Vomiting-related to Cancer

The most recent Cochrane review regarding acupuncture for chemotherapy-induced nausea or vomiting was published in 2006. It examined eleven randomized controlled trials, concluding that electroacupuncture helps reduce chemotherapy-induced nausea and vomiting, and that self-acupressure can help prevent nausea. However, manual acupuncture apparently was not effective, and cutaneous electrical stimulation in the setting of antiemetic drug use did not demonstrate a significant impact (Ezzo et al. 2006). A more recent Cochrane review examining acupuncture for nausea and vomiting for post-operative patients, regardless of the presence or absence of cancer, was published in 2009. After reviews of 40 randomized controlled trials involving stimulation of the PC6 acupuncture point, the reviewers concluded that this intervention does prevent post-operative nausea and vomiting, although significant differences between PC6 stimulation and antiemetic medications was not clearly demonstrated (Lee and Fan 2009). Subsequent trials that specifically addressed acupuncture for cancer patients but not previously discussed in the above reviews, are mentioned below.

A randomized, partially blinded, placebo-controlled trial (Jadad score = 5) by Wang et al. (2010) used the PC6 acupoint to investigate the ability of transcutaneous electrode stimulation to prevent post-operative nausea and vomiting within 24 h of craniotomy. Particularly in post-craniotomy patients, nausea control is critical for preventing increases in intracranial pressure, arterial pressure, lung aspiration, dehydration, and disturbance of electrolytes and acid-base status. Up to 60% of post-craniotomy patients continue to experience post-operative nausea and vomiting despite use of antiemetic medications.

The included patients ($n = 80$) were age 20–60 with supratentorial cerebral tumors undergoing craniotomy (mostly for gliomas and meningiomas), with body mass index <30 and no history of DM, smoking, motion sickness, or prior experience with electrodes or post-operative nausea and vomiting. True electrostimulation at 2 Hz alternating with 100 Hz was delivered to the right PC6 acupoint starting 30 min pre-operatively, continuing intra-operatively, and terminating six hours post-operatively. Sham control involved electrode placement at a non-acupoint on the dorsal forearm. All patients received pharmacological antiemetics, ondansetron and metoclopramide. Cumulative incidence of nausea at 24 h was significantly decreased by 40%, and the incidence of vomiting was decreased by 60% in the group randomized to electrostimulation of the PC6 acupoint.

This study was important not only because of the quality of its methodology and STRICTA reporting, but also because it demonstrated that a simple, non-puncturing acupoint intervention, administered by clinical staff untrained in acupuncture, was effective for nausea/vomiting control. It also demonstrated that pre-operative intervention at PC6 was extremely effective, whereas prior studies often found that post-operative stimulation at PC6 failed to produce adequate anti-emesis.

A randomized, double-blinded pragmatic trial of true *vs* sham acupuncture ($n = 215$, Jadad score $= 5$) at the PC6 point was undertaken by Enblom et al. (2012) to investigate the effect of acupuncture on treating radiation-induced nausea. Patients were at least 18 years of age, with various cancer diagnoses (i.e. gynecologic, anal, rectal, colonic, gastric, pancreatic, testicular), planned radiation of greater than $800\,\text{cm}^3$ and 25 Gy dose to the abdomen, without any acupuncture treatment ever for emesis or for any other indication in the past year, and without any persistent emesis or antiemetic treatment in the 24 h preceding the start of radiotherapy. The primary outcome measurement was number of patients with at least one episode of nausea. Ultimately, there was no statistically significant difference between the true and sham groups, although patients in both groups subjectively reported that they felt the treatment that they had received was effective (92–95% in the true group, 94–96% in the sham group).

Hence an additional analysis was published by Enblom et al. (2011) comparing true *vs* sham acupuncture against a third usual care group (i.e. a pragmatic and efficacy trial, Jadad score $= 3$) to investigate the degree to which non-specific anti-emetic effects are invoked during acupuncture used to treat radiation-induced nausea. This study was only partially randomized in that randomization occurred within an acupuncture group (i.e. to true or sham), but both the acupuncture and usual care groups were selected, apparently without randomization, from two partially overlapping populations of patients. Non-randomization led to the standard care cohort having significantly more men than the acupuncture cohort, more patients with testicular tumors, and fewer patients consuming antiemetics, serotonin-receptor antagonists, or corticosteroids. Nausea was assessed daily in the true/sham acupuncture cohort, and only once (after radiation) in the usual care group. Although nausea intensity was significantly lower in the true and sham acupuncture groups *vs* the usual care group, there were no statistical differences between the true and sham groups in terms of nausea frequency/intensity, vomiting or use of antiemetics in the preceding 24 h or week (at the time of questioning). However, patients' expectation of nausea was significantly correlated with actual development of nausea. Of note, a significant 30% cost savings per patient was also observed when comparing an equivalent number of acupuncture (true or sham) sessions to daily use of 8 mg of serotonin-receptor antagonists throughout a full course of radiation therapy.

An interesting variation of PC6 stimulation was examined by You et al. (2009) in a randomized, non-blinded trial (Jadad score = 3) examining treatment of cancer-related emesis using a combination of manual acupuncture plus simultaneous pyridoxine (vitamin B_6) 50 mg injection into the PC6 acupoints themselves, *vs* manual acupuncture alone *vs* pyridoxine 50 mg intramuscular injection twice daily for 21 days. Patients receiving acupuncture alone and acupuncture plus B6 injections were treated every other day for ten sessions. This study was conceived because pyridoxine has been demonstrated to be an inexpensive and effective treatment for cancer-related nausea/vomiting. Included patients ($n = 142$) were age 45–65 with stage 2–3 ovarian cancer, with mild-moderate nausea/vomiting, and utilizing an identical chemotherapy and antiemetic drug regimen, with no history of hepatitis or other gastrointestinal disease, mental illness, lymphedema or active infection. This trial demonstrated that, over the 21-day duration of the trial, subjects in the combination of acupuncture plus pyridoxine injections at PC6 group had significantly fewer total episodes of emesis per person and more emesis-free days than did subjects in either of the single-intervention groups.

A randomized, non-blinded, usual care-controlled crossover trial (Jadad score = 3) was recently performed by Gottschling et al. (2008) in pediatric cancer patients to investigate the utility of individualized acupuncture regimens in managing chemotherapy-induced nausea and vomiting. Most commonly employed points in these individualized regimens included PC6, Zusanli (ST36), Zhongwan (CV12) and Hegu (LI4). Included patients ($n = 23$) were age 6–18 with "solid malignant tumors" (the majority being Ewing's sarcoma and rhabdomyosarcoma) but without cerebral metastasis and with no prior acupuncture in the past 6 months, who were scheduled to receive at least three identical and consecutive chemotherapy courses with drugs that are considered "highly emetogenic." Patients who did not experience nausea and/or vomiting during the first course of chemotherapy were excluded from participation, and those who did were randomized to receive either acupuncture or usual care with standing prophylactic 5-HT_3 antagonists (i.e. ondansetron, tropisetron) as well as additional rescue antiemetics (i.e. dexamethasone, phenothiazines) during the second course of chemotherapy. For the third course of chemotherapy (each course is separated by at least 2 weeks) patients from the acupuncture group were switched to the usual care group, and *vice versa*.

While undergoing acupuncture, patients required significantly less phenothiazines as rescue antiemetics (though dexamethasone usage was not significantly different) and had significantly less episodes of retching or emesis. The only adverse effect noted was pain from needling (17%) and while six patients either died, stopped chemotherapy or were lost to follow-up, 71% of the remaining patients requested continuation of acupuncture for antiemesis when this option was offered at the conclusion of the study. This trial was significant because it demonstrated both safety and tolerability, and efficacy of acupuncture for treatment of cancer-related nausea/vomiting in pediatric patients. However, the publication's limited report of treatment details based on STRICTA criteria renders it difficult to examine critically or reproduce.

15.4 Acupuncture for Cancer-related Hot Flashes

15.4.1 Breast Cancer

Three recent review articles, including a Cochrane review, discussed nine randomized controlled trials examining acupuncture for treating hot flashes related to breast cancer, and concluded that evidence to date is not convincing that acupuncture is effective for this indication (Chao et al. 2009; Lee et al. 2009a; Rada et al. 2010). Four of the reviewed trials were performed within the 5-year scope of this chapter. The lone study showing clear benefit from acupuncture was an efficacy trial by Hervik and Mjaland (2008) ($n = 59$, Jadad score $= 3$) studying true *vs* sham acupuncture in post-surgical patients treated with tamoxifen, which showed significant improvement in both daytime and nighttime hot flash frequency in the true acupuncture group over 22 weeks (subsequent follow-up at 2 years is discussed below) (Hervik and Mjaland 2009). One efficacy trial by Deng et al. (2007) ($n = 72$, Jadad score $= 5$) demonstrated hot flash reduction with both true and sham acupuncture involving several acupuncture points, though no statistically significant difference was noted between groups.

A pragmatic trial by Frisk et al. (2008) ($n = 45$, Jadad score $= 3$) compared electroacupuncture (points unspecified) over 12 weeks with estrogen/progesterone hormone therapy for 24 months, and claimed that, while both treatments significantly reduced hot flash symptoms, hormone therapy was "more effective" than electroacupuncture at decreasing hot flash frequency and impact, although no inter-group statistical significance was cited (further analysis of other parameters was published later, see below). Notably, this trial represented a substudy of the larger Swedish HABITS trial that ultimately was discontinued because it showed higher rates of breast cancer recurrence in breast cancer patients treated with hormone therapy, with the final recommendation that hormone therapy be avoided in such patients (Holmberg et al. 2008).

Finally, results from a pragmatic trial by Walker et al. (2010) ($n = 50$, Jadad score $= 2$ with no mention of randomization method) comparing acupuncture to venlafaxine, an anti-depressant, showed that both therapies significantly reduced hot flashes, and although there was no statistical inter-group difference, acupuncture reportedly produced none of the venlafaxine-associated adverse effects, and more beneficial side effects, such as improvement in energy, clarity of thought, sex drive and overall sense of well-being. Following publication of these review articles, additional studies examining acupuncture for hot flashes in breast cancer were published and are discussed below.

A follow-up study published by Hervik and Mjaland (2010) ($n = 82$, Jadad score $= 3$ for previous design) re-evaluated patients from their initial 2008 efficacy trial (Hervik and Mjaland 2009) 2 years after completing true *vs* sham acupuncture treatment for post-surgical and tamoxifen-related hot flashes (Hervik and Mjaland 2010). Questionnaires soliciting open-ended thoughts about their breast cancer diagnosis and treatment were sent to living patients from the 2008 trial cohort, and to 31 additional women who were "treated and followed up in an identical manner to those included originally". Twenty eight of 61 respondents commented about hot flashes and acupuncture treatment. Of those who had been randomized to true acupuncture, 15 described positive experiences both during and after acupuncture treatment and ten stated that hot flashes were still "fewer and milder" than they were prior to the acupuncture treatment administered 2 years earlier, compared to only one patient from the sham acupuncture group. Among the sham group patients, nine women reported ongoing severe hot flashes at the 2-year follow-up interval, four stated that acupuncture had been ineffective, and one mentioned that acupuncture had been unpleasant. Limitations of the study include the fact that no statistical analysis of these qualitative results was performed, and an additional cohort of 31 patients was added who were not formally followed in the previous 2008 trial. However, these subjective results suggest that true acupuncture, if demonstrated to outperform sham acupuncture with statistical significance, may indeed induce long-lasting benefits that persist even for 2 years.

Frisk et al. (2012) ($n = 45$) published a re-analysis of their initial 2008 trial of electroacupuncture *vs* hormone therapy (Frisk et al. 2008) to examine other subjective measures of quality of life, sleep quality, distress level, and general well-being (Frisk et al. 2012). Modest but statistically significant improvement in these parameters was demonstrated in both the electroacupuncture and hormone therapy groups, although no statistically significant superiority of electroacupuncture was observed. These results are in accord with the original 2008 study's primary outcome measure of hot flash reduction. However, the authors make the case that, as closure of the HABITS trial renders hormone therapy a dubious first-line agent for treating hot flashes and associated symptoms in breast cancer patients, electroacupuncture may be considered an alternative of comparable efficacy that is perhaps better tolerated and safer than hormone therapy.

A randomized, single-blinded, sham-controlled efficacy trial (2010) ($n = 84$, Jadad score $= 3$) was published by Liljegren et al. (2010) examining the effect of true *vs* sham acupuncture on hot flashes in breast cancer, using a number of points. Included patients were age 36–80, at least one year following last menstruation, with history of completed medical and surgical treatment for breast cancer without recurrence, on adjuvant tamoxifen for at least two months, not on any other adjuvant chemotherapy or radiation, with significant vasomotor symptoms and with no acupuncture treatment within six months of the study. Although nighttime sweating alone was significantly improved in the true acupuncture group, no significant difference was observed in the primary outcome measures of hot flashes and sweating frequencies at one week after completion of the experimental course. Additionally, there were no significant differences between the groups in levels of follicle-stimulating hormone, luteinizing hormone, estradiol, progesterone, sex hormone-binding globulin, prolactin or testosterone.

15.4.2 *Prostate Cancer*

A recent review article discussed six studies investigating acupuncture for the treatment of hot flashes in prostate cancer patients (Lee et al. 2009b). Only one of the included trials was randomized and with a high quality Jadad score above 1, and conducted within the past five years. This trial, conducted by Frisk et al. (2009) ($n = 31$, Jadad score $= 5$), compared electroacupuncture *vs* traditional acupuncture at multiple points, for treating hot flashes in patients with prostate cancer. Patients had undergone castration therapy with either surgical or medical (i.e. gonadotropin-releasing hormone analogues) interventions. In brief, both groups demonstrated significant reduction in hot flashes following 12 weeks of treatment, although no significant difference was found between the electroacupuncture and traditional acupuncture groups. The authors recommended further investigation with sham or placebo controls, or with a usual care group.

15.5 Acupuncture for Xerostomia in Cancer Patients

A recent acupuncture neuroimaging study by Deng et al. (2008a) noted that acupuncture delivered with twisting manual stimulation at the Erjian (LI2) acupuncture point on the non-dominant side produced a distinct pattern of brain activation on fMRI that was not reproduced with sham acupuncture stimulation, and a corresponding significant increase in saliva secretion as compared to sham stimulation, with salivary flow measured at the bilateral parotid glands. These empiric objective findings suggest that acupuncture can be a useful modality for treating the complication of xerostomia that is often noted in cancer patients undergoing radiation treatment at the head and neck. A recent review by O'Sullivan and Higginson (2010) discussed three randomized trials examining acupuncture as treatment for radiation-induced xerostomia (RIX) in patients with head and neck cancer, and concluded that evidence to date was still inconclusive, yet justified further investigation of this modality. One of these trials was published in 1996 and falls outside of the timeframe of this review (Blom et al. 1996). One small, randomized, single-blind efficacy trial by Cho et al. (2008) ($n = 12$, Jadad score $= 2$ with no definite description of withdrawals or dropouts) examined true *vs* sham acupuncture at multiple points in patients with head and neck cancer following radiotherapy, noting significantly higher salivary flow rates and improved quality of life in the true acupuncture group after 6 weeks of treatment. A third randomized, non-blinded pragmatic trial by Pfister et al. (2010) ($n = 58$, Jadad score $= 3$) was extensively reviewed by multiple review papers (Capodice 2010; Lu and Rosenthal 2010; O'Sullivan and Higginson 2010). It investigated weekly acupuncture at multiple points (including LI2) *vs* usual care for xerostomia in patients who had undergone neck dissection for cancer at least three months prior to the study. Statistically significant improvement in xerostomia as measured on the Xerostomia Inventory, as well as pain and functional status as measured by the Constant-Murley scale, was noted in the acupuncture group as compared to the control group.

One other study was located during our literature search, which was not yet reviewed elsewhere. A randomized, non-blinded pragmatic trial of acupuncture *vs* usual care was recently undertaken by Meng et al. (2012) ($n = 86$, Jadad score = 3) to investigate the utility of acupuncture administered prior to and on the same days as radiation treatments for preventing RIX in patients with nasopharyngeal carcinoma. Included patients were over 18 years of age, with nasopharyngeal carcinoma but anatomically intact parotid and submandibular glands and no suspected or confirmed salivary duct closure, Zubrod performance status of 0–2, no history of xerostomia, no planned intensity-modulated radiation therapy, no bleeding disorder or anticoagulant use, no history of stroke or spinal cord injury, no saliva-modulating drug use in the preceding 30 days or during the study, and no contraindications for acupuncture at any of the studied acupuncture points. Seven weeks of acupuncture, three times each week, was performed. Statistically significant improvement in xerostomia and quality of life, as measured on the Xerostomia Questionnaire and the MD Anderson Symptom Inventory-Head and Neck, was noted starting at week 3, and persisted for 6 months. Additionally, significantly higher unstimulated salivary flow rates in the acupuncture group were noted from weeks 3–11, and significantly higher stimulated salivary flow rates were noted from week 7 through 6 months. This publication was important in that it was the first high-quality trial of its kind to demonstrate the preventive effects of acupuncture administered concurrent with active radiation therapy, indicated that future trials with larger sample sizes and a variety of control arms should be undertaken.

15.6 Acupuncture for Pain in Cancer Patients

Acupuncture appears to be a promising treatment for pain unrelated to cancer, with a review of recent Cochrane reviews published by Lee and Ernst (2010) discussing good evidence demonstrating that the modality is helpful for at least some types of pain (i.e. peripheral joint osteoarthritis, migraine treatment and prophylaxis, neck pain, low back pain), though they mentioned that definitive evidence has not yet been produced regarding some other pain indications (i.e. rheumatoid arthritis, shoulder pain, lateral elbow pain). The most recent Cochrane review by Paley et al. (2011b) examining acupuncture specifically for cancer pain in adults described only three high-quality randomized controlled trials for this indication, though a high-quality trial by Mehling et al. (2007) was also briefly mentioned. Of the three trials discussed, one was conducted in 1998 and one in 2003, which are effectively outside of the time scope of this chapter (Dang and Yang 1998; Alimi et al. 2003). The other trial cited from 2008 was not published in the English language, thus causing it to fall outside of the boundaries of this chapter, as well (Chen et al. 2008). Another recent review of acupuncture for cancer pain by Hopkins Hollis (2010) identified two of the above studies mentioned studies from the Paley Cochrane review (Dang and Yang 1998; Alimi et al. 2003), an older study from 1986 (Xia et al. 1986) and a more recent study from 2007 (Minton and Higginson 2007) examining electroacupuncture for neuropathic pain that was not peer-reviewed, but rather published as a letter to the editor. Both of these review articles concluded that evidence is currently insufficient to accurately judge whether acupuncture is helpful for cancer pain.

However, another review article by Capodice (2010) has in fact identified several other recent, high-quality trials examining acupuncture for cancer-related pain that were not mentioned in the Paley Cochrane review or the Hopkins Hollis review, and even concluded that acupuncture should be "recommended as a complementary therapy if pain is poorly controlled and may offer utility as a primary treatment for cancer-related pain" based on the "significant body of research" from these studies, with a level 1A recommendation. One high-quality randomized efficacy trial conducted by Crew et al. (2010) ($n = 43$, Jadad score $= 5$) compared true *vs* sham acupuncture at multiple body and auricular acupuncture points for the treatment of aromatase inhibitor-associated joint pain in women with stage 1–3 estrogen receptor-positive breast cancer, taking medications such as anastrozole, letrozole, or exemestane. Individualization of additional points according to the primary joint(s) involved was allowed, with the core protocol based on an earlier pilot study by the same principal author (Crew et al. 2007). Significant superiority of pain reduction at 6 weeks was observed in the true acupuncture group was noted, according to validated measures of cancer-related pain, as well as various indices of pain traditionally associated with osteoarthritis and rheumatoid arthritis (Crew et al. 2010). This trial was also favorably reviewed by Lu and Rosenthal (2010) and the initial pilot study was also reviewed positively by Chao et al. (2009) in their broad review of acupoint stimulation for the treatment of various adverse events in breast cancer patients.

Regarding post-operative cancer pain, two high-quality randomized studies have been reviewed by Capodice, including the Pfister trial for acupuncture for pain and xerostomia following neck dissection (Pfister et al. 2010), which has been reviewed extensively (Capodice 2010; Lu and Rosenthal 2010; O'Sullivan and Higginson 2010) and which was discussed in our xerostomia section above. The other such trial reviewed by Capodice includes a randomized, single-blind, sham-controlled efficacy trial by Deng et al. (2008b) ($n = 162$, Jadad score $= 3$) of intradermal needle studs at multiple true acupuncture points *vs* sham points for treatment of post-thoracotomy pain in patients with cancer requiring thoracotomy. Ultimately, no significant difference in pain scores between groups was noted at post-operative day 30. This negative finding was thought to be possibly related to lack of electrical stimulation, short depth of needle stud insertion, and acupuncture point selection, variables which were all different in previous prospective trials that had demonstrated adequate post-operative pain relief in patients undergoing thoracotomy and intra-abdominal surgery (Kotani et al. 2001; Wong et al. 2006).

Mehling et al. (2007) conducted another randomized, non-blinded pragmatic clinical trial ($n = 150$, Jadad score $= 3$) examining a combination of acupuncture and Swedish massage *vs* usual care for post-operative cancer pain, as well as mood symptoms and nausea/vomiting in a heterogeneous cancer patient population. This trial was reviewed in detail by Lu et al. (2008) and partially reviewed for its breast cancer subgroup by Chao et al. (2009) as well as briefly mentioned in the Cochrane review of acupuncture for cancer pain in adults by Paley et al. (2011b). Included patients were at least 18 years old and underwent surgery requiring at least 48 h of inpatient admission for procedures such as mastectomy or reconstructive breast surgery (for breast cancer), abdominal surgery (for intestinal or liver cancer), pelvic surgery (for ovarian, uterine or cervical cancer), urologic surgery (for cancer of the testicles, prostate, bladder or kidneys) and surgery for head and neck cancer. A 2:1 randomization scheme of intervention to usual care group was employed, to attempt to increase study attractiveness for enrollment purposes, which is expected to slightly decrease statistical power without compromising the overall impact of the study (Dumville et al. 2006). The combination of acupuncture points used on post-operative days 1 and 2 (i.e. LI4, Sanyinjiao (SP6) and various auricular points for pain, PC6 and ST36 for nausea, LI4, Taichong (LR3) and Yintang (EX-HN3) for anxiety, as well as 30 min Swedish massage sessions, ultimately produced significant reduction in pain scores by post-operative day 3 in the intervention group, though significant reduction as compared to the usual care control group was only achieved in the urologic cancer subgroup. Significant improvement in mood was also observed in comparison to the control group (see below), though no significant improvement in nausea/vomiting was observed with this particular intervention.

Regarding other forms of cancer-related pain, such as pain from metastatic disease, cancer-induced bone pain and neuropathic pain, no peer-reviewed, high-quality prospective randomized trials examining acupuncture as treatment have been located in the English language within the past 5 years (Robb et al. 2008; Capodice 2010; Hopkins Hollis 2010; Paley et al. 2011a,b).

15.7 Acupuncture for Fatigue in Cancer Patients

Evidence continues to accumulate that elucidates the multifactorial nature of fatigue often experienced by cancer patients undergoing treatment, as well as the potential of acupuncture as a therapeutic modality for this indication (Johnston et al. 2007a,b). Several high-quality clinical trials, albeit mostly pilot studies, were published in the past 5 years in order to examine the effectiveness of acupuncture for cancer-related fatigue.

One previously reviewed, randomized, double-blinded, sham-controlled efficacy trial was executed by Balk et al. (2009) ($n = 27$, Jadad score $= 5$) to examine the utility of electroacupuncture at Taixi (KI3), SP6, LI4, ST36 and (Qihai) CV6) *vs* sham electroacupuncture for treating fatigue in women with localized cancer (predominantly breast cancer, but one woman with endometrial cancer) that had been treated using surgery, with or without chemotherapy. A trend towards greater improvement in fatigue in the true electroacupuncture group was observed, but the study was apparently underpowered to detect statistical significance, a criticism that was raised by others who reviewed this study (Deng 2009; Capodice 2010). Furthermore, the study groups were observed to have differences in baseline fatigue that were not stratified during randomization, and the trial's method of double-blinding without actively seeking Deqi sensation was cited by its authors as a confounder that might diminish effect size of the true intervention. Additionally, a three-armed, randomized efficacy trial by Molassiotis et al. (2007) ($n = 47$, Jadad score = 3) was undertaken to investigate the effect of acupuncture *vs* true self-acupressure (at LI4, ST36 and SP6) *vs* sham self-acupressure on fatigue in patients who had completed chemotherapy for various types of cancer. This study was previously reviewed by Lu et al. (2008) as well as Escalante and Manzullo (2009) and demonstrated significant improvement in fatigue for the acupuncture and true self-acupressure groups, both after 2 weeks of treatment and persisting for 2 additional weeks following treatment completion. However, acupuncture was observed to be significantly more effective than either true or sham self-acupressure.

A more recent randomized, non-blinded, prospective feasibility study was conducted by Johnston et al. (2011) ($n = 13$, Jadad score = 3) to investigate the pragmatic value of acupuncture at multiple points (once weekly treatment for 8 weeks) and wellness education based on integrative medical and social cognitive theory (once weekly for the first 4 weeks) *vs* usual care in treating cancer-related fatigue. Included patients were female, aged 18–65, with no evidence of disease following completion of treatment for breast cancer, and with a fatigue score of >4 on the Brief Fatigue Inventory (BFI). Exclusion criteria included any history of depression with score of > 10 on the Hospital Anxiety and Depression Score (HADS), anemia with hemoglobin level < 9 g/dL or hematocrit <30%, decline in hemoglobin by more than 2 g/dL over the one month preceding the study, active treatment for anemia, or severe limitation in physical functioning (i.e. Karnofsky performance status (KPS) < 70); other potential causes of fatigue (i.e. hypothyroidism and hepatitis) were not criteria for exclusion. A combination of acupuncture and patient education was demonstrated to be beneficial for reducing by 66% according to BFI scores, though this effect did not reach statistical significance ($p < 0.10$), and changes in secondary outcomes of perceived cognitive impairment were not statistically significant. The lack of statistical significance can be attributed to the small sample size employed in this feasibility trial, and its non-blinded nature may have biased its results. However, the encouraging magnitude of fatigue reduction demonstrated by acupuncture and patient education in this study invites large-scale follow-up trials that are more adequately powered to detect statistical significance in this patient population.

Another recent pilot study employing a randomized, non-blinded pragmatic trial model was undertaken by Lim et al. (2011) ($n = 20$, Jadad score = 3) to examine the effect of weekly acupuncture *vs* supportive care guided by a palliative care nurse on multiple symptoms for cancer patients in palliative care. Included patients were age 31–81 with various types of cancer, undergoing palliative care and with at least three months of predicted lifespan remaining, and the interventions were delivered once weekly for 4 weeks. The acupuncture intervention was individualized based on patients' symptoms, which were reassessed each week with the acupuncture point regimen adjusted accordingly. The nurse-led supportive care involved 20–30 min weekly meetings in which nurses discussed with the patient details regarding symptoms, medications and other therapies, dietary adjustments and medication scheduling changes, and offered emotional support. Improvement in various symptoms (including pain, tiredness, nausea, depression, anxiety, drowsiness, appetite, feeling of well-being and dyspnea) was noted in both groups after each session, with improvement largely persisting at 6 weeks following completion of the 4-week treatment period. No calculations were performed to determine whether any of these changes were statistically significant. However, this study confirmed the feasibility of examining both this particular individualized acupuncture model and the palliative care nurse meeting model in larger scale future clinical trials.

15.8 Acupuncture for Depression, Anxiety, Insomnia and Other Mood-related Symptoms in Cancer Patients

A randomized, non-blinded, fluoxetine-controlled trial (Jadad score = 3) of acupuncture for depression in 80 patients with malignancy, (with 30 pulmonary, 16 gastric and 14 colorectal cancer patients comprising the majority of tumor types) was undertaken (Feng et al. 2011). There was no placebo control, and no overt description of blinding. Primary outcome measures were change in depression score on the Self-rating Depression Scale (SDS) and Hamilton Depression Rating Scale (HAMD), and change in sleep quality on the Pittsburgh Sleep Quality Index (PSQI). Inclusion criteria were age 18–75, baseline SDS > 50, HAMD > 7 and PSQI > 8, expected survival time > 3 months and absence of mental or intellectual disorders. Exclusion criteria were ongoing use of antidepressants, functional disorders of the heart, liver, kidney and spinal cord, dementia or low education level that precluded understanding of the questionnaires, or KPS < 30 (global assessment of function in cancer patients). Following 30 days of daily treatment with either acupuncture or fluoxetine 20 mg, the study authors reported significant improvement ($p < 0.05$) in all the measures of SDS, HAMD and PSQI in the acupuncture group. However, fluoxetine and other SSRIs usually require serial dose up-titration (maximal dose 80 mg for Fluoxetine) and a minimum of 4–5 weeks for maximal therapeutic efficacy to be achieved. Hence, a trial with longer follow-up duration and appropriate control dose titration should be attempted. Additionally, methodological reporting concerns regarding the nature of the acupuncture studied also render this study difficult to interpret or reproduce.

As mentioned above, the high-quality study by Mehling et al. (2007) investigating acupuncture and Swedish massage post-operatively for patients with various cancer types demonstrated a significant reduction in depression in comparison to the usual care group, as measured by the Profile of Mood States Short Form (POMS-SF) (Mehling et al. 2007; Lu et al. 2008; Chao et al. 2009). However, no significant improvement in anxiety between intervention and control groups was noted in the above study. The pilot study by Lim et al. (2011) for palliative care patients demonstrated improvement from acupuncture and palliative care nurse-led meetings in many domains of mood and psychological well-being (see above), though the study was not powered or designed to detect statistical significance in these parameters. Also as discussed above, the studies by Hervik and Walker (Hervik and Mjaland 2009, 2010; Walker et al. 2010) on acupuncture for reducing hot flash symptoms in breast cancer patients also showed a significant benefit on depression, sleep disturbance and other mood-related symptoms with adequate control of hot flashes.

15.9 Acupuncture for Chemotherapy-Induced Neutropenia

A randomized, blinded, sham acupuncture-controlled pilot study (Jadad score = 5) was undertaken to investigate the effects of acupuncture on leukopenia (WBC count), neutropenia (ANC count) and serum granulocyte-colony stimulating factor (G-CSF) levels in patients with ovarian cancer, which was the first sham-controlled trial of its kind (Lu et al. 2009). Post-chemotherapy neutropenia in gynecologic cancer patients often jeopardizes intended clinical outcomes by necessitating chemotherapy dose reduction, delayed treatment, inpatient hospitalization and the use of IV antibiotics. Current treatment with G-CSF and GM-CSF is expensive and includes adverse effects such as fever, bone pain, and the acceleration of possible myelodysplasia or acute myeloid leukemia. Patients in this study were over age 18, had newly diagnosed or recurrent ovarian cancer and were on myelo-suppressive chemotherapy (in 3-week cycles) but not on filgrastim or pegfilgrastim, with platelets > 100,000 cells/μL and ANC > 1,000 cells/μL, with regular use of acupuncture within 120 days of the study and no history of psychiatric or cardiac disorders, particularly those requiring a pacemaker.

Acupuncture was administered just prior to and until the end of chemotherapy #2. The study was conducted from the beginning of week 3 (one week prior to starting chemotherapy cycle #2, which is the predicted nadir of WBC/ANC count for cycle #1) to the end of week 6 (end of chemotherapy cycle #2, one week after the predicted WBC/ANC nadir for cycle #2). Significantly lower incidence of severe leukopenia (i.e. grade 2–4) was observed in the true acupuncture arm at the end of cycle #2 (i.e. 30 *vs* 90% in the sham arm), and the median leukocyte value at this time was significantly higher than that of the control arm (i.e. 8,600 cells/μL *vs* 4,800 cells/μL). A higher median leukocyte nadir, neutrophil nadir and recovering ANC were observed in the true group, but this trend did not reach statistical significance. Although a fourfold increase in G-CSF levels was noted in the true group at the beginning of cycle #2 (after three acupuncture sessions), this difference was not significant, and no further G-CSF differences were noted at the end of cycle #2 (Lu et al. 2009). This trial was remarkable as a pilot study because of its high quality of both methodological design and STRICTA reporting, and its results suggest that larger scale trials should be undertaken to further investigate the possible benefits of acupuncture on the immune system response during chemotherapy.

15.10 Discussion

In summary, applying rigorous criteria to evaluate the quality of acupuncture clinical trials, we found the most solid evidence came from studies of chemotherapy-related nausea and vomiting. Less strong and mixed evidence was demonstrated in trials on hot flashes, xerostomia and post-operative pain. There are not a sufficient number of trials of reasonable quality to evaluate other indications for acupuncture in cancer care.

As the majority of these trials were published prior to the publication of the new STRICTA guidelines in 2010, it is expected that many of these earlier trials would not conform to the reporting practices encouraged by the STRICTA criteria. However, we also expect that many more trials in the future will observe these reporting criteria, as familiarity with the STRICTA guidelines increases among acupuncture researchers. It is our hope that increased use of these criteria will expand the generalizability and reproducibility of future study results.

Price et al. (2011) have commented on the fact that reporting of acupuncture rationale has yet to be standardized and varies widely from paper to paper, even in the face of increasing conformity to STRICTA reporting guidelines. Design, execution and reporting acupuncture rationale in further clinical trial publications is mandatory to appropriately differentiate among different modes, styles and depths of needle stimulation in order to avoid inappropriate grouping of disparate acupuncture styles during systematic reviews and meta-analysis. And of course, general issues for all acupuncture trials remain regarding methodological variation (i.e. point selection, frequency of treatment, acupuncture style, operator skill and ancillary stimulation modalities such as manual force, moxibustion, electricity and massage), an incomplete understanding of the physiologic mechanisms through which the acupuncture encounter and the needles themselves exert their effects, the non-inert nature of sham acupuncture (as invoked by mechanoreceptor stimulation of even gentle touch such as is employed in Japanese styles) and the apparently larger non-specific effect size of acupuncture and other procedures (i.e. surgery, other devices or manual manipulations) in comparison to placebo pills used in drug trials. Such challenges may well continue to represent the most difficult obstacles to overcome in terms of future clinical trial design and distillation of evidence that will ultimately help guide clinical practice and reduce the suffering of patients with cancer.

The 2007 Society for Acupuncture Research (SAR) international symposium on acupuncture research was attended by 300 acupuncture researchers, practitioners, students, funding agency personnel, and health policy analysts from 20 countries (Park et al. 2008). Among the presentations and discussions, two paradoxes emerged. First, a number of well-designed clinical trials found that true acupuncture is superior to usual care, but did not significantly outperform sham acupuncture. Second, although many experimental studies showed that the mode of needling is associated with various physiological effects, whether these changes influence therapeutic outcomes in clinical trials is unclear. A White Paper was issued to identify gaps in knowledge underlying the paradoxes and proposes strategies for their resolution through translational research (Langevin et al. 2011). We endorse the recommendations in the White Paper that future research should focus on a "whole systems" approach and on mechanistic studies. The studies may incorporate consideration of efficacy and effectiveness and may include qualitative measures.

References

WHO. (1990). A standard international acupuncture nomenclature: Memorandum from a WHO meeting. *Bulletin of the World Health Organization, 68*, 165–169.

Alimi, D., Rubino, C., Pichard-Leandri, E., Fermand-Brule, S., Dubreuil-Lemaire, M. L., Hill, C. (2003). Analgesic effect of auricular acupuncture for cancer pain: A randomized, blinded, controlled trial. *Journal of Clinical Oncology, 21*, 4120–4126.

Balk, J., Day, R., Rosenzweig, M., Beriwal, S. (2009). Pilot, randomized, modified, double-blind, placebo-controlled trial of acupuncture for cancer-related fatigue. *Journal of the Society for Integrative Oncology, 7*, 4–11.

Blom, M., Dawidson, I., Fernberg, J. O., Johnson, G., Angmar-Mansson, B. (1996). Acupuncture treatment of patients with radiation-induced xerostomia. *European Journal of Cancer Part B, Oral Oncology, 32B*, 182–190.

Capodice, J. L. (2010). Acupuncture in the oncology setting: Clinical trial update. *Current Treatment Options in Oncology, 11*, 87–94.

Chao, L. F., Zhang, A. L., Liu, H. E., Cheng, M. H., Lam, H. B., Lo, S. K. (2009). The efficacy of acupoint stimulation for the management of therapy-related adverse events in patients with breast cancer: A systematic review. *Breast Cancer Research and Treatment, 118*, 255–267.

Chen, Z. J., Guo, Y. P., Wu, Z. C. (2008). Observation on the therapeutic effect of acupuncture at pain points on cancer pain. *Zhongguo Zhen Jiu, Chinese Acupuncture and Moxibustion, 28*, 251–253.

Cho, J. H., Chung, W. K., Kang, W., Choi, S. M., Cho, C. K., Son, C. G. (2008). Manual acupuncture improved quality of life in cancer patients with radiation-induced xerostomia. *Journal of Alternative and Complementary Medicine, 14*, 523–526.

Clark, H. D., Wells, G. A., Huet, C., Mc Alister, F. A., Salmi, L. R., Fergusson, D., Laupacis, A. (1999). Assessing the quality of randomized trials: Reliability of the Jadad scale. *Controlled Clinical Trials, 20*, 448–452.

Crew, K. D., Capodice, J. L., Greenlee, H., Apollo, A., Jacobson, J. S., Raptis, G., Blozie, K., Sierra, A., Hershman, D. L. (2007). Pilot study of acupuncture for the treatment of joint symptoms related to adjuvant aromatase inhibitor therapy in postmenopausal breast cancer patients. *Journal of Cancer Survivorship, 1*, 283–291.

Crew, K. D., Capodice, J. L., Greenlee, H., Brafman, L., Fuentes, D., Awad, D., Yann Tsai, W., Hershman, D. L. (2010). Randomized, blinded, sham-controlled trial of acupuncture for the management of aromatase inhibitor-associated joint symptoms in women with early-stage breast cancer. *Journal of Clinical Oncology, 28*, 1154–1160.

Dang, W., Yang, J. (1998). Clinical study on acupuncture treatment of stomach carcinoma pain. *Journal of Traditional Chinese Medicine, 18*, 31–38.

Deng, G. (2009). Acupuncture for fatigue during radiation therapy: Points made. *Journal of the Society for Integrative Oncology, 7*, 1–3.

Deng, G., Vickers, A., Simon Yeung, K., Cassileth, B. R. (2006). Acupuncture: Integration into cancer care. *Journal of the Society for Integrative Oncology, 4*, 86–92.

Deng, G., Vickers, A., Yeung, S., D'Andrea, G. M., Xiao, H., Heerdt, A. S., Sugarman, S., Troso-Sandoval, T., Seidman, A. D., Hudis, C. A., Cassileth, B. (2007). Randomized, controlled trial of acupuncture for the treatment of hot flashes in breast cancer patients. *Journal of Clinical Oncology, 25*, 5584–5590.

Deng, G., Hou, B. L., Holodny, A. I., Cassileth, B. R. (2008a) Functional magnetic resonance imaging (fMRI) changes and saliva production associated with acupuncture at LI-2 acupuncture point: A randomized controlled study. *BMC Complementary and Alternative Medicine, 8*, 37.

Deng, G., Rusch, V., Vickers, A., Malhotra, V., Ginex, P., Downey, R., Bains, M., Park, B., Rizk, N., Flores, R., Yeung, S., Cassiletha, B. (2008b). Randomized controlled trial of a special acupuncture technique for pain after thoracotomy. *The Journal of Thoracic and Cardiovascular Surgery, 136*, 1464—1469.

Dumville, J. C., Hahn, S., Miles, J. N., Torgerson, D. J. (2006). The use of unequal randomisation ratios in clinical trials: A review. *Contemporary Clinical Trials, 27*, 1–12.
Enblom, A., Johnsson, A., Hammar, M., Onelov, E., Steineck, G., Borjeson, S. (2012). Acupuncture compared with placebo acupuncture in radiotherapy-induced nausea—a randomized controlled study. *Annals of Oncology, 23*, 1353–1361.
Enblom, A., Lekander, M., Hammar, M., Johnsson, A., Onelov, E., Ingvar, M., Steineck. G., Borjeson, S. (2011). Getting the grip on nonspecific treatment effects: Emesis in patients randomized to acupuncture or sham compared to patients receiving standard care. *PloS One, 6*, e14766.
Ernst, E., Lee, M. S. (2010). Acupuncture for palliative and supportive cancer care: A systematic review of systematic reviews. *Journal of Pain and Symptom Management, 40*, e3–5.
Escalante, C. P., Manzullo, E. F. (2009). Cancer-related fatigue: The approach and treatment. *Journal of General Internal Medicine, 24*, S412–S416.
Ezzo, J. M., Richardson, M. A., Vickers, A., Allen, C., Dibble, S. L., Issell, B. F., Lao, L., Pearl, M., Ramirez, G., Roscoe, J., Shen, J., Shivnan, J. C., Streitberger, K., Treish, I., Zhang, G. (2006). Acupuncture-point stimulation for chemotherapy-induced nausea or vomiting. Cochrane Database System Review, 2, CD002285.
Feng, Y., Wang, X. Y., Li, S. D., Zhang, Y., Wang, H. M., Li, M., Cao, K., Ye, Y. F., Zhang, Z. (2011). Clinical research of acupuncture on malignant tumor patients for improving depression and sleep quality. *Journal of Traditional Chinese Medicine, 31*, 199–202.
Frisk, J., Carlhall, S., Kallstrom, A. C., Lindh-Astrand, L., Malmstrom, A., Hammar, M. (2008). Long-term follow-up of acupuncture and hormone therapy on hot flushes in women with breast cancer: A prospective, randomized, controlled multicenter trial. *Climacteric, 11*, 166–174.
Frisk, J., Kallstrom, A. C., Wall, N., Fredrikson, M., Hammar, M. (2012). Acupuncture improves health-related quality-of-life (HRQoL) and sleep in women with breast cancer and hot flushes. *Supportive Care in Cancer, 20*, 715–724.
Frisk, J., Spetz, A. C., Hjertberg, H., Petersson, B., Hammar, M. (2009). Two modes of acupuncture as a treatment for hot flushes in men with prostate cancer—a prospective multicenter study with long-term follow-up. *European Urology, 55*, 156–163.
Gottschling, S., Reindl, T. K., Meyer, S., Berrang, J., Henze, G., Graeber, S., Ong, M. F., Graf, N. (2008). Acupuncture to alleviate chemotherapy-induced nausea and vomiting in pediatric oncology—a randomized multicenter crossover pilot trial. *Klinische Padiatrie, 220*, 365–370.
Hervik, J., Mjaland, O. (2009). Acupuncture for the treatment of hot flashes in breast cancer patients, a randomized, controlled trial. *Breast Cancer Research and Treatment, 116*, 311–316.
Hervik, J., Mjaland, O. (2010). Quality of life of breast cancer patients medicated with anti-estrogens, 2 years after acupuncture treatment: A qualitative study. *International Journal of Women's Health, 2*, 319–325.
Holmberg, L., Iversen, O. E., Rudenstam, C. M., Hammar, M., Kumpulainen, E., Jaskiewicz, J., Jassem, J., Dobaczewska, D., Fjosne, H. E., Peralta, O., Arriagada, R., Holmqvist, M., Maenpaa, J. (2008). Increased risk of recurrence after hormone replacement therapy in breast cancer survivors. *Journal of the National Cancer Institute, 100*, 475–482.
Hopkins Hollis, A. S. (2010). Acupuncture as a treatment modality for the management of cancer pain: The state of the science. *Oncology Nursing Forum, 37*, E344–E348.
Jadad, A. R., Moore, R. A., Carroll, D., Jenkinson, C., Reynolds, D. J., Gavaghan, D. J., McQuay, H. J. (1996). Assessing the quality of reports of randomized clinical trials: Is blinding necessary? *Controlled Clinical Trials, 17*, 1–12.
Johnston, M. F., Xiao, B., Hui, K. K. (2007a). Acupuncture and fatigue: Current basis for shared communication between breast cancer survivors and providers. *Journal of Cancer Survivorship, 1*, 306–312.
Johnston, M. F., Yang, C., Hui, K. K., Xiao, B., Li, X. S., Rusiewicz, A. (2007b). Acupuncture for chemotherapy-associated cognitive dysfunction: A hypothesis-generating literature review to inform clinical advice. *Integrative Cancer Therapies, 6*, 36–41.

Johnston, M. F., Hays, R. D., Subramanian, S. K., Elashoff, R. M., Axe, E. K., Li, J. J., Kim, I., Vargas, R. B., Lee, J., Yang, L., Hui, K. K. (2011). Patient education integrated with acupuncture for relief of cancer-related fatigue randomized controlled feasibility study. *BMC Complementary and Alternative Medicine, 11,* 49.

Kotani, N., Hashimoto, H., Sato, Y., Sessler, D. I., Yoshioka, H., Kitayama, M., Yasuda, T., Matsuki, A. (2001). Preoperative intradermal acupuncture reduces postoperative pain, nausea and vomiting, analgesic requirement, and sympathoadrenal responses. *Anesthesiology, 95*, 349–356.

Langevin, H. M., Wayne, P. M., Macpherson, H., Schnyer, R., Milley, R. M., Napadow, V., Lao, L., Park, J., Harris, R. E., Cohen, M., Sherman, K. J., Haramati, A., Hammerschlag, R. (2011). Paradoxes in acupuncture research: Strategies for moving forward. *Evidence-based Complementary and Alternative Medicine, 2011,* 180805.

Lee, A., Fan, L. T. (2009). Stimulation of the wrist acupuncture point P6 for preventing postoperative nausea and vomiting. Cochrane Database System Review, *2*, CD003281.

Lee, M. S., Kim, K. H., Choi, S. M., Ernst, E. (2009a). Acupuncture for treating hot flashes in breast cancer patients: A systematic review. *Breast Cancer Research and Treatment, 115*, 497–503.

Lee, M. S., Kim, K. H., Shin, B. C., Choi, S. M., Ernst, E. (2009b). Acupuncture for treating hot flushes in men with prostate cancer: A systematic review. *Supportive Care in Cancer, 17*, 763–770.

Lekander, M., Hammar, M., Johnsson, A., Onelov, E., Ingvar, M., Steineck. G., Borjeson, S. (2011). Getting the grip on nonspecific treatment effects: Emesis in patients randomized to acupuncture or sham compared to patients receiving standard care. *PloS One, 6,* e14766.

Liljegren, A., Gunnarsson, P., Landgren, B. M., Robeus, N., Johansson, H., Rotstein, S. (2010). Reducing vasomotor symptoms with acupuncture in breast cancer patients treated with adjuvant tamoxifen: A randomized controlled trial. *Breast Cancer Research and Treatment*, doi: 10.1007/s10549-010-1283-3.

Lim, J. T., Wong, E. T., Aung, S. K. (2011). Is there a role for acupuncture in the symptom management of patients receiving palliative care for cancer? A pilot study of 20 patients comparing acupuncture with nurse-led supportive care. *Acupuncture in Medicine, 29*, 173–179.

Lu, W., Dean-Clower, E., Doherty-Gilman, A., Rosenthal, D. S. (2008). The value of acupuncture in cancer care. *Hematology/Oncology Clinics of North America, 22*, 631–648.

Lu, W., Matulonis, U. A., Doherty-Gilman, A., Lee, H., Dean-Clower, E., Rosulek, A., Gibson, C., Goodman, A., Davis, R. B., Buring, J. E., Wayne, P. M., Rosenthal, D. S., Penson, R. T. (2009). Acupuncture for chemotherapy-induced neutropenia in patients with gynecologic malignancies: A pilot randomized, sham-controlled clinical trial. *Journal of Alternative and Complementary Medicine, 15*, 745–753.

Lu, W., Rosenthal, D. S. (2010). Recent advances in oncology acupuncture and safety considerations in practice. *Current Treatment Options in Oncology, 11*, 141–146.

MacPherson, H., Altman, D. G., Hammerschlag, R., Youping, L., Taixiang, W., White, A., Moher, D. (2010). Revised standards for reporting interventions in clinical trials of acupuncture (STRICTA): Extending the CONSORT statement. *Journal of Evidence-Based Medicine, 3*, 140–155.

Mehling, W. E., Jacobs, B., Acree, M., Wilson, L., Bostrom, A., West, J., Acquah, J., Burns, B., Chapman, J., Hecht, F. M. (2007). Symptom management with massage and acupuncture in postoperative cancer patients: A randomized controlled trial. *Journal of Pain and Symptom Management, 33*, 258–266.

Meng, Z., Garcia, M. K., Hu, C., Chiang, J., Chambers, M., Rosenthal, D. I., Peng, H., Zhang, Y., Zhao, Q., Zhao, G., Liu, L., Spelman, A., Palmer, J. L., Wei, Q., Cohen, L. (2012). Randomized controlled trial of acupuncture for prevention of radiation-induced xerostomia among patients with nasopharyngeal carcinoma. *Cancer, 118,* 3337–3344.

Minton, O., Higginson, I. J. (2007). Electroacupuncture as an adjunctive treatment to control neuropathic pain in patients with cancer. *Journal of Pain and Symptom Management, 33*, 115–117.

Molassiotis, A., Sylt, P., Diggins, H. (2007). The management of cancer-related fatigue after chemotherapy with acupuncture and acupressure: A randomised controlled trial. *Complementary Therapies in Medicine, 15*, 228–237.

O'Sullivan, E. M., Higginson, I. J. (2010). Clinical effectiveness and safety of acupuncture in the treatment of irradiation-induced xerostomia in patients with head and neck cancer: A systematic review. *Acupuncture in Medicine, 28*, 191–199.

Paley, C. A., Bennett, M. I., Johnson, M. I. (2011a). Acupuncture for cancer-induced bone pain? *Evidence-Based Complementary and Alternative Medicine, 2011*, 671043.

Paley, C. A., Johnson, M. I., Tashani, O. A., Bagnall, A. M. (2011b). Acupuncture for cancer pain in adults. Cochrane Database System Review, *1*, CD007753.

Park, J., Linde, K., Manheimer, E., Molsberger, A., Sherman, K., Smith, C., Sung, J., Vickers, A., Schnyer, R. (2008). The status and future of acupuncture clinical research. *Journal of Alternative and Complementary Medicine, 14*, 871–881.

Pfister, D. G., Cassileth, B. R., Deng, G. E., Yeung, K. S., Lee, J. S., Garrity, D., Cronin, A., Lee, N., Kraus, D., Shaha, A. R., Shah, J., Vickers, A. J. (2010). Acupuncture for pain and dysfunction after neck dissection: Results of a randomized controlled trial. *Journal of Clinical Oncology, 28*, 2565–2570.

Price, S., Long, A. F., Godfrey, M., Thomas, K. J. (2011). Getting inside acupuncture trials—exploring intervention theory and rationale. *BMC Complementary and Alternative Medicine, 11*, 22.

Rada, G., Capurro, D., Pantoja, T., Corbalan, J., Moreno, G., Letelier, L. M., Vera, C. (2010). Non-hormonal interventions for hot flushes in women with a history of breast cancer. Cochrane Database System Review, *9*, CD004923.

Robb, K. A., Bennett, M. I., Johnson, M. I., Simpson, K. J., Oxberry, S. G. (2008). Transcutaneous electric nerve stimulation (TENS) for cancer pain in adults. Cochrane Database System Review, *3*, CD006276.

Sagar, S. M. (2008). Acupuncture as an evidence-based option for symptom control in cancer patients. *Current Treatment Options in Oncology, 9*, 117–126.

Stone, J. A., Johnstone, P. A. (2010). Mechanisms of action for acupuncture in the oncology setting. *Current Treatment Options in Oncology, 11*, 118–127.

Walker, E. M., Rodriguez, A. I., Kohn, B., Ball, R. M., Pegg, J., Pocock, J. R., Nunez, R., Peterson, E., Jakary, S., Levine, R. A. (2010). Acupuncture versus venlafaxine for the management of vasomotor symptoms in patients with hormone receptor-positive breast cancer: A randomized controlled trial. *Journal of Clinical Oncology, 28*, 634–640.

Wang, X. Q., Yu, J. L., Du, Z. Y., Xu, R., Jiang, C. C., Gao, X. (2010). Electroacupoint stimulation for postoperative nausea and vomiting in patients undergoing supratentorial craniotomy. *Journal of Neurosurgical Anesthesiology, 22*, 128–131.

Wong, R. H., Lee, T. W., Sihoe, A. D., Wan, I. Y., Ng, C. S., Chan, S. K., Wong, W. W., Liang, Y. M., Yim, A. P. (2006). Analgesic effect of electroacupuncture in postthoracotomy pain: A prospective randomized trial. *The Annals of Thoracic Surgery, 81*, 2031–2036.

Xia, Y. Q., Zhang, D., Yang, C. X., Xu, H. L., Li, Y., Ma, L. T. (1986). An approach to the effect on tumors of acupuncture in combination with radiotherapy or chemotherapy. *Journal of Traditional Chinese Medicine, 6*, 23–26.

You, Q., Yu, H., Wu, D., Zhang, Y., Zheng, J., Peng, C. (2009). Vitamin B6 points PC6 injection during acupuncture can relieve nausea and vomiting in patients with ovarian cancer. *International Journal of Gynecological Cancer, 19*, 567–571.

Index

W. C. S. Cho (ed.), *Acupuncture and Moxibustion as an Evidence-based Therapy for Cancer*, Evidence-based Anticancer Complementary and Alternative Medicine 3, DOI 10.1007/978-94-007-4833-0,